HUMAN BIOLOGY AND HEALTH:
AN EVOLUTIONARY APPROACH

Edited by Basiro Davey
and Tim Halliday

PUBLISHED BY THE OPEN UNIVERSITY PRESS
IN ASSOCIATION WITH THE OPEN UNIVERSITY

 OPEN UNIVERSITY PRESS

 The Open University Health and Disease Series, Book 4

The U205 Health and Disease Course Team

The following members of the Open University teaching staff and external consultants have collaborated with the authors in writing this book, or have commented extensively on it during its production. We accept collective responsibility for its overall academic and teaching content.

Basiro Davey (Course Team Chair, Lecturer in Health Studies, Biology)

Helen Dolk (Lecturer, Department of Environmental Epidemiology, London School of Hygiene and Tropical Medicine)

Geoff Einon (Lecturer, Department of Biology)

Gerald Elliott (Professor of Bio-physics)

Tim Halliday (Professor of Biology)

Richard Holmes (Senior Lecturer, Biology)

Heather McLannahan (Senior Counsellor, Biology)

Kevin McConway (Senior Lecturer in Statistics)

Judith Metcalfe (Staff Tutor, Biology)

Perry Morley (Senior Editor, Science)

Caroline Pond (Reader, Department of Biology)

The following people have contributed to the development of particular parts or aspects of this book.

Sylvia Abbey (course secretary)

Steve Best (graphic artist)

Debbie Crouch (cover designer)

Heather Davies (electronmicroscopist)

Alastair Gray (critical reader), Research Associate, Centre for Socio-legal Studies, Wolfson College, Oxford

John Greenwood (librarian)

Marion Hall (course manager)

Pam Higgins (designer)

Sarah Keer-Keer (picture researcher)

Jean Macqueen (indexer)

Philip Payne (critical reader), Professor of Human Nutrition, Centre for Human Nutrition, London School of Hygiene and Tropical Medicine

Rissa de la Paz (BBC producer)

Liz Sugden (BBC production assistant)

Doreen Tucker (text processing compositor)

Jenny Walker (independent television producer for the BBC)

Authors

The following people have acted as principal or co-authors for the chapters listed below.

Chapters 1, 3, 6 and 9

Basiro Davey, Lecturer in Health Studies, Department of Biology, The Open University.

Chapters 2 and 7

Caroline Pond, Reader, Department of Biology, The Open University.

Chapters 3 and 5

Tim Halliday, Professor of Biology, Department of Biology, The Open University.

Chapters 4 and 9

Judith Metcalfe, Regional Staff Tutor and member of the Department of Biology, The Open University.

Chapter 7

Geoff Einon, Lecturer in Biology, Department of Biology, The Open University.

Chapter 8

Heather McLannahan, Regional Senior Counsellor and member of the Department of Biology, The Open University.

Chapters 10 and 11

Helen Dolk, Lecturer in the Department of Environmental Epidemiology, London School of Hygiene and Tropical Medicine.

External assessors

Course assessor

Professor James McEwen, Henry Mechan Chair of Public Health and Head of Department of Public Health, University of Glasgow.

Book 4 assessor

Lewis Wolpert, Professor of Biology as Applied to Medicine, Department of Anatomy and Developmental Biology, University College and Middlesex School of Medicine, London.

Acknowledgements

The Course Team and the authors wish to thank the following people who, as contributors to *The Biology of Health and Disease*, made a lasting impact on the structure and philosophy of the present volume.

Nick Black, Rosemary Lennard, Jennie Popay, Rob Ransom, Steven Rose, Phil Strong

The Open University Press, Celtic Court, 22 Ballmore, Buckingham, MK18 1XW.

First published 1985. This completely revised edition first published 1994.

A catalogue record of the book is available from the British Library.

Library of Congress Cataloging-in-Publication Data

Human biology and health: an evolutionary approach/edited by Basiro Davey and Tim Halliday.

    p. cm. — (Health and disease series: Book 4)

    Completely rev. and updated version of The Biology of health and disease. 1985.

    Includes bibliographical references and index.

    ISBN 0-335-19253-X (pb.)

1. Human Biology. 2. Health. 3. Human evolution. 4. Pathology. I. Davey, Basiro. II. Halliday, Tim, 1945– . III. Open University. IV. The Biology of health and disease. V. Series.

[DNLM: 1. Disease. 2. Physiology. 3. Health. QZ 140 H918 1994]

QP34.H89 1994

612 — dc20   93–49558

CIP

Edited, designed and typeset by the Open University.

Printed in the United Kingdom by Butler & Tanner Ltd, Frome and London.

ISBN 0 335 19253 X

This text forms part of an Open University Second Level Course. If you would like a copy of *Studying with the Open University*, please write to the Central Enquiry Service, PO Box 200, The Open University, Walton Hall, Milton Keynes, MK7 2YZ.

2.1

8129C/u205b4i2.1

Contents

About this book   2

1   Why 'an evolutionary approach'?   5
Basiro Davey

2   The human biological heritage   8
Caroline Pond

3   The story of life in a few pages   31
Basiro Davey and Tim Halliday

4   Inheritance and variation   67
Judith Metcalfe

5   Living with other species   98
Tim Halliday

6   Surviving infectious disease   124
Basiro Davey

7   Digestion and dietary change   146
Caroline Pond and Geoff Einon

8   On living longer   173
Heather McLannahan

9   Tinkering with nature   188
Judith Metcalfe and Basiro Davey

10   Living with the chemical industrial
environment   211
Helen Dolk

11   The impact of modern culture   225
Helen Dolk

Appendix: Table of abbreviations used
in this book   233

References and further reading   234

Answers to self-assessment
questions   240

Acknowledgements   248

Index   249

About this book

A note for the general reader

Human Biology and Health: An Evolutionary Approach presents an evolutionary history of human health and disease, starting from the premise that patterns of resistance and susceptibility to illness and disability in twentieth-century human populations have been influenced by the biological and cultural evolution of the human species over the last five million years. The book focuses on the evolution of infectious, genetic and degenerative diseases and emphasises the degree of variation in susceptibility between individuals and between human populations. The authors are biologists who have written an introduction to human biology that is accessible to a general readership, but which aims to teach some fundamental aspects of the subject, from the structure of DNA and the nature of genes to the physiology of the whole organism and its interaction with the surrounding cultural and physical environment. However, this is not a book aimed exclusively at biology students, but at anyone with an interest in human social organisation and cultural development who wishes to add a biological dimension to their studies.

After an introductory chapter, Chapter 2 describes early human evolution and considers the impact of human cultural developments, such as the farming of grains and domestic animals, on human health. Chapter 3 is a speculative account of the origins of life on Earth, interwoven with a basic introduction to the structure and activity of human cells and the genetic code, and the theory of evolution by natural selection. Chapter 4 extends the discussion of normal genetic variation between individuals and populations and focuses on the inheritance of characteristics that affect health. In Chapter 5, we consider the long evolutionary history of close human contact with other organisms such as bacteria and larger parasites, and in Chapter 6 we describe the defence mechanisms which have evolved in response to the threat of infection. Chapter 7 describes human digestion and the absorption of nutrients and examines the interaction between cultural changes in the composition of the diet and the biological evolution of the digestive system. In Chapter 8, we investigate the mechanisms that underlie the ageing process and ask 'Why do we die?'.

In the final chapters of the book, the authors turn their attention towards the future. Biomedical technology promises to offer partial solutions to a few major health problems and Chapter 9 discusses the implications of transplanting cells and organs from person to person, and of the newest techniques aimed at manipulating human genes. Chapter 10 focuses on the chemical industrial environment and its possible impact on the global environment and on human health. The book ends in Chapter 11 with the suggestion that the pace of cultural change is now seriously challenging human capacity to evolve genetic and cultural adaptations to maintain and improve health.

The book is fully indexed and referenced and contains an appendix of abbreviations and an annotated guide to further reading.

Human Biology and Health: An Evolutionary Approach is the fourth in a series of eight books on the subject of health and disease. The book is designed so that it can be read on its own, like any other textbook, or studied as part of U205 *Health and Disease*, a second level course for Open University students. General readers do not need to make use of the study comments, learning objectives and other material inserted for OU students, although they may find these helpful. The text also contains references to a Reader of previously published material and specially commissioned articles[1] prepared in association with the OU course: it is quite possible to follow the text without reading the articles referred to, although doing so will enhance your understanding of the contents of *Human Biology and Health: An Evolutionary Approach*.

A guide for OU students

Human Biology and Health: An Evolutionary Approach presents the study of human biology as a dynamic evolutionary process which cannot be understood except in the context of human cultural evolution. It builds on knowledge of biomedical research methods discussed in *Studying Health and Disease,* and of human epidemiology described in *World Health and Disease*; in turn, it informs the development of biological themes in two later

---

[1] *Health and Disease: A Reader* (Open University Press, 1984; revised edition 1994).

books in this series, *Birth to Old Age: Health in Transition* and *Experiencing and Explaining Disease*. The structure of the book is outlined in the 'Note for the general reader' above, and is described further in Chapter 1.

Study comments, where appropriate, are given in a box at the start of chapters. These primarily direct you to important links to other components of the course, such as the other books in the course series, the Reader, and audiovisual components. Major learning objectives are listed at the end of each chapter, along with self-assessment questions that will enable you to check that you have achieved these objectives. The index includes key words in **bold** type (also printed in bold in the text), which can be looked up easily as an aid to revision as the course proceeds, and abbreviations are listed at the end of the book. There is also a list of further reading for those who wish to pursue aspects of study beyond the scope of this book.

The time allowed for studying *Human Biology and Health: An Evolutionary Approach* is five weeks, or about 50–60 hours. The following table gives a more detailed breakdown to help you to pace your study. You need not follow it slavishly, but try not to let yourself fall behind. Depending on your background and experience, you may well find some parts of this book much more familiar and straightforward than others. If you find a section of the work difficult, do what you can at this stage, and then return to the material when you reach the end of the book.

There is a tutor-marked assignment (TMA) associated with this book; about three hours have been allowed for completing it, *in addition to* the time spent studying the material it assesses.

Study Guide for Book 4 (total 50–60 hours, including time for the TMA, spread over 5 weeks). Chapters 1 and 11 are very short, but the other chapters vary considerably in length; Chapters 8 and 10 are the shortest of the central chapters and Chapters 3 and 4 the longest. The earlier chapters introduce the largest number of new terms and concepts; the later chapters extend and reinforce material taught earlier in the book. You should pace your study accordingly.

1st week

Chapter 1   **Why 'an evolutionary approach'?**

Chapter 2   **The human biological heritage**; *Reader* article by Bogin (1993)

Chapter 3   **The story of life in a few pages**; TV programme 'Blood lines', on haemoglobin and mutations in DNA

2nd week

Chapter 4   **Inheritance and variation**; the TV programme 'Blood lines' is relevant here too

Chapter 5   **Living with other species**

3rd week

Chapter 6   **Surviving infectious disease**; revise *Reader* article by Strassburg (1982) which was set reading for *World Health and Disease*

Chapter 7   **Digestion and dietary change**

4th week

Chapter 8   **On living longer**

Chapter 9   **Tinkering with nature**; *Reader* article by Müller-Hill (1993); audiotape 'Tinkering with nature'

5th week

Chapter 10   **Living with the chemical industrial environment**; *Reader* article by Leaf (1989)

Chapter 11   **The impact of modern culture**; *Reader* article by Jones (1993)

TMA completion

Cover photographs

Background: Haemophilus ducreyi bacterial cells associated with the tropical disease chancroid, or genital ulcers; the bacteria are growing in a laboratory culture inside a human cervical cancer cell and have been photographed with an electron microscope at a magnification of approximately 80 000 times life size (Photo: Heather Davies). *Middleground:* Human cultural and biological evolution has been persistently affected by warfare from the earliest times, as illustrated by this watercolour copy of a battle scene, originally painted in caves at Civil in Spain about 2 000 BC (Watercolour by J-B. Porcar, reproduced in Sandars, N. K., 1968, *Prehistoric Art in Europe*, Penguin Books, London). *Foreground:* The pace of change in modern industrial environments may have profound consequences for human health, for example through rising traffic pollution. (Photo: Mike Levers)

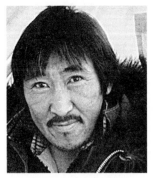

(Photo: Caroline Pond)

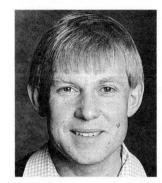

(Photo: Mike Levers)

Figure 1.1 *Humans display exceptional variation in their outward appearance, which is matched by invisible variations between individuals in the activity of the molecules, cells and organs of which their bodies are composed. Yet these varied individuals are members of a single species,* Homo sapiens.

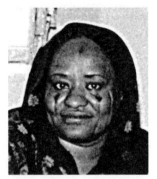

(Photo: Marion Hall)

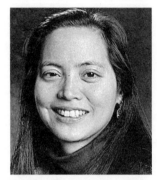

(Photo: Mike Levers)

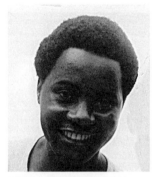

(Photo: Caroline Pond)

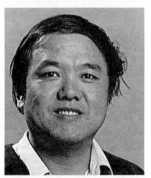

(Photo: Mike Levers)

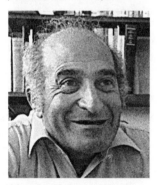

(Photo: Mike Levers)

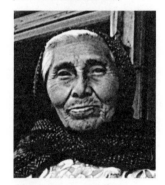

(Photo: Marion Hall)

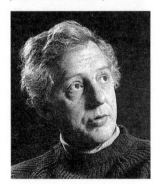

(Source: OU Open House magazine)

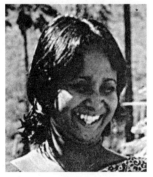

(Photo: Caroline Pond)

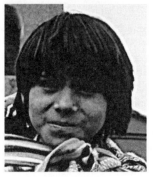

(Photo: Marion Hall)

1 Why 'an evolutionary approach'?

This book about human biology is rather unusual for several reasons. First, the authors have assumed that the readers don't know any biology beyond the most rudimentary general knowledge that organisms come in many different shapes and sizes and all are composed of cells made from lots of different chemicals. Anything else you need to know is taught within the pages of this book. We are aware that a minority of readers will already know a lot of biology, but we confidently expect that the unconventional structure of this book will shed a novel and interesting light on the presentation even of familiar terms and concepts.

Second, we have kept in the forefront of our minds the question 'Why does a non-biologist interested in human health need to know this bit of biology?'. With so much to choose from in the vast field of biological knowledge, what has guided our selection of certain aspects for attention here? To some extent our selection reflects the interests and expertise of the contributors, but our guiding principle has been to focus on the unique contribution that a study of biology can bring to a modern understanding of human health and disease. For example, it gives an important insight into the susceptibility and resistance to illness of individuals and populations. Biological explanations for fluctuations in the patterns of disease that human populations display across long time periods and between geographical locations, and during the span of each life from birth to old age, are among the most compelling.

For many people, biology is a daunting and impenetrable subject, principally because conventional teaching texts are crammed with new terms and fully-detailed explanations of complex mechanisms. We have attempted to side-step that approach by 'telling stories' wherever possible and keeping the terminology to an essential minimum. As a result, there are plenty of gaps in the details, but we hope this sacrifice ensures that you reach the end of the book with an understanding of the 'big picture' of human health and disease from a biological vantage-point.

Biology intrudes into people's lives constantly and in many diverse ways. When we catch a cold or suffer heart disease we are experiencing biological phenomena that are shared by at least some other animals, and understanding such events from a biological standpoint gives us insights that are not provided by a purely medical approach. There is a more general point here, too. The authors of this book believe that there is a need for greater 'scientific literacy' in our society. We find it odd that an 'educated' person is expected to know who wrote *Romeo and Juliet*, for example, but is not generally expected to understand the essential properties of DNA, the chemical that influences every aspect of our biology, and hence our lives, and about which you will read a great deal in this book.

The third unusual aspect of this book is that we have taken *evolution*, of humans and of other living things, as the 'backbone' of the story. It is a constant theme running through every chapter and the ultimate purpose of all the descriptions of mechanisms and molecules is to illuminate this theme. We are interested in discovering how and why the human species has arrived at the highly-successful body structure and internal activity that it presently enjoys and how and why that same body is prey to certain characteristic illnesses and disabilities. These are questions that biologists can only partially answer and about which there is much dispute, so you can expect to be challenged by uncertainty in this book as much as in others in the series. But there is one basic certainty among the authors: we believe that the humans we see today are the consequence of several million years of evolution from ancestral species. In adhering to this central dogma of modern biology, we mean no offence to readers who reject evolution in favour of divine creation, but we have to disagree.

However, we have broken with traditional biology by using a very broad definition of **human evolution**. We take it to mean 'gradual changes over successive generations in the biological and cultural development of the human species'. (Though biological and cultural evolution have both been very important in shaping modern humans, they are very different processes, as you will discover in later chapters of this book.) Note that this definition does not imply a linear progression from simple to complex, either in the form and function of human biology or human culture. Change does not march forward on a united front: as some aspects become more complex, so others simplify; the gains of one age can be reversed by the next. But like the Spanish-American philosopher and poet, George Santayana, we believe that

> The tide of evolution carries everything before it, thoughts no less than bodies, and persons no less than nations. (Santayana, *Little Essays*, number 44, quoted in Daintith and Isaacs, 1989, p. 68)

Finally, there is the question of ethics. As the pace of acquisition of new biological knowledge hots up and new techniques for manipulating human biology are developed, individual members of society are faced with the ethical implications of such developments. Moreover, cultural change continues to have profound effects on the environment and on human health which have provoked discussion of the ethics of industrialisation, deforestation, pollution and population growth. In this book, we join the ethical debate by identifying major causes of concern about the development of biological science and certain aspects of human culture (such as industrialisation) and their possible impact on the future health of the human species. We do not claim any special expertise in ethics, nor have we attempted to reach a judgement about the rights and wrongs of any issue. We have written simply from the viewpoint of biologists who are personally concerned to disseminate relevant information and encourage non-biologists to become engaged in the debate.

With that overview of the general approach taken in this book in mind, we can look briefly at the individual chapters in the sequence in which you will study them. Broadly speaking, the book begins in the distant past, considers the present situation of humans and, finally, looks forward to the future. Chapter 2, 'The human biological heritage', starts 60 million years ago and identifies some special features of the ancestors of present-day humans. It traces the evolution of some uniquely human characteristics, including upright posture and the ability to walk on two legs, the bodily changes we call *puberty* and the practice of cooking food. These features of human biology and culture have had major consequences for our health. For example, the backache that afflicts millions today may have had its origins in the move from a forested to a grassland environment made by early humans about 3 million years ago.

In Chapter 3 we go further back in time to tell 'The story of life in a few pages'. We start with the coalescence of *atoms* of certain *chemical elements* into *molecules* of *DNA* in the 'primeval soup' cooling on the surface of the newly-formed planet Earth. Then we sketch in the evolution of large creatures such as ourselves, composed of billions of cells organised into recognisable structural features such as the major organs, muscles and bones. For readers who are new to this series and new to science, the italicised terms earlier in this paragraph are likely to be familiar but may not be understood in their scientific sense.[1] Before moving on, we need to ensure that you know their scientific meaning.

All matter, whether it is in a living organism like a tree or a person, or in non-living material such as the rocks and the atmosphere, is composed of **chemical elements**. There are about 100 different elements in nature and among the most familiar are the most abundant constituents of living things: oxygen, carbon and hydrogen, which together form over 90 per cent of the mass of every organism. Under natural conditions on the surface of the Earth, one element cannot be turned into another, so you can think of them as the basic building blocks of the material world. (In the Earth's core and in the upper atmosphere, elements *are* transformed one into another, but this does not concern us here.) Each element exists in the form of extremely small 'particles' known as **atoms**, which can be joined together by energy fields known as chemical *bonds*. An assembly of two or more atoms is called a **molecule.**

Molecules often contain atoms of more than one element, so for example *water* molecules are formed from two atoms of hydrogen and one atom of oxygen, written in the familiar chemical notation of H_2O. Water is an extremely small molecule because it has only three atoms, but molecules can be millions of times larger than those of water and contain the atoms of several different elements. One of the largest is the 'thread of life', deoxyribonucleic acid or DNA. The structure and functions of DNA are major topics in Chapter 3.

In Chapter 4, 'Inheritance and variation', we describe the contribution of DNA to the variation we see between individuals and its role in passing on characteristics, such as height and susceptibility to a particular disease, from one generation to the next. Chapter 4 takes us into the realm of genetic disease and genetic resistance

---

[1] They were explained in an earlier book in this series, *Studying Health and Disease* (Open University Press, revised edition 1994), Chapter 9.

to disease, but it also emphasises the interaction of a person's genetic makeup and the environment in which they develop, in producing the normal variation between individuals we see all around us. The frontispiece to this book (Figure 1.1) illustrates the exceptional variation in the forms taken by members of the human species.

Chapter 5, 'Living with other species', considers the interaction between human populations and the organisms that have a major impact on our health. Most obvious among them are the *pathogenic* (disease-causing) species, which include some types of bacteria, viruses, single-celled animals, fungi and larger parasites like the tapeworms and liver flukes. This interaction has had a major impact on the evolution of larger organisms, including humans, and has played a role in fundamental aspects of their lives, including the fact that they reproduce sexually. But human survival also crucially depends on bacteria and other minute creatures such as the plankton in the sea, as Chapter 5 will reveal.

In Chapter 6, 'Surviving infectious disease', we examine the dynamic balancing act that goes on whenever a pathogenic organism invades the human body. Over the long time-scale of life on earth, pathogens have evolved numerous adaptations to evade the defensive strategies evolved by their 'hosts'. As a consequence of this evolutionary history, the human immune system is a network of mind-boggling complexity which has solved the problem of attacking infection without destroying the body itself. Chapter 6 gives a glimpse into this inner world of threat and counter-attack.

But there is more to survival than resisting infection. According to the English clergyman, W. R. Inge, 'the whole of nature is a conjugation of the verb to eat, in the active and in the passive' (from his *Outspoken Essays*, quoted in Daintith and Isaacs, 1989, p. 145). Chapter 7, 'Digestion and dietary change', is about the mechanisms of digestion and absorption and how they cope with the modern human diet. The chapter ends with a case study on variation in the ability to digest milk among different human populations.

In Chapter 8 we move more firmly into the present to examine the biological consequences of increased longevity. 'On living longer' describes the biological changes underlying the familiar signs of ageing and asks: Why, in evolutionary terms, do we grow old and die? Are we genetically programmed to grow old? The increased prevalence of degenerative diseases is one of the driving forces behind biological research aimed at improving human health in the future. Another is the desire to alleviate the hitherto intractable consequences of certain degenerative or genetic diseases. In Chapter 9, 'Tinkering with nature', we examine some of the most controversial methods that medical science is in the process of developing to increase the quantity and the quality of human life. These include organ transplant surgery, gene therapy and genetic screening. Some of these procedures have the potential not only to reduce human suffering but may also change the nature of human evolution. These topics are the subject of far-reaching ethical debates.

As it nears its conclusion, the book progresses steadily deeper into the vexed territory of modern life. In Chapter 10, 'Living with the chemical industrial environment', we turn from the intentional manipulation of human biology to the consequences of a prevalent feature of industrial development, the *unintentional* dissemination of chemicals. What evidence do we have that this activity is damaging human health in any general sense, or is human biology able to adapt sufficiently to defend the species from chemical pollution? The book closes in Chapter 11 by looking back over the sweep of human evolution and putting 'The impact of modern culture' in the context of this extensive timeframe. We consider the interaction of biological and cultural evolution and speculate about the future. We conclude by posing the question 'Is the pace of change too fast for human evolution to keep up?'.

2 The human biological heritage

This chapter outlines the biological back-ground to our modern human condition. The origins and incidence of many of the diseases discussed in the previous book in this series, **World Health and Disease,**[1] can be partly explained in terms of our evolutionary history and our interactions with other organisms. An understanding of how diseases have arisen in the past helps us to anticipate, and hence to control, new diseases that may appear and spread through the human population. You will find it helpful to look back at Chapters 5 and 11 of **World Health and Disease** to remind yourself of the general theory of evolution by natural selection and the meaning of the terms 'adaptation' and 'fitness'. We will be discussing the biological meaning of these terms later in the present book (Chapters 3 and 5), but for the moment a general grasp of the basic ideas is sufficient.

This chapter is written in the style of an essay, with few numerical data or elaborate diagrams. It is intended to be read straight through, to give you the 'big picture' rather than to teach detail. This text is a synthesis of information and points of view from a variety of different sources, so in most cases, it is not possible to attribute any particular fact or conclusion to a single author. Consequently, there are few specific references, but the 'Further Reading' list at the end of this book includes several sources that enlarge upon the various topics mentioned in the text.

The use of a few biological terms for kinds of organisms and parts of the body is unavoidable because there are no other unambiguous words for them. Many are mentioned in earlier books in this series and may already be familiar to readers who have studied some biology or anthropology; most are explained in greater detail in later chapters of this book.

There is one Reader article associated with this chapter, 'Why must I be a teenager at all?' by Barry Bogin, first published in 1993.[2]

Introduction

In many ways, humans are unique; some of our unique-ness arises from our evolutionary origin, some from our habits and culture. Many of our unique features and habits predispose us to certain diseases. Like all other animals, humans interact with many other organisms to obtain food and shelter. Although some modern city-dwellers seem to live largely isolated from their biological environment, the parasites and pathogens with which we came into contact when our recent ancestors lived as 'wild' creatures are still with us, and can be important causes of disease.

Parasites are organisms that spend part or all of their

---

[1]Another book in this series, *World Health and Disease* (Open University Press 1993).

[2]See *Health and Disease:* A Reader (Open University Press, revised edition 1994).

[3]The definition of 'species' is given in *Studying Health and Disease* (Open University Press, revised edition 1994), Chapter 9, as a population of organisms that usually interbreed in their natural habitat and produce fertile offspring. You do not need to memorise the Latinised names used in this book, which uniquely and unambiguously identify each species.

lives *on* (ectoparasites) or *in* (endoparasites) the body of another **species**[3] called the **host**. Many parasites do little harm to their hosts beyond minor irritation or taking small quantities of their food, but some may cause disease, either directly by poisoning the host or damaging its tissues, or indirectly by provoking damaging responses in the host, or by harbouring a third kind of organism that in turn causes disease. **Pathogen** is the term used in this book to refer to organisms that cause disease. The term refers not only to harmful **micro-organisms** which consist of a single cell and are only visible through a microscope, such as *bacteria*, *viruses* and single-celled animals like *Amoeba* (biologists call this group of organisms *protistans*), but also to **multicellular parasites** such as tapeworms, which consist of many cells and can be very large. (All these terms come up again many times in later chapters, where they are explained in greater biological detail. In particular, the meaning of 'a cell' is given in Chapter 3.)

In this book, we are concerned mainly with the pathogens that cause disease in *mammals*. All mammals are physiologically similar in a great many ways (for example, they all feed their young on milk), so experiments and observations on rats, guinea-pigs and other laboratory mammals can help us to understand the mechanisms of both normal and pathological processes in humans.[4] However, such studies tell us little about the origins or incidence of disease, or why people suffer frequently from disorders that are very rare in other kinds of animals. In this chapter, we look back into the distant past for clues about the origin of our anatomy, sensory and intellectual abilities, dietary requirements and diseases.

The evidence for human evolution is fragmentary, often only a few bones or stone tools; in spite of an intensive, world-wide search, we have very few human remains older than about 50 000 years, and those from earlier than 10 000 years ago are rare. Consequently, there are several contrasting theories, some of them mutually exclusive, about such crucial events as the evolution of sparse body hair, the origin of speech and conscious thought, and when and by what route people colonised the world's major continents. A thorough review of all the evidence is beyond the scope of this book, so we present a simplified picture, highlighting aspects of the story that clearly pertain to health and

disease. But you may find alternative accounts in other texts, and theories may be revised as new fossils and artefacts are discovered and existing remains are re-interpreted.

Humans as primates

Humans are **primates**, a distinctive group of mammals that first appeared more than 60 million years ago and which includes monkeys, apes, lemurs, lorises and many less familiar species. Most primates live in tropical forests, where they eat leaves, flowers, fruit, soft seeds and small animals such as insects. They have unspecialised teeth and guts and relatively long, flexible limbs that enable them to alternate between several different postures and modes of locomotion, including climbing and leaping. The five toes and fingers on each limb are relatively long and flexible, and are tipped with blunt, flat 'fingernails' in place of claws. Primates grip branches and grasp food between the fingers or toes rather than use sharp claws for

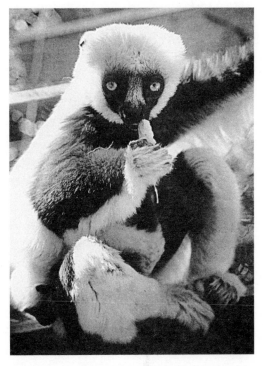

A ruff lemur Varecia variegata *with infant (whose head is visible at the lower left). Lemurs are primitive primates but they have most of the typical primate characters, including large, forward-pointing eyes, short nose and a large, rounded braincase. The limbs are long and mobile, with long flexible fingers and toes adapted to grasping. (Photo: Caroline Pond)*

[4] *Studying Health and Disease* (revised edition 1994), Chapter 9, discusses the practical and ethical advantages of, and constraints on, using laboratory animals as substitutes ('animal models') for humans in experiments to investigate human health and disease.

climbing and manipulating things. The brain is relatively large in all primates (compared to that of similar-sized mammals) and the eyes are prominent, forward pointing and, with the possible exception of some nocturnal species, capable of excellent colour vision and pattern discrimination. Hearing is also acute but, particularly in larger primates, the snout is relatively short and olfaction (the sense of smell) is not as sensitive as it is in most other mammals (e.g. dogs).

Nearly all monkeys and apes are social and most live in extended family groups led by a dominant adult, which in most species, but not all, is a male. Most species have frequent and elaborate social interactions between adults of both sexes as well as between infants and adults, and communicate by means of sounds (grunts, whistles, screams and more complex noises), facial expressions and gestures. Compared to other mammals of similar size, primates grow slowly, live a long time, and breed slowly, having only 1–4 babies at a time with many months, or, in large species, several years between pregnancies. In contrast to most other mammals, the young are not born in a permanent nest or den, and they cannot walk efficiently at birth. Instead, they are carried continually by one or both parents, giving the juveniles a 'front-seat' view of what their parents are eating, how they handle their food and how they detect and respond to danger and to other members of the group. Experiments in which infant monkeys are reared in isolation or by other species show that such experience is very important for successful foraging and for establishing normal social and sexual relations when adult.

The largest kinds of primates are the humans and the *apes* (two kinds of gibbons, orang-utans, gorillas, two kinds of chimpanzee and several extinct species), which differ from other primates in that the tail is greatly reduced, the chest is flattened from front to back instead of side to side, the lumbar region of the back (between the ribs and the pelvis) is shorter and stiffer and the shoulders and forelimbs are long and flexible. The apes are among the last major groups of primates to appear, the oldest fossils being about 30 million years old. As well as their fundamental anatomical differences, apes also differ from monkeys in intellectual and perceptual abilities; apes can monitor, and hence anticipate, each other's activities and are much better than monkeys at learning by observing the actions and experiences of other members of their species, as well as from their own experience. Gibbons and orang-utans

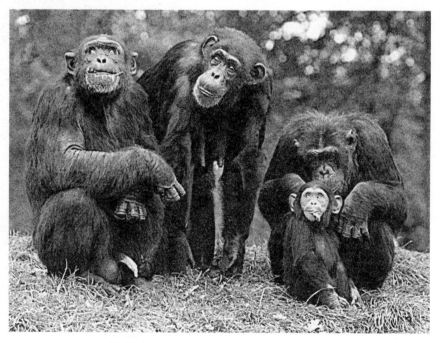

A chimpanzee family. Early hominids probably lived in family groups, as do most living species of apes. During their long juvenile period, infants associate closely with and learn from adult males (left) and other adult and subadult females, as well as their own mother (centre) on whom they are dependent for milk. They learn where to find food, how to detect and evade predators and how to deal with social and sexual interactions with other chimps. (Photo: Mike Levers)

live almost entirely in the crowns of tall trees but the other modern apes, although primarily forest-dwellers, can walk on the ground as well as climb trees.

All the basic features of apes are present, and in many cases enhanced, in humans. We live longer, grow more slowly and have still more elaborate forms of communication. Human ancestors probably lived in more open grasslands and savannah than other apes, and were almost certainly itinerant, walking from food source to food source over a large home range, carrying their infants with them. The prolonged contact between adults and children became increasingly important as foraging skills, social behaviour and communication became more elaborate, and so took longer to learn.

Some major features of human evolution

The direct ancestors of humans and their close relatives are collectively called **hominids**. Their remains can be recognised among fossils in central and east Africa from about 5 million years ago. Hominids are all primates belonging to several extinct species as well as the sole living species, *Homo sapiens*, which are the only hominids correctly referred to as 'people'. Hominid fossils are distinct from those of other ape lineages, so the last common ancestor of humans and modern apes lived well over 5 million years ago. Between about 3 and 1.8 million years ago, the climate became drier and possibly more variable, and in southeast Africa, dense rainforests gave way to grasslands and savannah. Fossil remains of hominids became more abundant (but still very rare compared to those of animals such as antelopes) and are found in south as well as east Africa. All known fossil hominids from 2 to 4 million years ago are found in sediments that contain animal remains and pollen typical of unforested areas, mostly grasslands, marshes and riversides, and many of the unique and fundamental features of our species may have evolved during this period.

◻ Compared to primates in general and to other apes, how recently have hominids appeared?

■ Very recently. The time since hominids took to living on grasslands is only about 5 per cent (3/60 million years) of that since primates first appeared, and only 10 per cent (3/30 million years) of the age of the oldest fossils of apes.

The evolution of hominids involved many anatomical changes that probably accompanied major changes in diet and foraging habits; hominids became more car-

nivorous than their tree-dwelling ancestors, eating carrion as well as animals that they killed for themselves. They probably lived and hunted in bands, cooperating to kill animals much larger than themselves (as do some carnivores, such as wolves and hyenas), and sharing or exchanging food with others. However, plant food almost certainly never disappeared completely from the diet and may have been the main source of nourishment at certain seasons.

Erect posture and bipedality

Upright posture is one of the most obvious and fundamental features of hominids. Although chimps and gorillas can stand erect and walk *bipedally* (on two legs) for a few metres, we are the only mammals that stand on our hind legs with straight knees and fully extended hips.

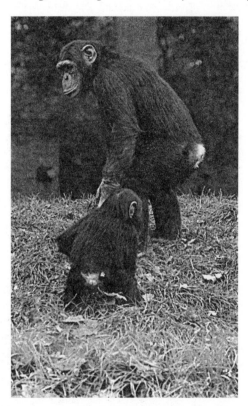

Chimpanzees walking bipedally. Note that like all non-human primates, these apes cannot straighten their knees or extend the hip fully, so they stand with a pronounced forward stoop. They do not go far in this posture: a four-legged gallop is faster and seems to be more comfortable for them. (Photo: Mike Levers)

Erect posture is among the first uniquely human characteristics to have evolved; analysis of skeletal remains and footprints indicate that, by 2–4 million years ago, hominids probably walked bipedally and stood erect, or nearly so.

The upright posture and **bipedality** involved several profound changes in the structure of the leg, foot, pelvis, spine and neck, which have had major consequences for human health and disease. Figure 2.1 is a summary of the main adaptations to erect posture. The leg became longer and the knee and hip joint almost fully extended, and the ankle flexed (Figure 2.1a), so that the foot is directly under the body. The foot (Figure 2.1b) became specialised for walking, almost completely losing the other functions it had in hominid ancestors and has in living apes, such as the capacity to grasp objects using opposable digits, in the same way as the hand does. Hominid toes are relatively shorter and more or less parallel, and the bones of the first ('big') toe are stout and strong because most of the weight of the body is carried on this toe. The foot becomes arched rather than flat as it is in apes; the tendons[5] strung between the bones of the middle of the foot absorb impact energy, cushioning the impact with the ground, and releasing the energy thus absorbed during the following stride.

The pelvis became shorter and more rounded, mainly due to the curving of the ilium and widening of the sacrum (Figure 2.1c) and greater curvature of the spine (Figure 2.1d). These changes are related to the enlargement of muscles that stabilise the hip on one side, while the other leg swings forward in a stride. Although they do not actually swing the legs, the contribution of these muscles is essential to long strides, and powerful, rhythmic walking and running. Chimpanzees, severely emaciated people (in whom the hip muscles are wasted and weakened), and those with paralysed hip muscles and people recovering from 'hip replacement' operations walk upright by shuffling rather than by striding, and cannot run at all.

Because it is stressed only in the fairly uniform forces of walking, rather than by the more variable forces generated by leaping and climbing, the head of the human femur (the thigh bone) is proportionately longer but less massive than in the tree-living apes, and has less efficient internal buttressing. These facts, and the importance for walking of correct coordination of the activity of the hip muscles (which may become weak or inefficient in old age), contribute to the tendency of the neck of the femur to break in old people. Such injuries often occur almost spontaneously, or following a very minor fall and, although much more effective treatment has been developed in the last 40 years, they are still fatal in roughly a quarter of cases. (The increased porosity of bone in old age, especially in women, is a contributory factor, as described in Chapter 8.)

The changes in the shape and size of the hip had important implications for the organisation of the soft tissues, and particularly for the process of *birth*. Although the anterior (upper) end of the pelvis is wider in hominids than in apes, the posterior (lower) end is narrow and the baby's head has to rotate in the birth canal as it is born. The problems of birth were probably much exacerbated by the increase in brain size among later hominids. The pelvis of modern humans is deeper from front to back, so the pelvic canal is more nearly round than that of early bipedal hominids. Some anthropologists believe that these changes actually reduced slightly the efficiency of walking and running. They are especially pronounced in adult women, who thus have a lower average maximum running speed than men.

Nonetheless, severe difficulties with childbirth are relatively common in humans, especially in very young women whose pelvis is not yet fully grown. Since mammalian births usually take place at night and in secluded nests or dens, there is very little detailed information about them, but so far as we can tell, the stress of giving birth is less severe, and perinatal and maternal mortality much less frequent in other mammals than they are in humans. Although labour is sometimes prolonged and apparently painful, maternal death is almost unknown among the few other primates in which many births have been observed.

In quadrupedal (four-footed) mammals, the head points forward and is attached to the neck by a stout ligament and strong muscles, which can be massive in animals such as wolves, pigs and bears. By comparison, the human neck is positively flimsy, and has so little muscle that large blood vessels and lymph nodes (sometimes called lymph 'glands') can be felt through the skin. Feel the crests of your own cervical (neck) vertebrae at the back of your neck. You may be able to locate all seven, although the first and last are often difficult to distinguish.

---

[5]In older biology and nursing textbooks, a rigid distinction between tendons and ligaments is often made (tendons connect muscle to bone and ligaments connect bones together); modern anatomists recognise that the composition and mechanical properties of these connective tissues are, in fact, almost identical and so, for simplicity, both are now often referred to as 'tendons', the term used in this book.

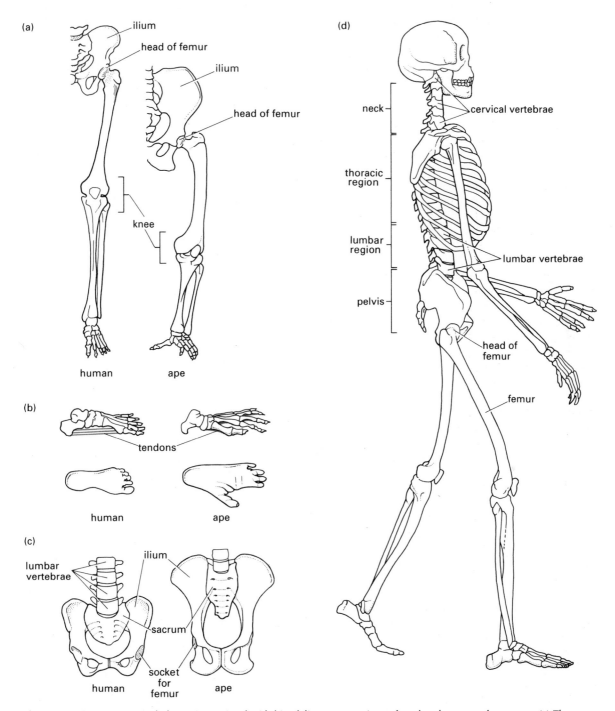

Figure 2.1 *Some anatomical changes associated with bipedality: a comparison of modern human and great ape. (a) The pelvis, leg and foot bones, (b) the foot bones and footprint, (c) the pelvis and lower spinal column, and (d) the human skeleton. (Based on Martin, R. D., 1992, Primate locomotion and posture, Chapter 2.8, p. 78, in Jones, S., Martin, R., Pilbeam, D. and Bunney, S. (eds) The Cambridge Encyclopedia of Human Evolution, Cambridge University Press, Cambridge.)*

In most other mammals, including dogs, horses and large apes such as chimps and gorillas, most of the cervical vertebrae are deeply buried in massive, powerful muscles so you could not feel them through the skin as you can your own.

Human heads are somewhat lighter than those of apes, because, although the brain is proportionately much heavier, the skull contains less bone and the jaw muscles are proportionately smaller and less powerful. However, the reduction in the neck muscles cannot be explained solely by the lighter head; it arises mainly from a fundamental change in posture made possible by bipedality. The human neck is almost vertical in all natural postures except lying down, and the skull is balanced on the cervical vertebrae, rather than braced against them (look back at Figure 2.1d). The occiput, the junction between the first cervical vertebra and the skull, is in the middle of the base of the skull and supports it from underneath, with the much smaller muscles just acting like 'guy ropes' around a flag pole. Areas of bone to which muscles were attached are easily identified on fossilised bones, so this integral feature of bipedality can often be identified even in small fragments of the skull.

The implications of walking upright

☐ What could have been the advantages to hominids living at this time of upright posture and walking bipedally?

■ The change from living in dense forest to open grassland may have promoted the shift from climber to walker. The erect posture is appropriate for walking and running on open ground, but much less suited to climbing or leaping in trees.

Although modern people, and presumably their anatomically similar hominid ancestors, can walk and run bipedally further and faster on flat ground than any other ape-like primate, humans still run slowly compared to quadrupedal mammals of similar size. Olympic races are won at average speeds of 6–10 metres per second (depending upon the distance), compared to 15–17 metres per second for racehorses and greyhounds. Bipedality also does not significantly improve the efficiency of locomotion; a person walking on two legs uses slightly less energy than a quadrupedal mammal covering the same distance at the same speed, but running requires proportionately more energy. So speed and efficiency of locomotion are unlikely to be explanations for why hominids adopted the upright posture.

Anthropologists have discussed several other suggestions for the circumstances that promoted the evolution of bipedality, for example: it enabled early humans to carry large items (tools, food, children, etc.), thereby promoting food sharing and improvements in hunting technology; erect hominids could feed in bushes and/or could see prey and enemies more efficiently, particularly on open savannah; upright hominids have a smaller proportion of the body exposed to direct sunlight, and hence heat up less rapidly under the tropical midday sun than quadrupedal animals of similar size, enabling them to run faster for longer without dangerous overheating.

Whatever the cause, a consequence of bipedality was to release the forelimb from direct involvement in locomotion. In other species in which comparable changes have taken place (e.g. kangaroos), the forelimbs became reduced, but in hominids the opposite happened. Tactile sensation and fine control of finger movement improved (though the length and maximum power output decreased compared to those of tree-climbing apes), making possible delicate manipulations of small objects, probably at first mostly food items such as seeds, and later tools.

The prevalence among modern people of lower back pain, arthritis of the hip and knee, and other skeletal disorders of the lower limb and pelvis is often attributed to incomplete or ineffective adaptation to the erect posture. However, when viewed on an evolutionary time-scale, this explanation is not convincing; relative to traits such as large brains, bipedality is ancient. Almost all the anatomical features that distinguish modern humans, *Homo sapiens,* from their probable direct ancestor, *Homo erectus,* relate to the skull, teeth and jaws; the rest of the skeleton has hardly changed for at least 2 to 2.5 million years, suggesting that an upright posture and bipedality were satisfactory for humans' habits. Any possible disadvantages arising in old age seem to be outweighed by advantages earlier in life, a subject to which we return in Chapters 5 and 8.

Human growth and life history

The development of humans, from a fertilised egg to a fully mature adult, is described elsewhere in this series.[6] Here, we take an overview of human growth, maturation and ageing across the lifespan. Humans live longer, take

[6]See *Birth to Old Age: Health in Transition* (Open University Press, revised edition 1995).

longer to reach sexual maturity and, in proportion to their size, grow more slowly than any other mammal. To understand how atypical the pattern of human growth is, we must compare it with that of a non-primate mammal such as a mouse and with another primate. In most mammals (Figure 2.2a), there is a steady growth rate between birth and maturity. In chimpanzees (Figure 2.2b), juveniles of both sexes grow at a rate of 4–6 kilograms per year for the first six years of life, but then the females continue to grow at a similar or declining rate. Growth in weight accelerates for the next 3–4 years in males, although by then their growth in height is almost complete.

□ List two features of growth rate that are peculiar to humans (Figure 2.2c).

■ Features unique to humans are the very slow growth in weight in childhood (1–9 years of age), and the later growth spurt in both sexes lasting about 3–4 years.

Human children grow at only 2–3 kilograms per year, compared to 4–6 kilograms per year for young chimps, although our average adult weight is similar to that of chimps. The acceleration in growth rate is called the **adolescent growth spurt**. It occurs about two years earlier in girls than in boys, with the result that for a brief period, the average height of girls is slightly greater than that of boys.

Secondary sexual characteristics (i.e. sex differences other than those of the reproductive organs) such as pubic hair, breasts, menstruation and adult voice appear during the adolescent growth spurt. But, whereas boys' sperm is fully fertile as soon as the testes and penis assume their adult form, girls cannot normally bear children until several years after acquiring other adult sexual characteristics. The adolescent growth spurt and this period of adolescent sterility in girls has no parallels in other mammals, which always become fertile and capable of adult sexual and parental behaviour in the next breeding season after they reach sexual maturity. Adolescence is associated with major changes in habits and desires as

Figure 2.2 *The average rates of growth in weight of (a) laboratory mice, (b) chimpanzees, (c) boys (solid circles) and girls (open circles) in the United Kingdom in the mid-twentieth century. (Based on Tanner, J. M.,1992, Human growth and development, Chapter 2.13, p. 100, in Jones, S., Martin, R., Pilbeam, D. and Bunney, S. (eds)* The Cambridge Encyclopedia of Human Evolution, *Cambridge University Press, Cambridge)*

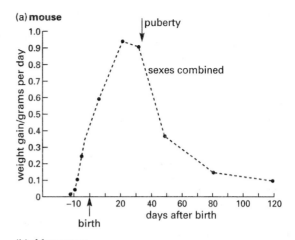

(a) **mouse**

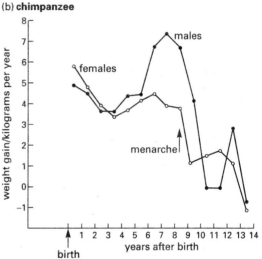

(b) **chimpanzee**

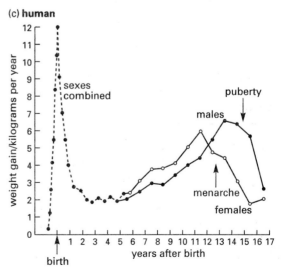

(c) **human**

well as in appearance and physical strength, some of which can lead to medical and social problems.[7] As Shakespeare put it:

> I would there were no age between ten and three-and-twenty...for there is nothing in the between but getting wenches with child, wronging the ancientry, stealing, fighting. (Shakespeare, 1610, *The Winter's Tale*, Act III, Scene 3)

Some recent scientific theories about the evolutionary origin and biological functions of human adolescence are discussed in a Reader article, 'Why must I be a teenager at all?', first published in 1993 by Barry Bogin, an American professor of anthropology. You should read it now. Bogin's account puts forward just one of several theories and is unlikely to be the last word on the topic; active research into human growth and sexual and social maturation is still in progress.

☐ Summarise the differences between the ages at which adolescent girls and boys begin to display secondary sexual characteristics, reach adult stature and achieve full reproductive capacity.

■ Girls develop secondary sexual characteristics first (around 11 years), then go on to reach adult stature (around 17 years), but only achieve full reproductive capacity at around 18 to 19 years of age. By contrast, boys develop secondary sexual characteristics and achieve full reproductive capacity at around the same age (roughly 14 years), but they don't reach adult stature until several years later.

☐ What does Bogin suggest are the advantages for human survival of these sex differences in the timing of growth and maturation?

■ Adolescent girls start to look like women long before they are reproductively mature, so they are invited into adult female society where they help with child-rearing and learn essential skills which later enhance their own children's chances of survival. Adolescent boys are excluded from many aspects of adult male society, even though they are reproductively mature, because they don't look like 'grown men'. This situation may enable boys to practise adult male behaviours, without running the

risk of injury in competition with mature men, until they become physically capable of fending for their dependents.

Another specifically human characteristic is *menopause*. At around age 45–50 years, women become infertile, secondary sexual characters such as breasts start to regress and a variety of changes in **metabolism** occur (metabolism refers to all the biochemical reactions going on in the body), including the turnover of calcium in the skeleton, and sexual and maternal habits generally decrease. After menopause, women usually remain in good health and may live for 30 years or more in the post-reproductive state. By contrast, female apes and monkeys continue to bear and rear young to the end of their lives, although the interval between births may increase a little with age, and profound metabolic changes comparable to those that are observed in women do not occur. Neither the fertility nor the capacity for sexual activity of men (and male apes) decrease any faster or more abruptly than the age-related decline in other physiological abilities such as running speed and maximum grip strength. In Chapter 8, we return to the subject of menopause and ask what its evolutionary significance might be. We also consider its effect on women's health.[8]

It is, of course, very difficult to be certain about the maximum lifespan of any wild mammal; elderly individuals are always a small proportion of natural populations, and their greater experience may enable them to avoid the attentions of intruding biologists more efficiently. But 70 years seems to be an absolute maximum for mammals, even for large species such as elephants, and few non-human primates live longer than 30–40 years. Thus both maximum and average human longevity are more than twice that of all modern apes. However, so far as can be determined, the average longevity of most female mammals is usually slightly greater than that of males, particularly in species such as baboons and polar bears where the adult males are much bigger than the females. On average, modern women live several years longer than men living under similar conditions,[9] a feature of the life history that we may have inherited almost unchanged from our primate ancestors.

Much effort has been directed to determining when in hominid evolution the peculiar features of human growth and longevity evolved, but since the analysis

---

[7]The health of British adolescents is discussed in *Birth to Old Age: Health in Transition* (Open University Press, 1985 and revised edition 1995).

[8]The social and personal consequences of the menopause among British women are discussed in *Birth to Old Age: Health in Transition* (1985 and revised edition 1995).

[9]See *World Health and Disease*, Chapter 9.

depends upon determining age independently of size and skeletal maturity, the subject is controversial, and there is little agreement beyond the conclusion that all the essential features of human growth and sexual maturation were in place by 1 million years ago. However, studies of tooth wear in skulls of Neanderthal people, an early subspecies (form) of *Homo sapiens* that lived in Europe between 130 000 and 40 000 years ago, suggests that few of them survived beyond the age of 40 years. Thus, until a few tens of thousands of years ago, menopause must have been a relatively rare occurrence.

In most long-lived species (e.g. elephants), organs such as teeth, eyes, ears, etc. 'wear out' before the end of the maximum lifespan and the failure of these structures often leads to starvation (because individuals cannot chew the available food) or increased vulnerability to predators (through lack of awareness of danger, or failure to keep up with the running herd).

☐ Defects of teeth, vision and hearing are an almost inevitable consequence of old age in humans. How are they now alleviated?

■ Technological advances such as cooking and the cultivation of plants that yield soft foods reduce the rate of tooth wear and offset the impairment of function once the teeth are worn. Much more recently, manufactured tools such as spectacles, hearing aids and false teeth partially correct loss of function. Living in social groups in which children and elderly people are protected reduces the dangers that arise from defects of vision and hearing.

All these aids and social habits greatly increase the life expectancy of elderly people, and impairment of function can be severe before the risks of external causes of death (e.g. starvation, predation and accidents) are substantially increased. Life expectancy for a few individuals may also be increased by 'spare-part' surgery to replace diseased or damaged organs and joints, a subject to which we return in Chapter 9.

Increased longevity has its drawbacks, however. Many parasites and pathogens that affect humans are rare and infection depends upon a chance encounter. Obviously, a longer lifespan increases the chance of exposure to a greater variety of such organisms and increases the probability of repeated infection. The human immune system has to be efficient to cope with the wide range of parasites and pathogens that it may encounter in its long life. These topics are taken up in much more detail in Chapters 5 and 6 of this book.

The evolution of soft tissues

Brain

The brain of the earliest hominids, as estimated from the volume of the braincase region of the skull, was about 0.4–0.5 litres, about the same size as that of modern apes, in a body that was a little smaller. For more than two million years, hominid brain size changed little, but about 2.2 million years ago, in *Homo erectus*, one of two distinct lineages of hominids called *Homo*, the teeth became smaller, the body lighter and more slender, and the brain larger (see Figure 2.3). The other lineage, *Australopithecus*, became taller and more massive, and

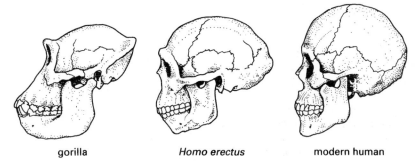

gorilla   *Homo erectus*   modern human

Figure 2.3 *Side views of some primate skulls. Left: a modern gorilla, whose last common ancestor with humans lived more than 5 million years ago. Centre: Homo erectus, an extinct hominid that lived about 1.4–2.0 million years ago and is probably ancestral to modern humans. The skull of Homo sapiens, modern human, is shown on the right. Note that in modern humans, the back of the skull enclosing the brain is taller and rounder than in Homo erectus, while the jaws are shorter and the face more flattened, with the eyebrow ridges greatly reduced. The volume of the brain, estimated from the capacity of the braincase region of the skull, averages 0.51 litres for adult gorillas, 0.95 litres for Homo erectus and 1.36 litres for modern humans. (Source: Open University S364 Course Team)*

evolved larger, stronger, more wear-resistant molar teeth (the grinding teeth at the sides of the jaw) but its brain changed very little. In *Homo*, the size of the brain relative to that of the body increased steadily for more than 1.5 million years, levelling off during the last few hundred thousand years at 1.0 to 1.6 litres (with an average of 1.36 litres), more than double the volume of the brain of early hominids. During the same period, molar tooth size decreased in *Homo*.

Fossils of both lineages of hominids occur in the same sediments in eastern and southern Africa, indicating that, for at least a million years, the large-brained and smaller-brained hominids coexisted. About 1 million years ago, *Australopithecus* disappeared without descendants and *Homo*, the lineage that eventually evolved into modern people, began to spread to southern Europe and Asia as well as expanding its range in Africa.

□ What can you conclude from this information about the advantages of a larger brain?

■ The advantages did not emerge immediately. The large-brained hominids have only become dominant within the last 1 million years. Small-brained but muscular hominids with large, powerful teeth coexisted for a long time with the smaller, lighter species that had relatively large brains.

Hair and fat

One of the most obvious differences between humans and all other primates is the peculiar condition of the hair: it is sparse or absent over much of the body, but grows thick and long on the head and in a few other patches, notably around the genitals. Almost nothing is known about when this arrangement evolved, and there is much controversy about its function. One likely theory is that hair reduction is an adaptation to prolonged, strenuous exercise that enabled people to run far and fast on tropical plains without overheating. Consistent with this idea are the facts that human sweat glands are much more numerous than those of apes, and people, especially light-skinned people, sweat more than apes.

The onset of the Pleistocene glaciations (the Ice Age), about 100 000 years ago, and the colonisation of central and eastern Asia and southern Europe meant that people began living in climates that were much cooler than those of Africa. There is no evidence that the body hair of such people became thicker or longer; instead, inhabitants of colder regions adopted the uniquely human habit of wearing the skins of other animals and, later, woven cloth.

Hair reduction reveals the skin and the tissues underlying it. Humans are almost unique among mammals in having pronounced, clearly visible sex differences in the distribution of fat (known to biologists as adipose tissue). These differences are minimal in children, develop rapidly at adolescence, are most pronounced in young adults and regress in old age. The breasts of adolescent girls and non-lactating women (i.e. those not producing milk) consist mostly of fat; the arrangement of adipose tissue on the thighs and buttocks accentuates the sex differences in bones of the pelvis and thigh. The distribution, texture and colour of the hair and superficial fat indicate a person's social and sexual status (i.e. distinguishing children, adolescents, mature adults and elderly people), and also help in the recognition of individual people from a distance, which would have been very important for nomadic hunters. Such minor but conspicuous sex differences in hair and superficial fat may have evolved as result of *sexual selection* (this important evolutionary process is explained in Chapter 5).

Cultural evolution

Culture can be defined as the habits, beliefs, values and knowledge transmitted between generations by observation and teaching rather than by genetic inheritance. It incorporates the religious, artistic and technological practices and social expression of a group of people with a shared tradition. Almost all theories about cultural change are based on the study of manufactured artefacts such as graves, tools and cave paintings, which provide some indirect information about hunting methods, living conditions and religious beliefs; very little data about cultural evolution can be obtained from the study of fossilised skeletons alone. It is impossible to pinpoint when cultural evolution began; deliberate human burials date from 100 000 years ago in Europe and Asia, and representational art and bone needles (suggesting manufacture of clothing) are known from about 40 000 years ago.

Tools

Manufactured tools are found only in association with remains of *Homo*, although earlier and contemporary hominids may have used sticks and unmodified stones as tools, as modern chimpanzees do. The first stone artefacts are dated at about 2 million years old, but manufacturing techniques and materials improved only slowly for the next 1.5 million years (see Figure 2.4). Nonetheless, such simple technology must have contributed greatly to hunting success, because the skeleton of *Homo* became less massive and the teeth smaller during this period, the

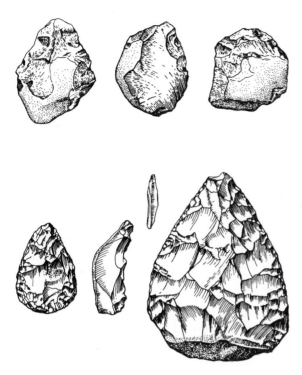

Figure 2.4 *Stone tools made by two different species of* Homo. Top row: *Simple chopping tools found in South Africa that were made about 1.7 million years ago, probably by* Homo habilis, *the first hominid to make stone tools.* Lower row: *More elaborate cutting and scraping tools made about 70 000 years ago by Neanderthal people, an early subspecies (form) of* Homo sapiens *living in western France. (Source: Open University S364 Course Team)*

opposite to expectations if teeth and brawn, rather than skilled manufacture and use of tools, determined hunting efficiency.

□ Should we conclude from such finds that all tools were made only of stone?

■ No. People may have made tools and other artefacts (e.g. clothing) out of other materials such as wood, shell, bone and leather, but they have all broken or rotted away. Only those made from very durable materials such as stone and pottery have survived long enough for us to study them.

Beginning about 0.5 million years ago, technology started to improve rapidly. A greater variety of more finely made stone tools (axes, choppers, scrapers and arrow heads) appeared, together with barbed fish-hooks, spear-throwers and, only a few tens of thousand years later,

bows and arrows, traps for catching fish and land animals, and tools for making tools. Some of these artefacts were composites of many different materials, including several kinds of wood and various grades of leather. In order to make such complex structures, people would have to plan ahead, assembling and preparing all the materials they would need to complete the article. It is possible that people obtained some of the rarer materials by trading with specialised suppliers, which gives us an important insight into the extent of cultural change taking place in this period.

It is important to emphasise that such elaborate artefacts are known only from the last 1–5 per cent of the time for which hominids have existed: they appeared *after* the brain reached its modern size and long after skeletal features such as erect posture, hands capable of fine manipulation, and reduced size of teeth were established.

Fire

The control of fire is a uniquely human achievement and is one of the major technological advances of the Palaeolithic.[10] Exactly when people acquired the ability is much disputed; there are definitely hearths 0.5 million years old, and the control of fires started naturally (e.g. by lightning or volcanoes) may have begun as long ago as 1.5 million years, long before people learnt how to light fires for themselves. Almost all animals are instinctively afraid of heat and flame, so fires near shelters and camps deter large predators, such as wolves and lions, thereby reducing losses of both people and stored food. However, managing and living close to fires doubtless caused many devastating injuries from burns and smoke inhalation in the Palaeolithic, as they still do today.

The earliest use of fire was probably deliberate burning of forests. This technique (which is still used) greatly increases the efficiency of hunting large animals by the creation and maintenance of open grassland instead of scrub or forest, in which prey are less plentiful and more difficult to see. Analysis of animal bones found near human settlements shows that hunting efficiency improved so much that, in many areas, some large mammals, including wild horses and mammoths, became extinct. Later people took to eating more small animals

[10]Archaeological terms like Palaeolithic (Old Stone Age) and Neolithic (New Stone Age) refer to stages in human *cultural* development, often characterised by the manufacture of particular kinds of tools or pottery. Different groups of people did not reach the same stage of cultural development simultaneously, so these terms do not indicate exact dates in the past.

(e.g. birds, rabbits), fish and shellfish, and, increasingly, plants. The control of fire also assisted the permanent colonisation of colder climates but its most far-reaching contribution to human culture was cooking.

□ How does cooking modify plant foods?

■ Many plants, especially roots and seeds, that are tough, toxic or unpalatable when raw can be made appetising and digestible by cooking, e.g. chestnuts, acorns, cassava, potatoes, turnips, rice, wheat, maize, beans, cabbage and many more.

Cooking meat also makes it easier to eat, and destroys the infective stages of most potentially harmful parasites, such as tapeworms (e.g. *Taenia* found in many large herbivores including cattle and pigs) and nematodes (e.g. *Trichinella spiralis,* which causes a debilitating disease called trichinosis). However, cooking also degrades the nutritional quality of many foods.

For example, early European explorers living off the land in the Arctic often suffered from scurvy, a disease caused by lack of vitamin C, characterised by anaemia, spongy gums and 'bleeds' under the skin. Scurvy is almost unknown among Eskimos,[11] even though they never ate potatoes or citrus fruit (which contain vitamin C and therefore prevent scurvy),[12] and indeed had no plant food at all except for a month or two in summer. The reason is that vitamin C occurs in meat, but is easily destroyed by cooking, smoking or drying. Eskimos traditionally ate meat raw (partly because there is little wood for fuel in the Arctic) and so obtained sufficient vitamin C from it. However, they suffered from trichinosis, particularly if they ate polar bears or arctic foxes, in which the parasite is very common. There are many other examples, some only recently revealed by modern chemical analysis, in which cooking improves or degrades the nutritional quality of foods. Clearly, the control of fire had far-reaching effects on both diet and health.

Clothing and shelters

Many early hominid remains are found in landscapes that include cliffs and caves, but it is far from certain that such

[11]Eskimo is the English word for the race of Arctic people probably descended from immigrants from Japan. In their own language, Inukitut, they call themselves 'Inuit' and some recent texts adopt this term.

[12]Treatment for scurvy is discussed in *World Health and Disease,* Chapter 11.

shelter was any more essential to humans than it is to modern apes. Colonisation of cooler climates led to the wearing of animal skins and, later, other forms of clothing and to the regular occupation of caves and (probably) other kinds of shelters. Leather and fur are rarely preserved, so we have little direct evidence about when or where these habits appeared, but the evolution of our ectoparasites tells us something about the change from naked nomads to fur-clad cave-dwellers.

Fleas are one such ectoparasite. They are wingless insects which, as adults, suck blood from mammals or, more rarely, birds, and attach themselves firmly to the host's fur (or feathers) by special hooks on the legs. Their flattened shape and remarkably tough outer covering enable them to scuttle quite fast through dense fur and to evade the most thorough grooming. The adults can live a long time between blood meals and can jump huge distances (relative to their minute size) from host to host. The eggs are laid in the host's nest, and the grub-like larvae feed for several weeks on detritus, dandruff and droppings deposited by the host. Nearly all mammals that breed or sleep in nests or dens are infested with fleas, often a unique species for each kind of mammal. Nomadic mammals, including nearly all primates other than humans, do not have their own species of fleas, although adult fleas from other species may feed on them transiently. Humans, however, are parasitised by a unique species of flea, *Pulex irritans*, that closely resembles the fleas that breed in the nests of badgers and foxes.

□ What can you deduce about human habits from these facts?

■ Humans have been occupying caves and other shelters regularly enough and for long enough for a species of flea that breeds only in association with humans to have evolved. The first human 'homes' may have been shared with, or formerly occupied by, ground-nesting mammals such as badgers and foxes. Early people were probably also more hairy or wore animal skins as clothes (or both).

Although their bite is little more than a nuisance, fleas, like other blood-sucking insects, can transmit disease-causing micro-organisms between species and from infected to uninfected members of the same species. Fleas that breed in the nests of other mammals, including those of rats, dogs and cats, often feed from each other's host, particularly when their normal host is absent. (Many readers may have experienced bites from cat fleas.) Many of the great plagues of the Middle Ages were caused by bacteria transmitted to humans by rat fleas.

Humans also harbour lice, another kind of blood-sucking insect that differs from fleas in many ways, among them the fact that the entire life cycle is completed in the host's fur. The human louse is similar to the species found on apes; we undoubtedly inherited the parasite from some distant common ancestor and have been troubled by their intensely irritating bites continually during the last 5 million years. The curvature of the louse's six legs closely follows that of its hosts' hair, enabling it to grip very tightly (and to resist combs and other forms of grooming). Each species is adapted to the shape of the hair of its own host. Humans have two kinds of lice, the head louse, *Pediculus humanus capitis*, which keeps strictly to the hair on the head, and the larger body louse, *Pediculus humanus humanus*, which seems to be happy to frequent, and lay its eggs upon, woven clothing and blankets as well as on body hair (e.g. pubic hair).

▫ What can you deduce from these facts about the evolution of human hair?

▪ The texture of head hair has been different from that of body hair for a long time.

Lice are still common in many parts of the world, especially where people live in close contact with each other or share unwashed bedding or clothing. Modern head lice resist regular shampooing and are now common among children in Western countries, including Britain.

Agriculture and pastoralism

Agriculture (the growing of crops) and **pastoralism** (herding and controlled breeding of animals as a food source) began about 10 000 years ago and continues to the present day. Instead of foraging for wild food and materials (the method of subsistence in *hunter-gatherer* societies),[13] people began to grow crops and herd or confine animals from which they obtained blood, milk, meat and non-edible products such as leather, fur, wool, horn, bone and (later) silk. Crops and livestock gradually became the main sources of nourishment, although many modern people still eat small quantities of wild food, e.g. wild mushrooms, truffles, berries, fish, whales, shellfish and game such as deer and grouse.

[13]Hunter-gatherers and the transition to agriculture and pastoralism are introduced in *World Health and Disease*, Chapter 5.

Many scores of different plants, but fewer than 20 species of animals have been *domesticated*, i.e. selectively bred in captivity for features and habits that suit human needs and desires. Agriculture and pastoralism have had profound effects on human diet, social organisation, health and the ecology of the organisms around human settlements; many wild animals have been hunted to extinction, or their habitat destroyed, to make space for agriculture and pastoralism. The process is by no means complete; as biological knowledge advances, more animals, plants and, increasingly, micro-organisms are being harnessed to human uses (for example by genetic engineering, a topic we discuss in Chapter 9).

Comparisons of seeds and other plant remains found in and around ancient human settlements before and after the development of agriculture reveal a drastic reduction in the variety of food eaten that has only been reversed in Western countries during the last hundred years. This reduced variety can in itself give rise to nutrient imbalances and deficiencies, and nutritional degradation from crop processing and storage. For example, cabbage (and related plants such as sprouts, cauliflower and broccoli) is in many ways an excellent food, but it interferes with iodine absorption, especially when eaten raw. This property does not matter if there is plenty of iodine in the diet and/or only moderate quantities of raw cabbage are eaten, but it can promote a condition called goitre (excessive growth of the thyroid gland, *see photo overleaf*), retarded growth and cretinism (severe, irreversible mental retardation) among people living away from the sea (the main source of iodine) in areas where the drinking water lacks iodine.

Animals and humans living in parts of the world where there are marked seasonal changes in climate face a severe problem; fresh food is abundant at some times of year but scarce at others. Some kinds of mammals, e.g. rodents such as squirrels, rats and mice, thrive on stored food such as seeds and dead leaves. Their bodies can synthesise many of the vitamins that would otherwise be obtained from a diet of fresh food.

▫ What basic habits of other primates indicate that they would need plenty of fresh food at all times of year?

▪ As explained at the beginning of this chapter, nearly all primates, including all the apes, live in the tropics, where there is less seasonality of plant growth than at higher latitudes, and they are nomadic, moving between food sources. With continuous access to fresh plants, they would not need the ability to survive on stored or dead plants as food.

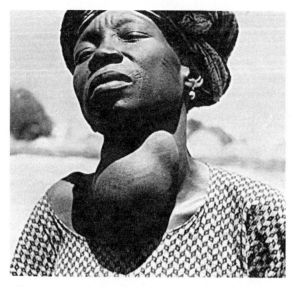

Goitre: a massive enlargement of the thyroid gland in the neck caused by prolonged deficiency of iodine in the diet. Seawater, and hence fish and other seafoods, are rich in iodine but some inland rivers, lakes and wells contain so little that goitre is common among people dependent upon such water. The disease, which can lead to mental retardation, was common in Derbyshire until the invention of the railways gave local people access to marine fish and whelks. (Photo: Wellcome Medical Foundation)

Unlike other primates, humans have colonised virtually every land habitat. Especially in mountains and semi-desert areas, only a few plants can be cultivated efficiently and almost all crops are seasonal, so much of the harvest has to be stored, often for many months. Modern people are the only primates to store food in large quantities or for longer than a few days and we cannot match the rodents' ability to compensate for absent or degraded vitamins and other essential nutrients in stored food. The less nutritious diet probably contributed to the reduction in stature and robustness following the adoption of agriculture that has been observed among skeletons found in various parts of southern Europe and Israel. Farming men were, on average, 3 cm, and women 4 cm, shorter than their hunter-gatherer ancestors. Analysis of skeletons and tooth enamel in cemeteries shows that life expectancy after the age of 15 declined in many parts of the world after the adoption of farming.

Although it later improved gradually, average life expectancy did not reach pre-agricultural levels until the eighteenth century.[14] Meanwhile, three (of more than 30)

[14]See *World Health and Disease*, Chapter 5.

species of mouse (*Mus*), and later several species of rats, evolved the habit of living in and near human dwellings, where they raided people's food stores and accompanied them wherever they travelled with their baggage and provisions. The consequences of this association for human health have been profound, as the epidemics of plague exemplify.

Cooking and farming

Grains (e.g. wheat, oats, barley, maize, rice), roots (e.g. taro, yams, manioc and potatoes) and pulses (e.g. peas, beans, lentils, soya) were among the first plants to be domesticated, and are still the most widely cultivated species. Such foods store very well, but must be cooked or otherwise processed before they can be eaten. They contain much more starch and starch-like nutrients, and much less protein than was normal in the diets of hunter-gatherers. Both wheat and maize lack certain nutrients that are present in pulses: long-established recipes and eating habits minimise the nutritional deficiencies of monotonous diets. Thus tortillas and beans, pea-soup and bread, and baked beans on toast are more satisfying and more nutritious eaten together than is either component separately.

Cooking and farming, particularly of cereals, also had other less direct, but equally profound, effects on people's well-being. The consequences of the new diet for dental health remain unsolved to the present day. Raw food, particularly leaves and nuts, are coarse and abrasive, and make the teeth wear rapidly, but the frequent abrasion prevents the accumulation on the teeth of the bacteria that cause dental caries (tooth decay). The teeth of ancient hunter-gatherers (and of some modern people who did not eat cereals, such as Eskimos) wore rapidly but rarely decayed. Grains such as wheat are among the stickiest of all foods, and, particularly when combined with sugar and fats, form a coating on the teeth that provides an ideal habitat for bacteria. Continual exposure to high concentrations of bacteria gradually corrode the hard surface of the teeth. Dental caries is now so widespread that we regard it as inevitable, but it was very rare among pre-agricultural people, and not common among the early farmers of ancient Egypt.

☐ Why do we know so much about dental health in these ancient people?

■ Teeth are very durable and remain intact for thousands of years after burial.

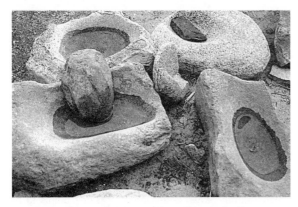

Grinding tools at Little Petra, Jordan, where agriculture was well established 8 000 years ago. Grain was ground, a handful at a time, in a hollowed-out bowl using hard stones such as the one in the left foreground, by the operator kneeling in front and pushing and pulling with both arms. Very similar apparatus has been in use in remote areas until the middle of this century. (Photo: Caroline Pond)

Surface scratches and cavities in teeth are easily identified in human remains, as is evidence of surgical extraction or natural loss of adult teeth. The practice of burying the dead in specially prepared tombs, first performed on a large scale by the ancient Egyptians about 5 000 years ago, further facilitates such studies.

Cooking makes most foods easier to chew and more digestible and thus more suitable for infants (and elderly people). Babies could be weaned onto cereal gruels and meat or vegetable soups at a much earlier age than was possible when the only soft food available was that pre-chewed by the mother. In humans, lactation partially (though not completely) inhibits conception, but once she stops breast-feeding, the mother's fertility increases quickly. By facilitating early weaning, cooking and cereal production promoted shorter average intervals between births, but the physiological stress to the mother of each pregnancy and of caring for infants remained much the same. So more frequent pregnancies, combined with caring for numerous dependent children, increased the burden of reproduction for most women.

The development of dairy farming permitted even earlier weaning onto goats', ewes' or cows' milk, and further reduced the minimum time between births from about 4 years to less than 2 years. This reduction doubled the potential number of children a woman could rear in her life-time (i.e. her **fecundity**) from 5 to 6 children to more than 10. Cereal gruels and animal milk are less easily digested by very young infants, and are often less nutritious than breast milk. The artificial diet is also much more easily contaminated with pathogens or pollutants, so infants weaned at a young age often suffer more ill-health and grow more slowly than breast-fed children. Consequently, infant mortality was probably higher among farmers than among hunter-gatherers, but such losses were more than offset by the greatly increased number of children they produced.

The costs and benefits of working the land

Wherever hunter-gatherer and primitive agricultural lifestyles have been compared, the latter is much harder work, involving longer hours of strenuous physical activity, and more repetitive actions and unnatural postures (e.g. planting crops, grinding corn), which involve physiological stress. For example, comparison of the incidence of arthritis in skeletons from pre-agricultural and post-agricultural deposits suggest that the disease is largely restricted to elderly people in hunter-gatherer societies, but becomes much more common in younger farming people.

To be able to reap where they have sown, farming people are much more sedentary than hunter-gatherers. Many forms of animal husbandry also require people to live in permanent settlements, although some pastoralists remain nomadic to the present day, moving between good grazing areas with their flocks and herds.

☐ How would sedentary habits affect the incidence of infectious diseases?

■ Sedentary habits mean living continuously near one's own refuse and that of the livestock, which, together with more disturbance of soil and water, promotes transmission of infectious diseases. A settled home also favours the breeding of ectoparasites such as fleas and lice, and stored food supports rats and mice, some of which may harbour infectious diseases.

On the other hand, agriculturalists came into contact with wild animals less frequently, so accidents and hunting injuries may have become rarer.

Compared with hunting, agriculture and pastoralism are much harder work and do not produce a healthier diet, and unforeseen and uncontrollable failures in supply are no more easily avoided, so why did people abandon hunting and gathering in favour of the new technology? The most plausible answer is that the practices enabled people to live at higher densities and, because one family could produce enough food for several others, more people were able to devote themselves full-time to activities unrelated to food acquisition, such as religion, arts, manufacturing, building, commerce and politics. Agriculture made possible the political infrastructure and labour needed to raise an army or undertake major projects such as building irrigation systems, ramparts, temples and pyramids.

Wherever they come into direct conflict, people living in such complex communities defeat hunter-gatherer groups who have no tradition of centralised political leadership. For example, the main reason why Eskimos are confined to the tundra is that the more numerous, better-armed and politically better-organised Amerindians could (and frequently did) defeat small bands of Eskimos that entered forested areas in search of wood. Except in Australia, all modern hunter-gatherers are confined to the Arctic, deserts, inaccessible rainforest and other areas that are useless for agriculture. In short, agriculture produced modern society and enabled the human population to increase very rapidly; it is estimated

that there are now at least 1 500 times as many people as there were about 9 000 years ago, when agriculture and animal husbandry began.[15]

Comparisons between the few remaining modern hunter-gatherer societies and agricultural societies suggest that, although the changes brought about by agriculture diversified and extended men's activities, on the whole they reduced the social status and opportunities of women. Ownership of agricultural land and other resources increased the importance of inheritance and hence of paternity, which restricted women's choice in marriage and promoted more severe penalties for infidelity and low fertility. More of their lives was spent pregnant or caring for small children, many of whom would die young, and food production, preparation and storage became more onerous. Women became more tied to the home, and had less opportunity to collaborate with the men in artistic, commercial and political activities.

The origins of infectious diseases

As you will see later in this book (Chapter 5) many of the most dangerous and debilitating human diseases are caused by pathogens. They fall into two main groups: **endemic human diseases** in which the pathogens are transmitted from person to person (e.g. dysentery, typhoid, influenza, syphilis) and **zoonoses** in which the pathogens either spend part of their life cycle in or on another species (the secondary host), or were originally diseases of other animals that incidentally or occasionally infected people.[16] The prevalence of endemic diseases depends very much upon the habits of the people themselves, such as their mobility, hygiene and group size. The life cycles and abundance of zoonoses are largely independent of human population density, although our habits, particularly diet, may greatly influence their transmission from the other species to humans. While working as a vet at the London Zoo in the 1950s and 1960s, Richard Fiennes demonstrated **cross-infection** of parasites and infectious diseases between different species of animals and between animals and people, and developed the theory of the animal origins of many human infectious diseases. (The standard text is

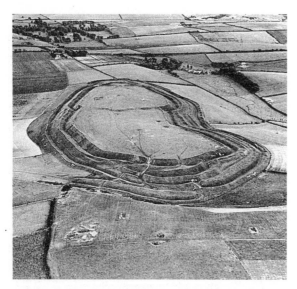

Maiden Castle near Dorchester in Dorset. This impressive structure, fortified with several rows of dykes and ditches, was built by people who became numerous and had established a highly organised society more than 2 000 years ago (long before the Romans invaded Britain). It may have been a religious centre or a military fort, or both, for the surrounding population, who kept sheep and other livestock, grew crops and made a rich variety of metal and wooden tools, pottery, clothes and ornaments. (Photo: Aerofilms Ltd)

[15]See *World Health and Disease,* Figure 5.2, estimated population of the world from 40 000 BC to AD 2 025.

[16]*World Health and Disease,* Chapter 3, introduces endemic diseases, zoonoses, primary and secondary hosts, and vector-born diseases.

listed under Fiennes, 1978, in the Further Reading list at the end of this book.) In the final part of this chapter, we will illustrate this theory in a brief review of some major infectious diseases, starting with those involving larger parasites which are generally visible with the naked eye for at least part of their life cycle. (You are not expected to memorise the details; most are mentioned again in Chapters 5 and 6 of this book.)

Multicellular parasites

Most flatworms (which include tapeworms and flukes) and unsegmented roundworms (known to biologists as *nematodes*) cannot be transmitted from person to person, but require a secondary host to complete their life cycle. Most such life cycles are very complex and often variable. The following examples give you an idea of the number and variety of interactions between people and their biological environment.

Schistosomiasis (or bilharzia), a complex and debilitating disease, is caused by *Schistosoma*, a fluke for which the secondary host is a freshwater snail; river blindness and elephantiasis are caused by several species of nematode and are transmitted by various biting flies including blackflies (*Simulium* species) that breed in freshwater; the guinea worm, *Dracunculus medinensis*, is also a nematode that proliferates in a small freshwater shrimp-like animal. All these parasites also infect other mammals, including dogs, horses, cattle, apes and monkeys and have probably troubled hominids for millennia. But the parasites probably became more common when, as mentioned earlier, fish became an important food many thousands of years ago. People spent more time standing or swimming in freshwater (and defaecating in or near it) than would have been necessary when they hunted land mammals. More recently, artificial irrigation systems created additional habitat for the snails that serve as the secondary host for the fluke.

The adult stages of the tapeworm *Taenia* (and of the nematode *Trichinella*, mentioned earlier as a problem among Eskimo peoples) occur only in mammals that eat the flesh of other mammals so are very rare in other primates. These parasites have probably been an occasional cause of illness ever since hominids became hunters, but *Taenia* did not become common until people began living in close association with domesticated pigs. The use of human and animal excreta as manure increases crop yields and reduces the need for chemical fertilisers, but it also facilitates the transmission of parasites. In fact, in central China, lavatories were sometimes built over pigsties, enabling the pigs to eat the freshly deposited human faeces. While these arrangements recycle the faecal nutrients as pig food and hence eventually as food for humans, they also maximised the efficiency of transfer of tapeworm eggs from humans to pigs.

☐ How can the spread of the parasites from pigs to humans be limited?

■ Cooking the pork kills the infective stages of the tapeworm in the pigs' muscle, and thereby limits the spread of the parasite.

However, one meal of incompletely cooked meat is often enough to establish infection, so in practice a high proportion of people who eat pork from pigs reared in this way harbour tapeworms. People have probably been troubled by tapeworms for many thousands of years, but many parasites, some of which cause serious disease, have apparently spread into the human population quite recently, as a direct result of people's habits and their associations with domesticated animals.

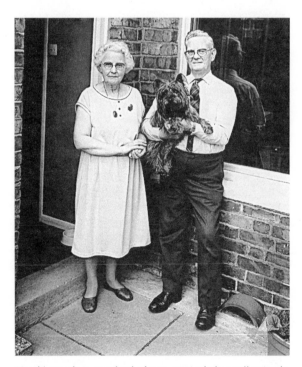

People are often very fond of pets, particularly small animals with 'baby' features such as relatively large eyes and head, short limbs, and soft fluffy fur. (Photo: Mike Levers)

For example, *Toxocara* nematodes are normally parasites of dogs and cats. The larvae infest the lungs, liver, muscles and uterus (whence nearly all puppies acquire them from their mother before birth) and eventually migrate to the gut where they mature. The ripe eggs are eliminated with the faeces and may be eaten by a rat or mouse, in which they become larvae that burrow into the rodent tissues. Dogs and cats are normally re-infected by eating infested prey. Humans, particularly children, may acquire *Toxocara* eggs from contact with contaminated dog or cat faeces or from handling puppies. The resulting larvae wander through the human tissues, causing abdominal and muscular pains. More rarely, but more seriously, they infest the eye, and cause blindness. Clearly, the use of cats to kill the rodents that eat our stored food, and the keeping of cats and dogs as pets, greatly facilitate the transmission of *Toxocara,* increasing its abundance and turning what were formerly rare, isolated cases of cross-infection into a significant medical problem.

Micro-organisms

Malaria and yellow fever are zoonoses endemic to Africa that we probably inherited from our primate ancestors. At least four different species of the single-celled animal, *Plasmodium,* cause malaria, and a virus causes yellow fever. These pathogens cannot pass directly from person to person but are transmitted by a *vector*, in both cases blood-sucking mosquitoes. Although the micro-organisms live for some time in the secondary host, their presence does no apparent harm to the mosquitoes, which continue to feed from any thin-skinned mammal they find, including humans. An opportunity for the pathogenic micro-organisms to invade another host is created each time an infected insect pierces a host's skin to take a blood meal. The malaria-carrying *Anopheles* mosquitoes breed in warm, stagnant water, so shallow pools and ditches created by artificial irrigation systems in the tropics provide ideal habitats for them.

Sleeping sickness is caused by several different kinds of the protistan, *Trypanosoma,* which also parasitise many species of birds, reptiles, amphibians and mammals, including deer, horses, antelope, buffalo and cattle. *Trypanosoma* is transmitted by tsetse flies between people and between humans and other animals, many of which appear not to suffer any serious symptoms of disease. Because such wild animals can harbour the pathogen for a long time without becoming ill, they act as a reservoir from which humans and their domesticated livestock can acquire the infection.

☐ Is it likely that sleeping sickness would have occurred among our hunter-gatherer ancestors?

■ Yes, probably. Hunters had frequent contact with the large mammals in which the pathogens occur, and people may have followed the herds, sleeping and eating near their grazing grounds, thereby exposing themselves to tsetse flies.

Diseases such as sleeping sickness, yellow fever and malaria are rare outside the tropics because their insect vectors cannot breed in cold climates. Rabies is a zoonosis that is transmitted by one mammal biting another and so is world-wide in distribution, even occurring among foxes and seals in the high Arctic. People can acquire the infection from many kinds of mammal, most often bats, foxes and dogs (but, curiously, not from other humans), and so this fatal disease almost certainly afflicted hunter-gatherers who shared the caves that these animals used as dens or roosts, and may also have caught them as food.

Some bacteria and viral diseases that are now endemic to humans appear to have originally been zoonoses that underwent a physiological transformation that enabled them to transfer directly from person to person. We will look at the evolutionary process more closely in Chapter 5; here we focus on the interaction between human culture and the biological environment that increased the likelihood of transmission between people and other animals. Many of these infectious diseases originated in domestic animals and therefore must have spread to people only since the rise of animal husbandry. For example, the microscopic structure of the measles virus closely resembles that of the canine distemper virus (which causes a 'flu-like disease in wolves and dogs) and the rinderpest virus, which causes debilitating disease in many kinds of hoofed mammals, including domestic cattle. Measles may have become a human disease after domestication of the dog about 12 000 years ago, or when people took up pastoralism about 8 000 years ago, but there were no known serious epidemics of the disease until the middle of the first millennium AD. It was a major cause of death among children in Europe and Asia until the middle of this century and is still a hazard among Third World children.

Smallpox is probably a mutant form of cowpox, a relatively benign disease of cattle. The first recorded major smallpox epidemic occurred in the eastern Roman

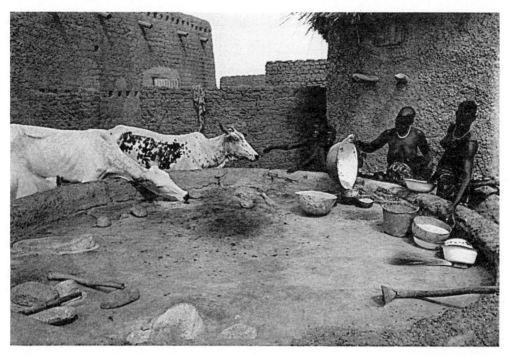

People and their domestic animals have lived in close proximity since animal husbandry started to replace hunting more than 8 000 years ago. Parasites and infectious diseases derived from, or shared with, livestock are very common in pastoral societies, like this one in the West African state of Burkina Faso, often affecting almost the entire population. (Photo: Panos Pictures/Jeremy Hartley)

empire (Syria, Turkey, Cyprus) in the second century AD, and there were scores more outbreaks of the disease before its similarity to cowpox was exploited. Vaccination with matter from cowpox pustules gave some protection against later infection with smallpox.[17] Diphtheria is another major disease derived from cattle husbandry and milk drinking. It is caused by toxins secreted by the bacterium *Corynebacterium diphtheriae* that proliferates on cow udders, where it produces minor ulcers, but no serious disease. Diphtheria is a relatively new disease; it is mentioned in writings from the 6th century AD but did not become widespread until the sixteenth century in Spain, by which time it could be transmitted directly from person to person as well as from cattle to people.[18]

Cattle (and many related hoofed animals) suffer from tuberculosis, caused by the bacterium *Mycobacterium tuberculosis bovis*. People who drink raw (i.e. unpasteurised or unboiled) milk risk infection with the bacterium, which enters the body via the bowel and thence travels to the spleen, kidneys, bones and joints, where it produces characteristic deformations. Such evidence for bovine tuberculosis is observed in a few Neolithic human skeletons from 7 000 years ago and in some Egyptian mummies. Much more recently, probably within the last 1 000 years, a new strain of bacteria called *Mycobacterium tuberculosis hominis* has appeared; it can live for short periods in air and so can be transmitted directly from person to

[17]The early history of vaccination against smallpox is described in another book in this series, *Caring for Health: History and Diversity* (Open University Press, revised edition 1993), Chapters 3 and 4. The global eradication of smallpox achieved in 1980 is the subject of a Reader article by Marc Strassburg, studied with *World Health and Disease*, Chapter 3, and revised later in the present book (Chapter 6).

[18]Diphtheria was common in Europe until immunisation was developed. It is one of the few infectious diseases that have been almost eliminated by immunisation. The relatively small contribution of immunisation and medical therapy to control of other infectious diseases is the subject of a Reader article by Thomas McKeown, studied with *World Health and Disease*, Chapter 6.

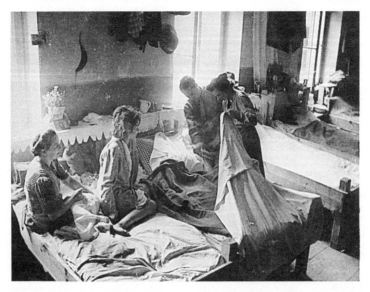

The human body louse flourishes in refugee camps like this one in Poland in 1945, where people are forced to live in overcrowded and insanitary conditions. Here bedding is being treated with anti-louse powder. As well as being an irritant, numerous lice can lead to epidemics of typhus fever, which took thousands of lives in refugee and army camps all over continental Europe at the end of World War II. (Photo: Hulton–Deutsch Collection Ltd)

person in their breath. This form of tuberculosis mainly affects the lungs and has become a serious endemic disease.[19] There is more about the physiological and evolutionary consequences of people drinking animal milk in Chapter 7.

Horses are the only animals other than humans to harbour the rhinoviruses ('nose' viruses) that cause colds. Rhinoviruses undergo frequent changes in microscopic structure and properties and numerous variant forms of the virus probably spread into the human population after horses were domesticated about 6 000 years ago. The large number of variants of rhinovirus means that people 'catch a cold' many times in their lives, as new variants are encountered.

Earlier, we mentioned plague and the association with rats living in human settlements, but we can take the story back even further in time. The plague bacterium originated among burrowing rodents and their fleas on the dry plains of central Asia. Gerbils were probably the original host, but the organism proliferates in dozens of related species, including ground squirrels, marmots, hamsters and rats. By 1940, it had been described in 34 different rodents and 35 species of fleas in the USA alone. Disturbance of the land by agriculture brought gerbils and their fleas into contact with the rats that lived in close association with people, eating their stored food. Where mammals mix, their fleas do as well, and thus plague became a disease of rats and then of people, probably during the first century AD. There were numerous outbreaks of plague, particularly in the densely populated agricultural areas of India, northern China, southern Russia, parts of Africa, and, from the fifth century AD onwards, in western Asia and Europe.

Typhus also originated from rodents, in this case mice. It is caused by a kind of very small bacterium called rickettsia. Mouse typhus is transmitted by lice and, although widespread, is not very dangerous to mice nor to people who, since ancient times, have sometimes contracted this form of the disease from mouse lice. Early in the fifteenth century, probably in Europe, a new form of the rickettsia arose that is much more lethal both to people and to the human lice that transmit it.

☐ What would be the consequences of the lice becoming ill?

■ They probably stop searching out new hosts and sucking their blood, thereby ceasing to be effective as vectors of the disease, and they may fail to breed.

[19]Tuberculosis is the subject of a major case study in the first book in this series, *Medical Knowledge: Doubt and Certainty* (Open University Press, revised edition 1993), Chapter 4.

Failure to feed and abnormal lethargy are probably the only ways that scientists know that the lice are adversely affected by infestation with the rickettsia. Lice infected with the typhus rickettsia never survive longer than a fortnight, and louse morbidity and mortality usually contribute more than human mortality to terminating epidemics of typhus that were (and in some areas still are) frequent and severe, especially in overcrowded cities, ships and army encampments.

This example illustrates the *instability* of the balance between survival of the host species and survival of the pathogens that infest them. The constantly changing relationship between environmental conditions and the evolution of pathogens and their hosts is discussed further in Chapter 5.

Conclusions

Humans are primates and much of our anatomical structure and sensory abilities, our social habits and dietary needs, arise directly from that heritage. Some of the anatomical and physiological features that make humans unique among primates still have medical repercussions. The demands of giving birth to large-brained infants compete with those of bipedality and walking efficiency in shaping the pelvis. The hip and thigh of modern women are significantly less efficient for walking and running than those of hominids of 3 million years ago, and mechanical difficulties in giving birth are much more frequent and severe than in any other mammal for which there is adequate information.

It is important to realise that evolution cannot be arrested; human anatomy, physiology, reproductive habits and longevity will change in the future in ways shaped by agriculture, industrialisation, modern medical practice and much more. The fossil record of humans and other species clearly shows that the rate of change of a structure usually accelerates when habits and habitat are changing rapidly. Human culture and technology are now changing faster than ever.

The course and incidence of infectious diseases are profoundly affected by our biological heritage and by interactions with other species, both ancient or recent. One striking feature of the biology of 'new' human infections is the variable, often very long, interval between their first appearance and becoming widespread or serious. Measles, tuberculosis, plague, and perhaps smallpox probably affected people occasionally for centuries, even millennia, before they became a cause of serious epidemics (and hence were mentioned in official records). The same may be true of AIDS.

The evolutionary processes described in this chapter (and expanded in Chapters 3 to 5) are still in operation and will continue in the future. Diseases have been acquired from 'new' foods such as cows' milk, and from animals such as cattle, pigs and rats with which we came into frequent contact relatively recently, and, although most of these diseases are now controllable, new ones can, and probably will, emerge by similar mechanisms. We add new 'unnatural' components to our diet (e.g. novel foods, synthetic drugs and hormones), acquire new stressful habits (e.g. driving fast cars in dense traffic) and expose ourselves to new infections derived from animals (e.g. psittacosis, a kind of bird pneumonia that is common in pigeons, named after the Latin word for parrot, *psittacus*). It is important to emphasise that most such habits and most pets and livestock pose little threat to the health of their owners. The half a dozen cases of psittacosis each year may attract attention, but the rest of the millions of people who live for years in close contact with poultry, pigeons, budgerigars and parrots do not develop the disease (though such contact may contribute, along with smoking, to susceptibility to lung cancer).

However, when people's habits favour their development and transmission, new diseases can become common. AIDs (caused by a virus that may have originated in monkeys) is just the latest in a long series of diseases that have arisen apparently *de novo*, and spread alarmingly rapidly through populations who are unused to dealing with them.

There is also no reason to conclude that humans are inherently more susceptible to disease than other animals. Human diseases have been far more intensively studied than those of any other species, so we know something about even very rare diseases that affect perhaps one person in a million. Among wild animals, only the commonest and most lethal diseases have been investigated scientifically; rare or chronic diseases go unnoticed among all the other causes of mortality such as starvation and predation. Other animals, particularly large, long-lived species, probably have similarly complex relationships with their biological environment about which we know very little. Indeed, disturbance of such disease patterns may be behind the unexplained decline and extinction of some species.

Finally, we should avoid idealising primeval humans and should not underestimate the enormous benefits that agriculture, animal husbandry and other aspects of civilisation have brought to human health. Would you swap a comfortable home for a damp, dark, smoky cave infested with lice, fleas and rabies-carrying bats and rats, in constant danger of injury from both large prey and other predators?

OBJECTIVES FOR CHAPTER 2

When you have studied this chapter, you should be able to:

2.1 Describe some anatomical and physiological similarities and differences between modern humans and other living kinds of primates, and comment on their possible consequences for human health and survival.

2.2 Outline the evolutionary origin and main implications for human health of: bipedality; enlarged brains; hair reduction; adolescent growth spurt; menopause.

2.3 Outline the main implications for human health of: the control of fire; living in caves and shelters; wearing clothes; cultivation of crops; animal husbandry.

2.4 Illustrate the interaction between human culture and the biological environment with examples of some zoonotic human diseases.

QUESTIONS FOR CHAPTER 2

Question 1 (*Objective 2.1*)

Which features and habits of non-human primates are associated with the evolution of the following?
(a) large, forward pointing eyes, good colour vision and reduced sense of smell;

(b) relatively small jaws and unspecialised teeth;

(c) good balance, agile, flexible limbs and flat, blunt fingernails and toenails.

Question 2 (*Objective 2.2*)

Describe in a few sentences the main changes to the pelvis and spinal column that have evolved in humans. How do these adaptations to locomotion affect the process of giving birth? How does the growth and mature shape of the female pelvis affect locomotion?

Question 3 (*Objective 2.3*)

What adverse effects did (a) occupying caves and shelters, and (b) living permanently in one place, have on human health?

Question 4 (*Objective 2.4*)

Describe in a few sentences the roles of: (a) insects, (b) freshwater animals, and (c) dogs in the transmission of human infectious diseases.

3 The story of life in a few pages

This chapter builds on an understanding of the hierarchy of biological organisation, from the molecular level to the multicellular organism, which is described in Chapter 9 of Studying Health and Disease.[1] That chapter also describes methods of staining thin sections of biological material for magnification and viewing through various kinds of microscope, including very powerful electron microscopes; several photographs taken with the aid of this technology appear in the present chapter.

The theory of natural selection and the biological meaning of 'adaptation' and 'fitness' were introduced in Chapters 5 and 11 of World Health and Disease, and are expanded here.

The present chapter introduces a considerable number of new biological terms and concepts, which will be reinforced and illustrated further in later chapters and in other books in this series. Some terms (for example, cell, protein and DNA) will already be familiar to readers who have never studied biology, but a more detailed biological description is given here. We suggest that you read right through the whole chapter once (it will take two to three hours), and then return to re-read any sections that you feel uncertain about. In particular, you will need to study the sections on DNA and protein synthesis again carefully; they are quite difficult for newcomers to biology, but you will find that later chapters in this book refer back to them very frequently.

There is a television programme 'Blood lines', associated with this chapter, which shows how the genetic code for the blood protein, haemoglobin, is contained in the structure of DNA. It will help you to visualise DNA and understand its central role in evolution.

[1] Studying Health and Disease (revised edition 1994). Figure 9.1 is particularly relevant.

The time-scale of evolutionary biology

Biology is the study of living things. All living things, or **organisms**, share two fundamental properties that distinguish them from inanimate objects. They have the capacity, first, for self-maintenance and, second, for reproduction. *Self-maintenance* refers to the fact that organisms grow, they have a limited capacity to repair or replace parts that wear out, and they can protect themselves to some extent against threats to their survival. *Reproduction* refers to the ability of organisms to leave progeny that are replicas of themselves. These properties are shared not only by all the organisms that co-exist on Earth today, but by every successful life-form that has ever existed. In this context, 'success' simply means that the organism survived long enough to reproduce.

This chapter introduces some basic biological concepts that provide a framework in which the **evolution** of large, complex animals such as ourselves can be examined. Evolution can be defined as:

> All the changes that have transformed life on Earth from its earliest beginnings to the diversity that characterises it today. (Campbell, 1993, Glossary, p. G–11)

In Chapter 2, we turned back the 'evolutionary clock' just a fraction, to the appearance of primates about 60 million years ago. But there is evidence to suggest that the Earth was formed very approximately 4 500 million years ago and that the most primitive life-forms evolved sometime within the next 1 000 million years. What happened in the unimaginably vast period between the first life-forms appearing and the evolution of modern humans, *Homo sapiens*? This time-scale may be easier to grasp if you think of the history of the Earth as being represented by a single year: the Earth formed on the first of January and the earliest single-celled organisms appeared around the end of March, but it took until early November before simple, worm-like multicellular creatures evolved; reptiles appeared about the middle of December and humans at about teatime on New Year's Eve.

On this time-scale, we have some reasonably well-accepted theories (as told in Chapter 2) about what went on in the last week of December, but little more than a number of interesting hypotheses about the nature or sequence of events for the first 95 per cent of the time for which life has existed on Earth. We begin this chapter by sketching in some of the ideas that are currently being discussed among evolutionary biologists, noting that it is highly unlikely that a definitive version will ever be agreed.

In describing the possible circumstances of the origins of life-forms, we inevitably have to use some new biological terms. Our intention in this chapter is first to 'tell the story' of the origins of life (in so far as we can guess at it) and then go back and unpack the important terms and concepts, piece by piece. The middle of the chapter therefore describes a number of processes that take place within living things that are so basic they are common to all, from bacteria to people. Then we look at the kind of organisational features that accompany an increase in complexity, as multicellular (many-celled) organisms evolved from their single-celled ancestors. Finally, the chapter examines the meaning of such words as 'simple', 'complex', 'primitive' and 'advanced' in the context of evolution.

In the beginning?

As the crust of the newly-formed Earth cooled, the surface seems to have been a slurry of muddy water which gradually formed into pools of liquid and expanses of soft clay. This has often been called the 'primeval soup'. The Earth's surface was subject to violent electrical storms, intense ultraviolet radiation, very high temperatures and volcanic eruptions on a massive scale. The surface layers contained a rich variety of molecules but, unlike the Earth today, neither the crust nor the atmosphere above it contained more than a trace of 'free' oxygen (oxygen that is not bound to other chemical substances).

As noted in Chapter 1, *molecules* are assemblies of *atoms*, which in turn are the basic units of matter from which each of the unique chemical *elements* (such as carbon, oxygen, hydrogen and nitrogen) are made. Some molecules are very simple and very small; for example, carbon monoxide (a constituent of volcanic vapours and of modern car exhausts) consists of just one atom of the element carbon (denoted by the letter C) and one of another element, oxygen (O)—hence its chemical symbol, CO.[2] Small molecules such as this may have been

present in the interior of the newly-formed planet and were thrown up by volcanic activity, or they may have arrived from outer space in meteors and the dust-tails of comets.

We have limited knowledge of which molecules were actually dissolved in the pools and clays of the early Earth environment, or were part of its atmosphere. What biologists think may have been present has been deduced partly from observations of conditions on Earth today. For example it is widely assumed that there must have been some simple compounds containing carbon and oxygen, such as carbon monoxide and carbon dioxide (CO_2), plus some nitrogen gas (two atoms of the element nitrogen joined together, N_2), lots of hydrogen gas (H_2) and some ammonia, sulphur dioxide and methane, because these gases are found in the emissions of present-day volcanoes.

The other strand of reasoning has been to work backwards from the molecules found in present-day organisms and deduce how they might have been formed from simpler precursors under the conditions believed to exist on the primitive Earth. In the 1950s, biologists began to try to recreate the 'primeval soup' in laboratory apparatus; various mixtures of small molecules that were believed to be present in the earliest times were subjected to heat, electrical activity and ultraviolet radiation to see if they would fuse to form larger molecules under these conditions. It was established that so-called **organic molecules** could be induced to form; these are molecules containing mainly the elements carbon, hydrogen, oxygen and nitrogen, arranged in configurations that resemble the molecules of living organisms today.

Experimental manipulation of conditions in the test-tube showed that these organic molecules can be induced to 'coalesce' into droplets (rather like tiny globules of liquid fat in water), creating a primitive structure that *may* have been the forerunner of the cell. Whether or not the laboratory experiments actually recreated what went on 4 000 million years ago we shall never know, but the theoretical principle has been established: little molecules can be made to fuse into bigger ones which resemble the building blocks from which organisms are made, and these in turn can form structures with a surface boundary that have a passing resemblance to cells. The 'giant leap' in the evolution of life on Earth was the formation of a cell with the ability to *replicate*, that is, produce more cells just like itself.

Building on success: from RNA to protein

However, no progress towards the evolution of a cell could be made unless, among the larger molecules that formed in the primeval soup, there was one that had the

---

[2] We do not expect you to become fluent in, or memorise, any chemical symbols used in this book; all you need to know is that each element has a unique symbol (such as C or O) and these can be joined together to give a chemical symbol for a molecule formed from atoms of those elements (as in CO, carbon monoxide).

capability to reproduce itself. In the absence of such a molecule, the processes that were building and demolishing molecules would have remained random. Imagine that, by chance, some molecules came together in an assembly that had the potential to form part of a living structure; this assembly would have to be stabilised, retained and 'built on' before a living cell could evolve. But in the chaotic world of random encounters between molecules, potentially useful assemblies would be demolished in the next electrical storm, *unless* some process developed that not only preserved useful molecules but also made lots more.

The prime candidate for such a key stabilising role in early evolution is a large molecule called **RNA** (ribonucleic acid), which is a single strand of much smaller organic molecules called *nucleotides,* joined end-to-end like beads on a necklace.[3] RNA consists of only four different kinds of nucleotides, but they can join up in any order (Figure 3.1), to form a strand anywhere between a few hundred and a few thousand nucleotides long. This generates a huge number of *variants* of RNA, each molecule made of the same four nucleotides, but differing in their number and sequence.

One of the most important points to remember about this very simple, repeating structure is that it lends itself to being *copied*. If whole molecules of RNA are placed into a test-tube with a mixture of *separate* nucleotides of all four types, under certain conditions each of the original strands of RNA can act as a sort of 'template' or pattern for the construction of new copies just like itself, built from the nucleotides in the surrounding mixture. Thus, a single strand of a particular RNA variant can rapidly 'reproduce' to give hundreds, even thousands, of identical copies of the 'parent' strand. This process is known as **RNA replication**.

RNA is a vital component of all living cells today; in essence you can think of an RNA molecule as a set of coded instructions for how to make **proteins**. All life forms use proteins for a huge variety of tasks (we shall discuss some of them later). The ability to produce proteins with the help of RNA has to have been an important stage in the evolution of an ordered living cell from a random molecular soup. We don't know exactly how this happened, so what follows is simply the best guess around at the moment (and some biologists would dispute even this statement).

[3]Later in this chapter you will learn about the structure of nucleotides when we discuss DNA (deoxyribonucleic acid), which probably evolved *after* RNA and is also built from nucleotides; for the moment, just think of them as the 'blocks' from which RNA is constructed.

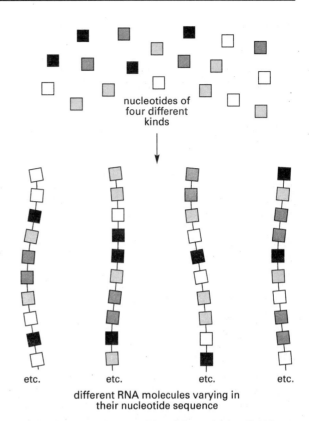

nucleotides of four different kinds

different RNA molecules varying in their nucleotide sequence

Figure 3.1 *RNA consists of four different kinds of building blocks called nucleotides, which can join up in any sequence to form a huge number of variant RNA molecules.*

The four nucleotides from which RNA is constructed have a weak affinity for another kind of molecule known as an **amino acid**, which may have formed in early Earth environments. In the present day, there are only 20 different kinds of amino acids in living things and (like the nucleotides in RNA) they can be joined together in long strings in any sequence. Since there are 20 different kinds, endless permutations are possible in a string of several hundred amino acids. Each unique sequence of joined-up amino acids constitutes a different *protein*, and each protein has a unique function. A tentative idea about how primitive proteins may have been formed with the help of RNA is summarised in Figure 3.2 (*overleaf*). The hypothesis runs thus:

• First came RNA in a huge number of variants, differing in the sequence of their nucleotides (only one variant is shown in Figure 3.2).

• Each of these RNA variants attracted a particular, unique sequence of amino acids, which joined up with each other to give a unique protein.

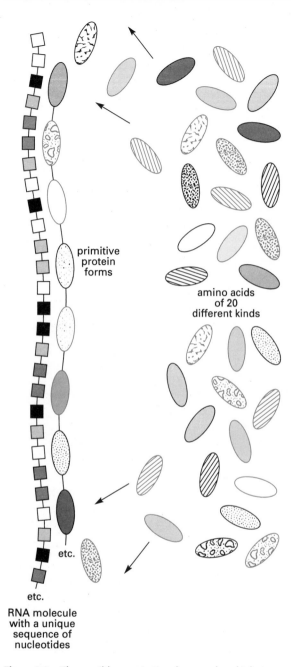

primitive
protein
forms

amino acids
of 20
different kinds

etc.

etc.

RNA molecule
with a unique
sequence of
nucleotides

Figure 3.2 *The possible organisational process by which primitive proteins were formed with the help of RNA. Amino acids exist in 20 different kinds; they are attracted to a particular RNA molecule and join together in a precise sequence, which is determined by the sequence of nucleotides in that variant of RNA. Thus, RNA carries in its structure the 'coded' instructions for making a particular protein.*

• Once the protein had formed, it floated off into the 'soup', leaving the strand of RNA free to attract more of the same amino acids in the same sequence, and hence make another copy of the same protein, and so on.

Some of the RNA variants would, in theory, be more successful than others at attracting amino acids and, by the same token, some of the resulting proteins would be more useful than others in constructing primitive cells. Later in this chapter, we will look at the processes by which most biologists believe these more useful RNA variants might have been 'selected' and as a consequence made more and more copies of themselves, while other less useful variants died out. As you will see, this selection process is thought to operate not only at the level of molecules, but on whole organisms: you may have heard of it referred to as *natural selection* in the context of Charles Darwin's theory of evolution. For the moment, we ask you to focus on the notion that a primitive molecule that has the ability to replicate itself and to 'instruct' the building of numerous different proteins is an essential component of the origins of life. Whether this primitive molecule was indeed RNA, we may never know.

The next step in the story is even more clouded in speculation. Where did the other sorts of molecules found in life-forms, such as carbohydrates and fats, come from? They must also have been assembled from simpler molecules found in the 'soup'. Some of them may have required complex interactions with primitive proteins before this could take place. Certain proteins in the modern cell (described below) have the property of aiding the fusion of small molecules into larger ones, or conversely breaking down larger molecules into smaller components. These proteins are called *enzymes* and we will give them more attention later, but you should get the general idea at this point that enzymes *might* have been produced in the primeval soup (along with other proteins), and these in turn *might* have helped to build carbohydrates, fats and all the other molecular components needed to make a cell.

So, assuming that all the necessary building blocks of a primitive cell gradually appeared in the primeval soup and coalesced into droplets with a surface boundary, how did the first living cell arise? We have no answer to this except to say that the time-scale from 'soup' to cell may be 500–1 000 million years. In this vastness, primitive structures with some cell-like features may have evolved and died out many times, until by chance a variation on the theme arose which was stable enough to survive and, more importantly, *reproduce*. The distinguishing features of living organisms are (as we said at the outset) self-maintenance and reproduction. The key to the reproduction of a whole cell is *DNA* (deoxyribonucleic acid), a molecule with certain similarities to RNA (and from which it may have evolved). Just as RNA contains the coded instructions for making certain proteins, so DNA contains the coded instructions for making whole new cells. You will find out later how it does this fabulous trick. Our next task is to look at the cell in some detail, since it is the building block from which all living organisms are made.

Cells: variations on a common theme

Organisms are enormously diverse, but they also show uniformity; that is, they all share a number of features and fundamental properties that differentiate them from non-living things. As described above, all organisms are capable of self-maintenance and reproduction in appropriate environments. Another aspect of the uniformity of organisms is that they are all made up of similar basic units, called **cells**.

In this book, we are concerned primarily with human biology and evolution, including the interaction of humans with other organisms that have the potential to cause us harm. We can't get much further without stopping to look in more detail at the characteristics of the cells from which we are made, but note that the *basic* structure of all *animal* cells is very nearly the same, and they also have a great deal in common with the cells of all plants, fungi and protistans. In describing the basic features of a 'typical' cell, we have to introduce several new technical terms. This 'naming of parts' is one of the aspects of biology that many people find off-putting, but we have kept the terms to an essential minimum and they will come up again many times later in this book, so be reassured that by the time you get to the last chapter you will be using them fluently!

Cells come in a huge variety of shapes and sizes (see Figure 3.3); the variations in structure reflect the specialised functions of that type of cell. However, the basic life processes carried out in each cell type show remarkable similarities. All cells are built on one of only two basic plans. The simpler of the two is found in all **bacteria** (Figure 3.3a), which are believed to have evolved before other cells. The more complex is found in all animal cells (Figure 3.3b) as well as all plants and fungi, and in single-celled organisms which are known collectively as **protistans** (Figure 3.3c shows one kind of protistan, an

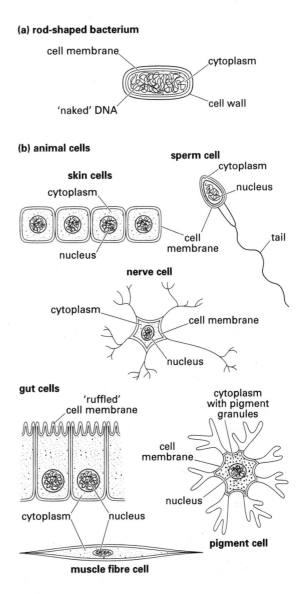

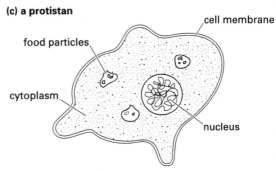

Figure 3.3 *Diversity in the structure of cells is revealed in these drawings. (a) A bacterium. (b) A selection of animal cells. (c) A protistan, a single-celled organism capable of independent life.*

amoeba). Protistans are capable of independent life and, although most are harmless, they include several species that cause diseases in humans; for example some kinds of amoeba cause dysentery and other important protistans cause malaria and sleeping sickness.

    □ Compare the bacterial cell (Figure 3.3a) with the other cells in Figure 3.3. What are the most obvious differences?

    ■ You probably noticed that the bacterium does not have a *nucleus* whereas all the other cells do, and that it is unique in having a protective *cell wall* outside the cell membrane.[4]

You may have wondered why we left out **viruses**, but viruses are not true cells at all and are generally referred to as virus *particles*. They are minute 'boxes' containing little more than one or two strands of genetic material. They are not capable of independent life but survive by invading a true cell and taking control of the basic life processes going on in that cell, subverting them to produce new virus particles. (It is debatable therefore whether viruses can be described as 'living organisms'.) Figure 3.4 shows the relative sizes of various types of true cells. Even if magnified 100 times, virus particles would be too small to see; look at the magnifications necessary to visualise the viruses in the photographs.

A typical **animal cell** is shown in Figure 3.5 (*over-leaf*); compare the drawing with the photograph and see if you can identify all the structures. All cells are bounded by an outer layer, the *cell membrane*. Shortly, we will look at membranes in more detail but, for the moment, it is enough to know that the cell membrane is a highly complex structure that allows the passage of certain substances into the cell and lets other substances pass out of it. The contents of the cell can be distinguished as the **cytoplasm**, a watery fluid rich in dissolved molecules, and a variety of solid structures called **organelles**, each bounded by a membrane very similar to the one around the outer margin of the cell.

There are many different kinds of organelle; here we will do no more than point out some of the principal ones and give a 'thumbnail sketch' of their main functions.

You should be aware that this is a vastly simplified account: each of these organelles would have a whole chapter to itself in a textbook of cell biology.

The largest organelle in any cell is usually the *nucleus*, where most of the DNA in the cell can be found. Cells typically have one nucleus, though certain kinds of cell have more than one and others, notably the red blood cells of mammals, have none. Other organelles, of which there are usually many in each cell, that can be identified in Figure 3.5 are the *ribosomes*, the *mitochondria* (singular, mitochondrion), the *endoplasmic reticulum*, the *vesicles* and the *lysosomes*.[5]

Ribosomes are tiny structures where proteins are assembled from their constituent amino acids, with the help of RNA. Ribosomes are often attached to the endoplasmic reticulum.

The endoplasmic reticulum is a vast canal system of membranes, on the surfaces of which an unimaginable number of chemical reactions takes place—some creating new molecules, others breaking old ones down.

Mitochondria are the sites where most of the energy is generated from chemical reactions to fuel all the processes going on inside the cell.

Lysosomes are fluid-filled 'bags' of membrane, which contain a cocktail of enzymes for breaking down complex molecules and providing the cell with the simpler nutrients it requires (they also have a role in defence against infection, as you will see in Chapter 6).

Vesicles are also bags of membrane, containing substances being transported into or out of the cell.

If you look back at Figure 3.3, you would perhaps be amazed to be told that all the cells shown there had the structural features described above, because they *appear* to be so different. Certainly, they each have special characteristics that are reflections of the different lives they lead (or, put in a more biological manner, their structures reflect their functions), but these specialisations are superimposed on a common basic plan. What goes on at the chemical level inside these cells is also remarkably similar, as you will see shortly. First, we want to look more closely at an often neglected aspect of cell structure which is, in reality, crucially important.

[4]Biologists call the bacterial cell type a *prokaryote*, pronounced 'pro-carry-oat', from the Greek meaning 'before kernel' (no nucleus). All other cells belong to the *eukaryote* type, pronounced 'you-carry-oat', meaning 'true kernel'. There is no need to remember these terms, but you may come across them in other textbooks.

[5]You may need some help with pronouncing some of the terms in this paragraph: cytoplasm ('sight-oh-plasm'); organelles ('organ-ells'); nucleus ('new-clee-us'); ribosomes ('rye-boh-somes'); mitochondria ('might-oh-kon-dree-a'); endoplasmic reticulum ('end-oh-plaz-mik ret-ik-you-lum'); vesicles ('vee-sickles'); lysosomes ('lye-soh-somes').

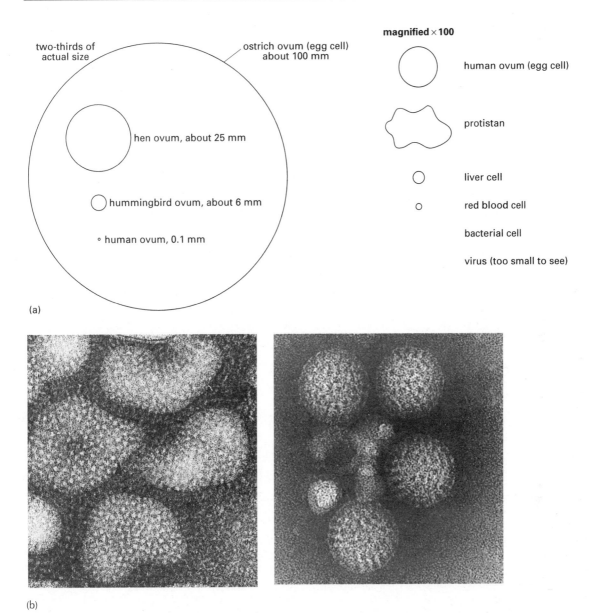

(a)

magnified × 100

two-thirds of
actual size

ostrich ovum (egg cell)
about 100 mm

hen ovum, about 25 mm

hummingbird ovum, about 6 mm

human ovum, 0.1 mm

human ovum (egg cell)

protistan

liver cell

red blood cell

bacterial cell

virus (too small to see)

(b)

Figure 3.4 *(a) The relative sizes of various cell types; you may get some idea of the actual dimensions of these cells by considering that a fully-grown human finger contains about one billion (one thousand million) cells. Even if magnified 100 times, virus particles would be too small to see. (b) Influenza virus particles (left) and rotavirus particles (right), photographed at a magnification of 350 000 with an electron microscope. The outer layer of virus particles generally displays a regular geometric pattern because it is formed from identical repeating structures, as shown in these examples. Rotaviruses are a common cause of diarrhoea in humans. (Photos: Heather Davies)*

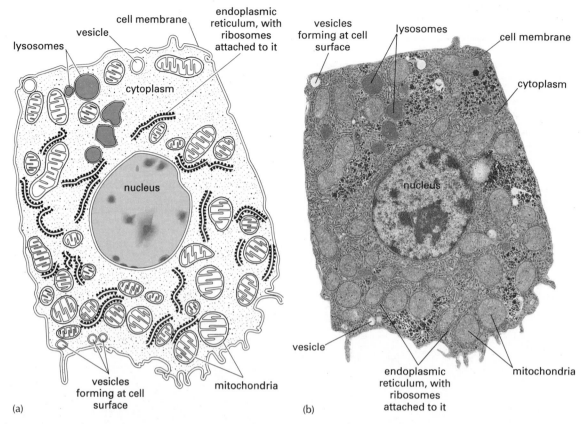

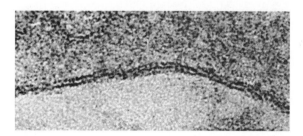

Figure 3.5 *(a) Schematic drawing of a typical animal cell, showing some of the common structural features. Compare this with (b) a photograph of a liver cell taken through an electron microscope and magnified 8 000 times. (Photo: Heather Davies)*

Cell membranes: a dynamic interface

All the organelles mentioned above, as well as the cell itself, are bounded by **membranes** (see Figure 3.6). They give the cell its inner and outer organisation and act as the

Figure 3.6 *Part of an animal cell, photographed through an electron microscope and enlarged 300 000 times, showing the outer cell membrane, which can clearly be seen to consist of a double layer. (Source: Open University Electron Microscopy Unit)*

semi-solid 'platform' on which many of the chemical reactions inside the cell take place. In addition, as you will see from later parts of this book, membranes play a vital role in many life processes that affect the whole organism: for example, in the immune system which protects us against infection (Chapter 6) and in the digestive system which provides us with the nutrients required to sustain life (Chapter 7).

Figure 3.7 shows a schematic diagram of the basic structure of the membranes found in all cell types, both around the outer margin of the cell and around the organelles within the cell. Two parallel sheets of fatty molecules known as *phospholipids* (pronounced 'fosfoh-lipids') form the regular framework of the membrane: you can see from the diagram that the 'heads' of these molecules are packed together to form the inner and outer layers of the membrane, with their 'tails' pointing towards each other like the jam in a sandwich. The two sheets are not fixed together, but can move laterally (from

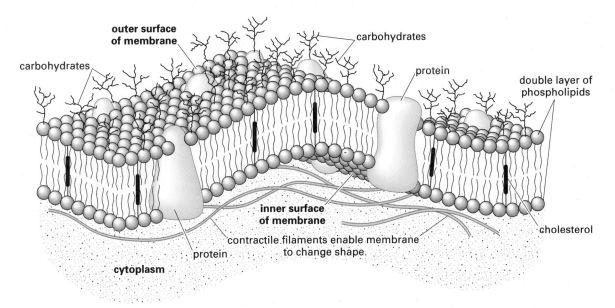

Figure 3.7 *The basic structure of the outer membrane of all cells. This structure is known as a 'fluid mosaic'. Membranes surrounding the organelles within cells are also built on this basic plan.*

side to side), slipping across each other. This would be a highly unstable situation but for the presence of molecules of another fatty substance, *cholesterol,* which are dotted about between the phospholipids and stop the sheets from sliding too far.

Until now, you may only have thought of cholesterol as a harmful constituent of certain foods, which until quite recently was believed to be the main culprit in the causation of heart disease. In the 1990s, this view has been radically revised and it is accepted that for the great majority of people moderate amounts of cholesterol in the diet contribute to the construction of new membranes within and surrounding all cells.[6] The high fat content of biological membranes means that substances which can dissolve in fats can very easily pass into and out of cells; membranes also act as 'reservoirs' for fat-soluble substances, such as some vitamins.

Look at Figure 3.7 again. Bobbing about in the regular two-layer framework of phospholipids are lumps of *protein*, which can move laterally in all directions and can also 'bob up' so that sometimes they poke out of the membrane and at other times they 'bob down' below the

surface. A vast number of small *carbohydrate* molecules also cover the outer surface of the membrane, standing up like trees in a forest; carbohydrates consist of strings of small sugar molecules, like glucose. On the inner surface, the cell membrane is in contact with filaments of proteins, which can contract and relax in a coordinated manner, changing the overall shape of the membrane. They can pull it into folds or push it outwards, creating 'fingers' of membrane which reach out and can enclose material outside the cell. In some cells, this primitive musculature attached to the underside of the membrane can enable the cell to 'crawl' about. The highly mobile structure of biological membranes has been aptly named a **fluid mosaic**.

Biological membranes have three main functions, which can be thought of (metaphorically) in terms of a *barrier*, a *gate* and a *switchboard*. Membranes are barriers in that they prevent both the entry and the exit of certain substances, some of which are never allowed transit, but most are kept in or kept out only at certain times. When the 'internal world' of the cell begins to run short of a certain substance in order to maintain life processes, or when the concentration of waste rises too high, the barrier of the membrane turns into a highly selective 'gate' across which certain substances can enter or leave, while maintaining a barrier to others. It is also a 'switchboard' through which a great many chemical messages are transmitted to and from the cell.

[6]A discussion of heart disease and the debate about cholesterol as a contributing factor occurs in another book in this series, *Dilemmas in Health Care* (Open University Press, 1993), Chapter 10.

Crossing a membrane

We will look first at the membrane as a barrier and as a gate. There are several different ways that substances can cross a biological membrane, but we will focus on three general methods, all of which will come up again later in the book. They are (a) *passive diffusion,* (b) *active transport* and (c) *endocytosis* and *exocytosis* (pronounced 'end-oh-sight-oh-sis' and 'ex-oh-sight-oh-sis'; *endo* signifies movement into the cell, and *exo* signifies movement outwards).

Passive diffusion refers to the free movement across biological membranes of molecules to which the membrane is *permeable* (that is, it cannot act as a barrier against them). These include very small molecules, like water, oxygen, carbon dioxide and dissolved salts, and larger molecules that are soluble in fats (remember the membrane is formed from sheets of fats). Movement of these molecules into or out of the cell occurs by passive diffusion whenever the concentration of that molecule is greater on one side of the membrane than it is on the other (see Figure 3.8). In this situation, a *concentration gradient* is said to exist; you could think of molecules 'rolling down' the gradient from the high side to the low side. Unless other forces oppose them, molecules will always 'spread out' or diffuse *evenly* through any available space (like a drop of ink in water) until any concentration gradient is abolished. This process is known as *passive* diffusion because it does not require the expenditure of energy.

□ If there is a higher concentration of molecules of substance X on one side of a membrane than on the other (as in Figure 3.8), and the membrane cannot act as a barrier to those molecules, what will happen?

■ Molecules of substance X will move by passive diffusion across the membrane from the high concentration side to the low concentration side, until the concentrations are equal on both sides of the membrane. The molecules are then dispersed evenly through the available space.

Single-celled organisms, such as bacteria and protistans, have a relatively large surface area of cell membrane in contact with the outside world, so they can get a lot of the water, oxygen and salts they need by passive diffusion of these substances into the cell from the external environment. As they are used up *inside* the cell, the concentration falls lower than the concentration in the fluids *outside* the cell; this creates a concentration gradient which 'sucks' more of these molecules across the membrane into the cell.

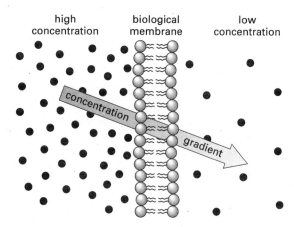

Figure 3.8 *Schematic representation of a concentration gradient across a biological membrane.*

□ What will happen to a waste product such as carbon dioxide, which builds up in the cell as life processes go on?

■ When it reaches a higher concentration than the carbon dioxide in the outside world, it will leave the cell by passive diffusion across the cell membrane.

Multicellular animals have very few of their cells on the outer surface of the body, but passive diffusion is still a vitally important method of obtaining the necessities of life. For example, oxygen enters the bloodstream by passive diffusion across the membranes of blood vessels lying very close to the surface of the lungs; as the blood circulates around the body, oxygen leaves the bloodstream by passive diffusion out of the blood vessels into nearby cells. In Chapter 7 you will learn about digestion in the human gut and the absorption of small molecules, broken down from our food, which pass across the wall of the gut by passive diffusion into nearby blood vessels.

However, passive diffusion works only for very small molecules (like oxygen) to which biological membranes are permeable. What about the rest? One option is **active transport**, which relies on the proteins bobbing about in the membrane (look back at Figure 3.7). The function of many of these proteins is to transport across the membrane (in either direction) molecules which the membrane would otherwise exclude. This process requires the expenditure of energy, hence it is called *active* transport.

Transport proteins either form 'tunnels' through which the transported molecule can pass, or they act as 'carriers' by binding temporarily to the molecule and moving it physically through the membrane. These transport proteins are highly selective: each one will only transport a certain kind of molecule. For example, in mammals excess glucose molecules are 'mopped up' from the bloodstream for storage in the liver with the help of transport proteins in the outer membranes of liver cells; these proteins are so selective that they cannot transport other sugars into the liver cell, even those that are structurally very similar to glucose. (You will learn more about the regulation of blood glucose levels in Chapter 7.)

Before moving on, you should note that although we have discussed passive diffusion and active transport mainly in terms of the *outer* cell membrane, these processes are also going on across all the membranes *inside* the cell. Every organelle, including the nucleus, is bounded by a membrane constructed on the same basic plan as that outlined above.

The third method of getting large molecules across biological membranes also illustrates the extreme fluidity of membrane structure. In **endocytosis**, the outer membrane of the cell is thrown into a cup-shaped depression, which gradually closes over and seals within itself a portion of the 'outside world' (see Figure 3.9a and b). This bag of membrane is called a *vesicle*. It separates from the cell surface and drifts into the interior of the cell. It may simply contain water and dissolved nutrients, or it may contain very large molecules such as certain proteins which are too big to get in by active transport. It may even contain whole cells: certain kinds of cell in the immune

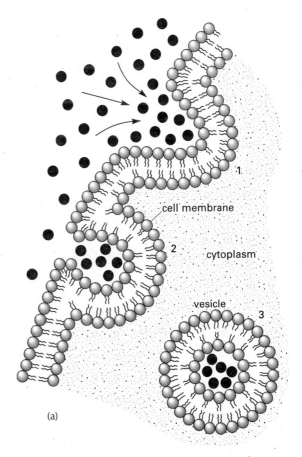

(a)

Figure 3.9 *(a) The basic sequence of events by which material is taken into a cell by endocytosis. (b) Photograph taken with an electron microscope showing a vesicle of membrane being drawn into the interior of the cell. (Source: Perry, M. M. and Gilbert, A. B., 1979, Yolk transport in the ovarian follicle of the hen,* Journal of Cell Science, **39**, p. 266).

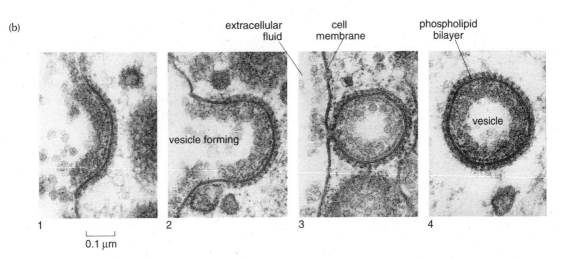

(b)

extracellular fluid

cell membrane

phospholipid bilayer

vesicle forming

vesicle

1   2   3   4

0.1 μm

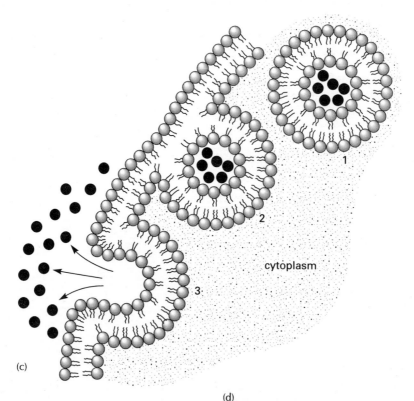

cytoplasm

(c)

Figure 3.9 *(c) The events in exocytosis, which culminate in material being ejected or secreted from the cell.*
(d) Photograph taken with an electron microscope of a secretory vesicle emptying its contents outside the cell. (Source: Herzog, V., Sies, H. and Miller, F., 1976, Exocytosis in secretory cells of rat lacrimal gland, Journal of Cell Biology, **70**, *p. 698; reproduced by copyright permission of the Rockefeller University Press)*

(d)

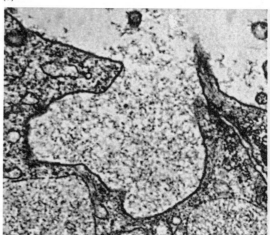

system can engulf bacteria and protistans by endocytosis, drawing them into the cell for destruction (a subject we return to in Chapter 6).

In the opposite process, **exocytosis**, substances are transported *out* of the cell by first packaging them in a vesicle (bag of membrane), which travels to the cell-surface and fuses with the outer membrane of the cell. The contents of the vesicle are then dumped outside (see Figure 3.9c and d). The contents might be waste products, but this is also the method used by cells to *secrete* many essential molecules into the environment outside the cell. Examples of major groups of molecules which are secreted from cells by exocytosis include: *hormones,* signalling molecules transported in the bloodstream in many animal species, and *neurotransmitters,* signalling molecules that pass between active nerve cells and

between nerves and muscles (both of which are mentioned again later in this chapter); *enzymes,* proteins that speed up the construction and breaking down of other molecules in all the chemical reactions taking place in living organisms (to which we return shortly); and *antibodies,* proteins produced by cells in the immune system as part of our defence against infection (discussed further in Chapter 6). Note that enzymes and antibodies are all proteins, and so are some hormones and neurotransmitters.

Lock-and-key interactions in membranes

Thus far, we have discussed the function of biological membranes in terms of barriers and gates, which leaves the other main function: the switchboard. Membranes act as switchboards in a communication network of daunting complexity. Cells are constantly sending and receiving signals across the outer cell membrane, which either modify the activity inside the cell or change the conditions outside, and membranes around organelles inside the cell act similarly. You will meet examples of highly specific communication pathways later in this book, so here we will simply sketch in the basic principles.

As described above, cells can secrete a variety of different **signalling molecules**, such as hormones and neurotransmitters, into the fluid outside the cell. Each of these molecules has a highly specific three-dimensional shape, part of which is known as the *active site* (see Figure 3.10a). It exactly fits a 'mirror image' of itself known as the *binding site* on the surface of a **receptor molecule** (often shortened simply to 'receptor'). The two surfaces fit together so precisely that, like a key in a lock, no other combination will result in the transmission of the correct signal; these are commonly known as **lock-and-key interactions**.

Many of the proteins that bob about in the outer membrane of every cell, and most of the carbohydrates that stick out into 'space', are actually receptor molecules. When a receptor encounters a signalling molecule to which it can *bind* (that is, form a very close, though transient contact), the binding event sets off a chain reaction which leads ultimately to a change in the activity of the cell displaying that receptor (Figure 3.10b). In this example, only the receptor molecule is part of the structure of a membrane and the signalling molecule is 'free-floating'; but both receptor and signalling molecule can be part of a membrane and this provides a mechanism to transmit messages between adjacent cells (Figure 3.10c).

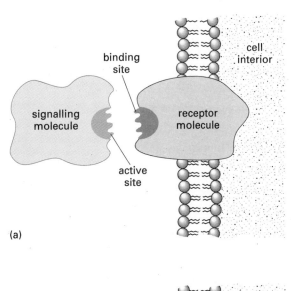

(a)

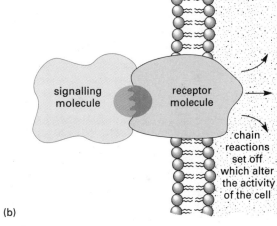

(b)

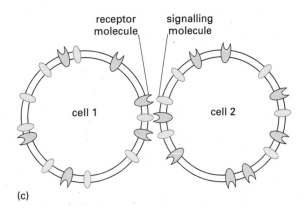

(c)

Figure 3.10 *(a) and (b) Stages in a lock-and-key interaction between the active site of a 'free-floating' signalling molecule and the binding site of a receptor protein embedded in a cell membrane. (c) Cells in close contact can send and receive signals simultaneously when signalling molecules in the membrane of each cell bind to receptors on the other cell.*

☐ Can you suggest an example of a lock-and-key interaction which was mentioned a little earlier in this chapter?

■ The transport protein that picks up excess glucose from the bloodstream and carries it across the outer membrane of liver cells will transport only glucose; it cannot transport other similar sugars. The transport protein appears to 'select' glucose from among a host of other molecules, but in reality its selectivity relies on an accurate lock-and-key fit between part of the transport molecule and part of the glucose molecule.

This glimpse into the 'working life' of a biological membrane should have convinced you that membranes are essential to maintain not only the structure but also the correct functioning of every living cell, from the simplest bacterium to the most complex animal cell, and hence are vital to the life of the whole organism. Several fast-acting poisons, such as the toxin produced by cholera bacteria, work simply by disrupting the 'traffic' across cell membranes, and medical science exploits the highly selective transport mechanisms across membranes in the delivery of certain drugs.

Cell metabolism

The wealth of *molecular interactions* associated with the inner and outer membranes of the cell, and occurring 'free' in the fluid-filled interior of the cell (the cytoplasm), is known collectively as **cell metabolism**. The term covers all the chemical reactions that go on from moment to moment, either building up molecules or breaking them down. In an organism made up of many cells (such as a human) it is conventional to speak of 'the metabolism' or 'metabolic activity', meaning the sum total of all the chemical reactions going on in all the cells of the body.

The metabolic activity of a cell has varying time-scales. Interactions between very small molecules, such as the fusion of water (H_2O) and carbon dioxide (CO_2) to make simple sugars such as glucose, take place in fractions of a second; but it can take many minutes to string together the hundreds of small sugar molecules required to make a long-chain carbohydrate such as starch. Similarly, individual amino acids can be made in seconds, but joining them together to make a coherent protein can take hours. You may get an insight into why it takes a relatively long time to make a protein if we take a specific example.

Haemoglobin, the substance that makes our blood red and which carries oxygen around the body, is a protein molecule which (in the commonest form found in adults) is made from 574 amino acids linked together in a precise sequence. One critical amino acid out of place and it ceases to function properly as haemoglobin (as you will learn in Chapter 4). The scale of the 'manufacturing output' of just this one type of protein gives some idea of the total metabolic work going on in the human body: your body contains about six thousand million million million molecules of haemoglobin, which are constantly being used up and replenished.

All cells require *energy* to fuel the huge number of chemical reactions necessary to maintain life. In Chapter 7, we will spend some time looking at the breakdown of food molecules (particularly carbohydrates and fats) that yield energy, but at this point we simply want to emphasise the fact that all cells that live in an oxygen-rich environment get their energy in much the same way. Carbohydrates and fats, which are large and complex chains of smaller molecules, are broken down step by step in a complex sequence of hundreds of individual chemical reactions, yielding carbon dioxide, water and energy. The energy is 'trapped' in the structure of a molecule called **ATP** (adenosine triphosphate, a name you need not remember). ATP can be transported anywhere in the cell and energy can be released from it in controlled amounts wherever energy is required to drive a chemical reaction. Millions of different interlinked reactions are taking place in every cell all the time. If you tried to draw a map of all these chemical reactions (biochemists have done this) it looks a bit like the bus, rail, road and underground networks of the London transport system superimposed on top of one another.

You may be wondering what *regulates* these complex chemical reactions. The short answer is **enzymes**. These are proteins that catalyse (speed up) biochemical reactions in living organisms. As a general rule, each enzyme can only catalyse a specific reaction (as in Figure 3.11) and the presence or absence of the enzyme acts as a regulator on the extent to which that reaction occurs. In Chapter 7, you will meet an example in the enzyme *lactase,* which regulates the breakdown of *lactose,* the principal sugar found in milk. Each enzyme is restricted to act on a given biochemical reaction because an essential step in the catalytic process involves a lock-and-key fit between the enzyme and the other molecular participants in the reaction. We are used to thinking of enzymes digesting food in the cavity of the gut (as described in Chapter 7), but the fluid interior of all cells (the cytoplasm) is rich in enzymes and some of the proteins embedded in the cell membrane and in the membranes surrounding organelles are also enzymes, each one regulating a highly specific biochemical reaction inside the cell.

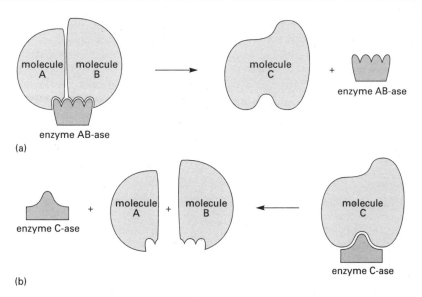

Figure 3.11 *(a) Molecules A and B can only combine to form molecule C at a biologically useful rate with the help of a highly specific enzyme, which we have called AB-ase (enzymes are named after the constituents of the reaction they speed up and all names end in the syllable 'ase'). (b) The reverse reaction, in which molecule C is broken down into A and B again, requires a different enzyme, this time called C-ase. Note that in both these reactions the enzyme is not used up and is released to participate in another identical reaction.*

Enzymes are just one category of proteins found in the cell, or in the fluids between cells in multicellular animals. In passing, we have mentioned several other categories of protein molecules earlier in this chapter.

☐ Can you recall any examples?

■ Transport proteins, some hormones and neurotransmitters, antibodies, haemoglobin and certain receptor molecules in cell membranes have all been mentioned.

There are a great many other types of protein, which we shall not attempt to catalogue, but you should understand that much of the variation between cells of different types stems from *differences in the nature of the proteins they contain*. Although many of the metabolic processes are very similar in all cells, the end-products may have characteristic differences. So, for example, a 'cell-specific' protein with a familiar name is the hormone *insulin*, which is made only by certain cells in the pancreas (more on this follows in Chapter 7).

So, in one sense, proteins hold the key to the unique character of each living cell, both in terms of the cell's structure and functions, and (crucially) in the nature of its enzymes and hence the whole of its metabolism. Yet if you think back to our speculative account of how life may

have begun on Earth, you will recall that proteins are assembled according to a 'template' carried in the structure of *RNA*. Amino acids do not join together in the absence of RNA, much less join up in the precise sequences that give each protein its characteristic form and function. So should we rewrite the first sentence of this paragraph to read 'RNA holds the key to the unique character of each living cell'? In fact we have to step back one stage further and look at the molecule that directs the production of RNA, its larger and more complex molecular 'cousin', DNA.

DNA: the double helix

Perhaps the most important aspect of the uniformity of all true cells is that all possess the same genetic material, **DNA** (deoxyribonucleic acid). This 'icon of the twentieth century' holds the key not only to RNA production (and hence to the assembly of proteins), but also the key to *inheritance*: the passing on of meaningful instructions about making RNA (and hence proteins) from one cell to another, and from one generation of organisms to the next. DNA plays a fundamental role in the life of organisms, providing the 'instructions' by which they develop, grow, survive and reproduce; hence, it is often referred to as the 'genetic code', or the 'blueprint' of an organism. You may already have noticed that biologists with an interest in the early evolution of life on Earth are faced with a 'chicken-and-egg' conundrum about the relationship between DNA and RNA. Most believe that RNA evolved *first* (as we suggested at the start of this chapter), but in modern cells RNA is made *under the direction* of DNA. The solution to this puzzle may lie in the discovery in the 1980s that some variants of RNA can act like enzymes, speeding up the construction of much bigger molecules which resemble DNA. Maybe these RNA catalysts were involved in assembling primitive molecules of DNA, which in turn directed the assembly of more RNA? This is a circular argument which may reflect a circular process: perhaps RNA directed the assembly of some DNA, which then directed the assembly of more RNA; this in turn could have helped to make more DNA, and so on, until the DNA structure we recognise today was produced. Biologists can only make plausible guesses about the sequence of events, but quite a lot is known about the end-product, DNA. No twenty-first century adult should consider themselves literate without some knowledge of how DNA works; fortunately, the essential aspects of the 'story' are fascinating and relatively straightforward to describe.

DNA is a remarkable molecule, breathtakingly simple in its structure and yet capable of directing all the living processes of a cell, including the reproduction of new cells and new generations of organisms. Most of the DNA in a cell is in the nucleus, coiled around cores of protein in structures called **chromosomes** (you might like to glance ahead to Figure 3.20b to see what they look like; they are described in a little more detail later in this chapter and are a major topic in Chapter 4). Each species has a characteristic number of chromosomes in its cells; there are 46 of them in most human cells and 48 in the cells of chimpanzees. If all the DNA in the nucleus of a single human body cell were uncoiled and stretched out straight, it would measure about two metres (see Figure 3.12, which is actually the DNA of a bacterium). If all the DNA in all of your cells were stretched out end-to-end, it would reach to the Moon and back about 10 000 times!

Since the structure of DNA was worked out by James Watson and Francis Crick in 1953, the study of biology and human understanding of the nature of life have been revolutionised. In order to explain how this has come about, we must briefly describe the structure of DNA and its most important properties.

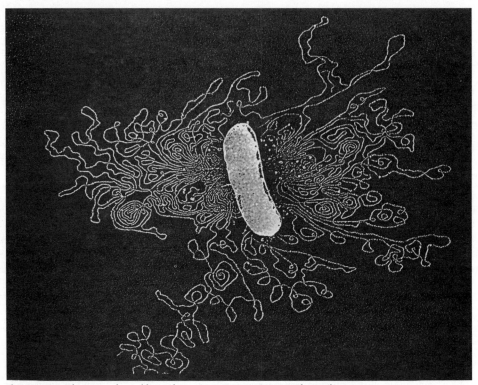

Figure 3.12 *The DNA released from a bacterium. (Source: Science Photo Library)*

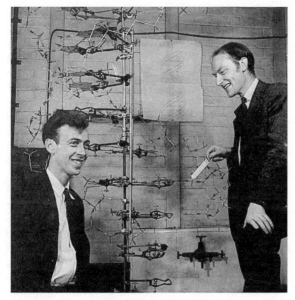

James Watson (left) *and Francis Crick in 1953 with the 'double-helix' model of deoxyribonucleic acid, DNA, which they built to help them determine its structure; the model was assembled from metal clamps used to hold test-tubes and other bits of laboratory apparatus. (Photo: A. Barrington-Brown)*

DNA structure and replication

The basic structure of DNA is provided by two helical strands (like two spiral staircases), each coiled around one another; hence its name 'the double helix' (Figure 3.13a). The two strands are linked by cross-pieces like the rungs of a ladder; Figure 3.13b shows this structure straightened out so that we can more easily describe its chemical composition.

Like RNA, each molecule of DNA is constructed from building blocks called **nucleotides**; now is the time to describe them in more detail. There are just four kinds of nucleotide in DNA (they differ from those in RNA in ways that need not concern us here), each one consisting of a section of the 'backbone' of a DNA strand, joined to a nitrogen-containing molecule called a *base* (a single nucleotide has been drawn separately in Figure 3.13b).

Figure 3.13 *The structure of DNA. (a) The DNA molecule consists of two helical chains coiled around one another; (chemically, the 'backbone' of each chain consists of alternating sugar and phosphate molecules, not shown here). (b) A section of the double-helix has been 'uncoiled' to show the two chains linked together by pairs of molecules called bases, of which there are four types, denoted by the letters A, T, C and G.*

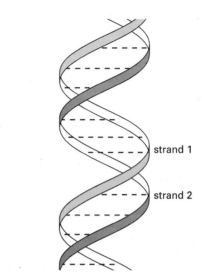

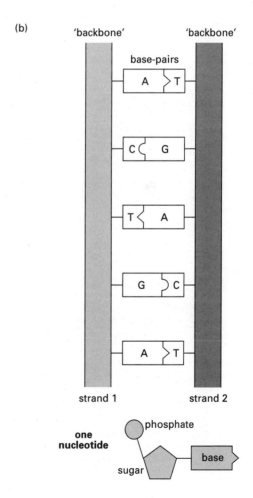

The important feature of the DNA double helix from our viewpoint is that each rung of the ladder consists of a *pair* of different bases joining the two strands.

The bases are what distinguish one nucleotide from another; there are four kinds, known by the initial letters of their chemical names: A (adenine), C (cytosine), G (guanine) and T (thymine). There is no need to remember these names; all you need to know is that the pairs of bases are not arranged randomly. The rungs across the DNA ladder are formed from unvarying pairs of bases: A can only bind to T, and C can only bind to G. This **base-pairing rule**, as you will see, gives the DNA molecule its unique ability to replicate exact copies of itself. Watson and Crick ended the research paper in which they published the long-sought after structure of DNA with a classic understatement to this effect:

> It has not escaped our notice that the specific pairing we have postulated immediately suggests a possible copying mechanism for the genetic material. (Watson and Crick, 1953, p. 738)

When a molecule of DNA makes copies of itself—a process known as **DNA replication**—the two chains within the DNA molecule separate (Figure 3.14), each rung of the ladder breaking where the two bases are normally joined together. This leaves *exposed* bases on each of the separated DNA chains, which then attract 'free' nucleotides present abundantly in the fluids inside the cell nucleus. Each of these free nucleotides has one of the four bases (A, T, C or G) as part of its structure; an exposed base on the original DNA chain can only attract and bind to a free nucleotide with the 'correct' base in its structure, in accordance with the base-pairing rule.

☐ Suppose that, at a particular point on the separated DNA chain there is an unattached base of type C. What kind of nucleotide is attracted to it?

■ One containing the base G (remember the base-pairing rule is that C can only bind to G, and vice versa).

As the bases on the 'naked' DNA chain bind to the 'free' nucleotides they have attracted, a second, new, complete DNA chain forms alongside the original one. When it is complete and the two chains coil around one another, the result is a double helix, a complete DNA molecule in which one chain is 'original' and the other is 'new'. Exactly the same process occurs alongside the *other* original DNA chain, so that ultimately there are two DNA double helices where formerly there was only one.

☐ How do these two DNA molecules compare with the original one?

■ They are each identical to it, because of the base-pairing rule that restricts the assembly of the new DNA chains: nucleotides with base A always pair with T (and vice versa), and those with base C always pair with G (and vice versa).

The order along one strand exactly defines the order on the other; the new strand is a kind of 'inverse image' of the original strand (look at Figure 3.13b again if you are unsure).

DNA and the genetic code

So this is how DNA replicates, but how does it direct the metabolism of the cell and pass on these instructions to 'daughter' cells each time a cell reproduces by dividing in two? The answer lies in the *sequence* of nucleotides from which each molecule of DNA is constructed; the sequence is a form of coded message.

We have already said that DNA is constructed from four types of nucleotide, each characterised by the nature of its *base*. Analysis of the *linear* sequence in which the nucleotides occur in a single DNA strand reveals that they can be arranged in any order. The linear sequence can be written down as a series of letters corresponding to the four bases, 'read' from one end of the strand to the other. For example, an extremely small sequence of only 18 nucleotides might 'read'

AAGATGCCGAGTTAAGAT

but it could equally well exist in any other sequence you care to think of.

☐ How many different permutations of four nucleotides in a series of 18 'items' do you think there are?

■ If you have a powerful enough calculator you may have worked out that the answer is 68 719 476 736 (or 4 to the power of 18), not far short of seventy billion (thousand million) possible different permutations of four nucleotides in a sequence of DNA that is only 18 nucleotides long.

The nucleus of most of your cells contains 46 molecules of DNA (one in each chromosome), which together contain about 6 *billion* nucleotides, each base paired with its opposite number. It is impossible to imagine the possible different permutations of 6 billion 'items' of four different types. This gives DNA one of its crucial properties; it can

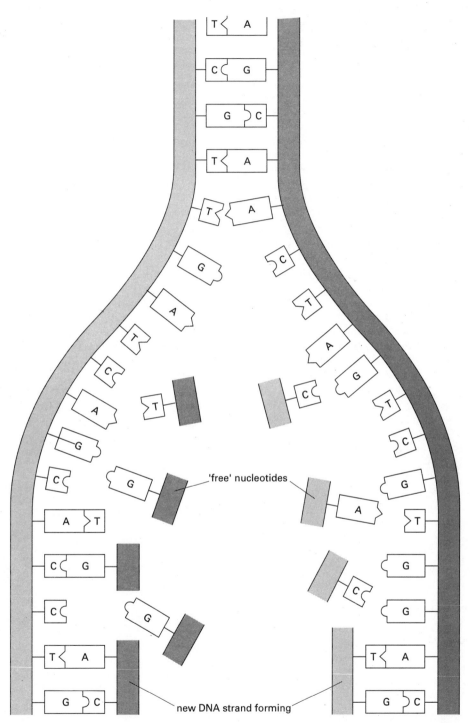

Figure 3.14 *Diagram of DNA replication. A molecule of DNA separates into two chains, exposing unpaired bases (top of diagram). Each exposed base attracts a free nucleotide containing the 'opposite' base (centre of diagram), to which it binds in accordance with the base-pairing rule (A pairs with T; C pairs with G). Two new DNA chains form alongside the original chains (bottom), leading to the formation of two identical double-helix molecules of DNA.*

exist in an infinite number of different forms, each one specified by the linear sequence in which the four bases appear along each strand.

Within the 6 billion nucleotides in the DNA of a single human cell, there are 'meaningful' sequences which biologists call **genes**. A gene can be defined in two ways: either *chemically*, as a sequence of nucleotides which contains the coded instructions for making a specific *protein*; or it can be defined in *evolutionary* terms as a 'unit of inheritance', coded information about making a protein that can be passed on to future generations of cells or organisms. Later in the chapter we will look at how a sequence of DNA nucleotides can be 'translated' into a sequence of amino acids to give rise to a specific protein; you already have most of the story, so just a few additional details are required to complete it. In Chapter 4, we reveal how genes are passed on from parent to offspring, and how the proteins 'encoded' by those genes affect the way that the offspring turns out.

There are about 100 000 different genes (meaningful sequences of nucleotides) scattered through the 46 molecules of DNA in a human cell. Only about 5 per cent of the total nucleotides in human DNA are involved in these genes; at present, scientists have absolutely no idea what (if anything) the other 95 per cent is doing there.

DNA, mutation and variation

Let us return to the primeval soup and the speculative story of how life might have evolved on Earth. Imagine that a primitive cell has formed, which contains molecules of some ancestral form of DNA, busily replicating more copies of itself, as shown in Figure 3.14. The environmental factors that probably helped DNA to form in the first place, like radiation, high temperature or lightning, are also likely to produce *random changes* in the sequence of its nucleotides, that is to produce **mutations**.

We can have some confidence in this hypothesis because ultraviolet light, X-rays and other forms of radiation are among the factors known to produce mutations in DNA today; they are *mutagens*. If you have ever had an X-ray, you are probably aware that considerable precautions are taken to protect your reproductive organs, and those of the radiographer, from the mutagenic effects of X-rays. This is primarily to prevent mutations occurring in the DNA of your sperm or egg cells, which might be passed on to future generations. There is currently much concern about the mutagenic effects of increased levels of ultraviolet light resulting from the thinning of the ozone layer, which is predicted to cause an increase in certain

cancers.[7] Far more extreme conditions existed when ancestral DNA molecules first appeared on Earth, so we can predict that random changes to the structure of primitive DNA molecules could have happened very frequently.

Mutations can be of three general kinds:

1   A section of DNA double helix might mutate by acquiring an additional pair of nucleotides, inserted into the original sequence. For example, a section of DNA with the following base-pairs (across the 'rungs' of the ladder):

A ··· T
G ··· C
T ··· A

might acquire an additional pair of nucleotides to become

A ··· T
G ··· C
C ··· G
T ··· A

It is still DNA, but it is a *different version* of DNA, which nonetheless retains the essential property of exact self-replication. When the mutant version of DNA replicates, it will copy the additional pair of bases along with the rest. Mutation is a source of new *inheritable* variants of DNA (there are other sources of variation, which are discussed in Chapter 4), and inheritability is essential to evolutionary change, as you will see shortly.

2   The reverse process might equally well occur; a section of DNA might *lose* a pair of nucleotides. In fact, mutation might result in more than one pair of nucleotides being lost or gained.

3   Alternatively, a section of DNA might be chopped out of the sequence and stuck back in elsewhere, that is, some nucleotides might be *relocated* in the DNA molecule.

Each time a mutation takes place, a different version of DNA is created. The variants might have slightly different properties from each other. Suppose that a new DNA variant, created by mutation, has the property of being able to replicate faster than the original version of DNA. For any DNA molecule to be able to replicate, it needs raw materials in the form of nucleotides. That version of DNA which could assemble the necessary nucleotides fastest and thus replicate fastest would, over time, produce more copies of itself, that survive to replicate

---

[7] Chemical mutagens, radiation and the thinning of the ozone layer are discussed further in Chapter 10 of this book.

faster in their turn, than slower-replicating versions. In other words, if there was *competition* among DNA variants for the resources that they required in order to replicate themselves, then a consequence of this competition is that certain versions would become more numerous than others. This, in essence, is what *natural selection* is all about. Mutation and natural selection are essential driving forces behind the evolution of all the diverse life forms we see on Earth today.

Natural selection and DNA

Most people think they know what **natural selection**[8] is about and will express it in such phrases as 'the survival of the fittest' or 'nature red in tooth and claw'. In fact, such phrases are misleading in many ways. The theory of natural selection, as set out by Charles Darwin, is a series of logical statements that explains how, over the course of time (to be exact, over the course of a number of generations), the form of a given species can change. The species could be mouse, mango, or indeed, a certain kind of molecule. As our 'story of life' is still focused on molecules, the theory is set out here as it might apply to ancestral DNA molecules but, if you substitute 'mouse' or 'mango' for 'molecules', the same arguments hold true. There are four propositions in the theory of natural selection:

1   Reproduction generates more individuals (of molecules, or mice, or mangos) than are able to survive until they themselves reproduce, because there are insufficient resources for all individuals to survive and reproduce.

2   There is a 'struggle for existence', because of the disparity between the number of individuals generated by reproduction and the number that can survive.

3   Individuals are not identical; they show variation one from another, arising at least partly from mutations in their DNA. Those variants with advantageous features have a greater chance of survival in the struggle for existence and thus have a greater chance of reproducing. There is thus *selection* of those molecules (or mice or mangos) that are more *fit* than others. (**Fitness** is a relative term; within a population of individuals, whether molecules, mice or mangos, an individual that produces the largest number of offspring who, in their

turn, survive to reproduce themselves, is said to have the highest fitness.)

4   Since the fittest varieties of molecule (or mice or mango) tend to produce offspring that are similar to themselves (that is, the variations are *inherited* by their offspring), these better-adapted varieties become more abundant in subsequent generations. As a result, over many generations, the characteristics that gave them an advantage spread throughout the population. Conversely, less-well adapted varieties are at a disadvantage in the competition for resources, and so will produce fewer offspring with that inherited 'defect', who in turn are also disadvantaged by it; in time, the maladaptive characteristic will disappear from the population.

The conditions under which natural selection occurs: reproduction, variation, competition for resources and inheritance, existed in the environment in which life-forms first evolved on Earth. DNA molecules reproduce by replication, they vary because the order of base-pairs can change, they compete because they need smaller molecules in order to make copies of themselves, and they show inheritance because they can replicate themselves exactly. Thus, the natural selection of increasingly useful variants of DNA could take place and, with them, increasingly complex forms of life on Earth evolved.

As we said earlier, ancestral DNA molecules would have been exposed to an environment which was highly likely to cause mutations (changes in the sequence of nucleotides) and hence increase the number of different variant forms of DNA. While some mutations would inevitably produce more successful (fitter) forms of DNA, others would have been deleterious, and thus would have produced forms of DNA that were less successful. This variation is the 'raw material' on which evolution by natural selection acts. As Steve Jones, a leading British geneticist, says on the audiotape associated with Chapter 9 of this book:

> If everything was perfect, we'd still be living in the primeval ooze, because you know without mutation ... most of which is inevitably damaging, we couldn't evolve.

☐ Explain this statement, based on your understanding of natural selection.

■ It involves competition between variants (whether they be different molecules of DNA, or mice, or moose), which results in only the best adapted to survival under the prevailing conditions being able to reproduce and thus expand their numbers in the next generation.

[8]The theory of natural selection and the biological meaning of 'adaptation' and 'fitness' were introduced in Chapters 5 and 11 of *World Health and Disease*.

We have one more stop to make on this tour round the structure and functions of DNA, to fill in a blank we left earlier in the chapter. How does the cell make all the various proteins it either needs for its own maintenance and reproduction, or pumps out into the surrounding fluid to fulfil other functions at a distance in the organism's body? You already know a great deal about the three molecules involved: DNA, RNA and amino acids, so it should not take much more effort to piece them together.

Protein synthesis and the genetic code

First a reminder: there are 20 common amino acids which, when linked together in specific combinations and sequences, form specific proteins. The instructions about which of the 20 possible amino acids contribute to a given protein, and in what sequence they are joined together, are contained in a coded form in the structure of DNA. We mentioned earlier that all the DNA in a human cell contains about 6 billion nucleotides, and that only about 5 per cent of these sequences contain instructions about how to make a protein. Those sequences that can be 'translated' into functioning proteins are termed *genes*.

Same genes: different cells

All the genes that an organism contains in its DNA are collectively referred to as the **genotype** of the organism. Nearly all the cells in an organism's body contain *exactly the same genes*; the principle exceptions are sperm and egg cells, and certain cells involved in the immune system of complex animals such as ourselves.[9] This raises an interesting question: if nearly all the cells in an individual have identical genes, how is it that such a huge variety of different kinds of cells exist in that organism's body? (Look back at Figure 3.3b to remind yourself of just a few of the different cell types found in the human body.)

In an earlier part of this chapter, we stated that variation between cells of different types stems from differences in the *nature of the proteins* they contain. Genes contain the coded instructions for making proteins and each unique gene carries the specification for a unique protein. To use the shorthand of genetics, human DNA contains a 'gene for haemoglobin' and 'a gene for insulin', and so forth—about 100 000 different genes in all, each one unique. But they are not all active all of the time: there are mechanisms for switching genes on and off. A

switched-on gene is actively engaged in the production of whatever protein it 'codes for' (another useful phrase, much in use among biologists), and synthesis of that protein ceases when the gene is switched off. The protein is often described by biologists as the **gene product**, that is, the *product* of the active gene.

☐ Can you suggest how the same set of genes can determine the variety of structures and functions of all the different cell types found in a human body?

■ The kinds of protein that a cell contains can be altered by switching on certain genes and keeping others switched off; for example, the gene containing the code for insulin is switched on in the hormone-producing cells in the pancreas, but switched off in all other cell types.

So, most cells in an individual carry the same set of genes, but not all of the genes are active all of the time. Differences in the structure and functions of cells of different types result from differences in which genes are switched on (actively engaged in producing certain proteins) and which genes are switched off.

From active gene to functioning protein

We will follow through the events that occur when a gene becomes active and its protein product is synthesised; the process from start to finish is known as **protein synthesis**. The following account of how the DNA code in a particular gene is 'translated' into a specific protein is greatly simplified, but you need only remember the general idea.

First, the section of the DNA double helix corresponding to the gene uncoils and the two strands separate, like a weak zip popping open in the middle (see Figure 3.15; in fact, the gene 'unzips' in several places at once, but we have simplified the story here). This exposes the bases which contain the coded instructions that lead ultimately to the production of a particular protein. However, DNA is a huge molecule, containing about 100 000 different genes in humans, which remains in the nucleus throughout the cell's life; the amino acids from which all the proteins are constructed are found *outside* the nucleus, in the cytoplasm of the cell. How is the coded instruction from just one gene to be carried from the DNA out to the cytoplasm where the protein can be made? The answer is that *RNA* carries the message from nucleus to cytoplasm.

The sequence of nucleotides in the 'unzipped' section of DNA is used as a template against which a new strand of RNA is built from the kinds of nucleotides

[9]The production of sperm and egg cells and the reasons why their DNA differs from that in all the other cells in the body are discussed in Chapter 4 of this book. The cells of the immune system are described in Chapter 6.

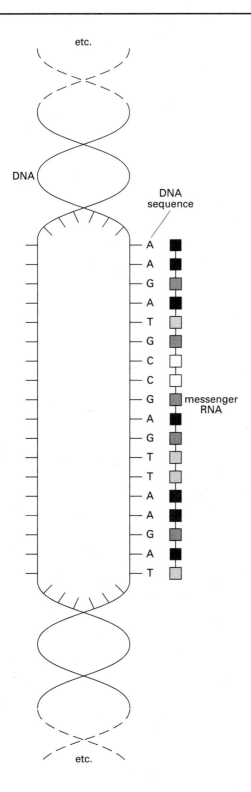

etc.

DNA

DNA
sequence

messenger
RNA

A
A
G
A
T
G
C
C
G
A
G
T
T
A
A
G
A
T

etc.

Figure 3.15 *A simplified version of the first stage in protein synthesis. The DNA sequence corresponding to a gene 'unzips' and becomes the template against which a new strand of messenger RNA is built.*

unique to RNA. Similar sorts of base-pairing rules apply when the exposed DNA bases attract RNA nucleotides, as those described earlier when DNA replicates and the exposed DNA bases attract DNA nucleotides. As a consequence of these DNA–RNA base-pairing rules, the new molecule of RNA reproduces in its structure the coded instructions that existed in the original section of DNA (the gene); the code has simply been transcribed into a slightly different RNA nucleotide 'language'. Appropriately enough, this type of RNA is called *messenger RNA.* The details of the messenger RNA code need not concern us here; it is enough to note that it carries the DNA 'message' out of the nucleus to the organelles where proteins can be assembled. (These organelles are called *ribosomes,* and you can just about see some if you look back at Figure 3.5b). However, we should spend a moment looking at the relationship between the original code in the DNA and the structure of the resultant protein, ignoring the intervening messenger RNA for simplicity.

Imagine that a sequence of DNA bases in a tiny part of a gene has been exposed on one of the two 'unzipped' DNA strands (as in Figure 3.15). The letters by which we know these bases could be written down, reading along the strand from left to right:

AAGATGCCGAGTTAAGAT

Now imagine that this 'message' forms a series of three-letter words; in this example they would be:

AAG–ATG–CCG–AGT–TAA–GAT

Biologists call these groups of three bases a *triplet* and sometimes refer to the genetic code as being 'written in triplets'. Next, imagine that each unique triplet is a command-word which means 'get a certain kind of amino acid'. For example, the triplet formed from adjacent nucleotides with the bases AAG (the first triplet in the sequence above) is an instruction to get an amino acid called *phenylalanine,* whereas the next triplet along, ATG, is an instruction to bring a different amino acid, *tyrosine.*[10] There are 20 different kinds of amino acids, so there have to be at least 20 different triplets. (If you work

[10]Don't try to memorise these triplets or their corresponding amino acids; the general idea is enough. In Chapter 4, you will meet the two amino acids named here again in the context of a genetic disease known as PKU. Phenylalanine is pronounced 'fee-nile-alan-een'; tyrosine is pronounced 'tie-roh-seen'.

out how many different three-letter combinations of C, G, A and T you could make, the answer is 64, so there are plenty to spare.)

Finally, think of the series of triplets in the gene as instructions which say (in effect) 'join together these particular amino acids in the order specified by the triplets in this piece of DNA'. So, in our example, the first two amino acids joined together in this piece of the protein would be phenylalanine and tyrosine.

As we said earlier, DNA cannot leave the nucleus, so first the complete message contained in the gene, written in hundreds of triplets of bases, is transcribed into the structure of a new strand of messenger RNA. This passes out of the nucleus and attaches to the ribosomes, where proteins are actually assembled. Amino acids are brought to the ribosomes and joined together into a protein along-

side the strand of RNA, in the order that corresponds to the triplets of bases in the gene (see Figure 3.16). When that protein is complete, it is released to do its work in the cell, and the strand of messenger RNA is available to act as a template for assembling another strand of the identical protein, and so on.

This whole sequence is often abbreviated to 'DNA makes RNA makes protein' and it brings us back more or less to where we began this chapter. Take a look back at Figure 3.2 and you will see that we have gradually built up a much more detailed picture of the way in which proteins are synthesised in modern cells. Remember that the ability to synthesise thousands of *different* proteins is the key to the variety and complexity of modern cells, and hence to the variety and complexity of present-day organisms.

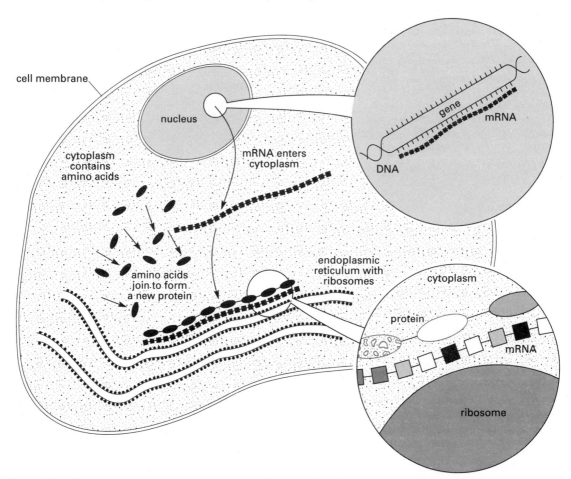

Figure 3.16 *The genetic code for a particular protein is first transcribed from a piece of DNA (a gene) into a new molecule of messenger RNA (mRNA), and this in turn specifies the sequence of amino acids that are assembled into a new protein. (Nothing in this diagram has been drawn to scale!)*

A brief reflection on immortality

It is worth pausing for a moment to reflect on how an understanding of how DNA works affects our perception of life. You have just read a quite detailed account of protein synthesis, though you should be aware that it is a greatly simplified one. Why is DNA so important, and why has the discovery of its structure and properties had such a profound effect on the study of biology?

It should be obvious to you that understanding the substance that controls the way that our cells, and hence our bodies, are built is pretty important in itself, but we can go further than that. At some stage in the evolution of early life-forms, DNA acquired the property of making proteins, which in their turn protected the DNA to some extent as it became 'packaged' ever more securely within cells. This enhanced its chance of survival. The Oxford biologist Richard Dawkins, in his book *The Selfish Gene*, calls organisms 'survival machines'. Organisms are mechanisms, he argues, built by DNA to promote its own survival and reproduction; organisms are DNA's way of making more DNA. In terms of the old chicken and egg problem, a chicken is an egg's way of making more eggs. Such a view of living things places DNA at the very centre of our understanding of evolution.

It may come as a surprise to learn that a very small fraction of your DNA is *potentially* immortal and could continue to contribute to human evolution until humans become extinct, whereas the bulk of your DNA will die with you. The DNA with a chance of immortality is referred to by biologists as **germline DNA** and is contained in the **germline cells**; these are the **gametes** (sperm or egg cells) and the cells in the testes or ovaries which give rise to sperm or eggs. Some of your germline DNA will be passed on to the next generation in a sperm or egg if you have a child, and your offspring's gametes will contain some of *your* germline DNA, which could be passed on to your grandchildren, and so on from one generation to the next. By the same token, you inherited your germline DNA from your parents, and they got it from *their* parents, and so on back in time. All the other cells in your body are collectively called **somatic cells** (from the Greek word 'soma' meaning 'the body') to distinguish them from the gametes and gamete-producing cells; the DNA in these somatic cells is called **somatic DNA** and it is not passed on to your descendants.

Later in this chapter, we will describe how somatic cells divide to make more somatic cells for growth and repair of the body. In Chapter 4, we describe the rather different process by which germline cells divide to make sperm and egg cells.

Self-maintenance and reproduction

We can now return to the speculative story of life and identify some of the features of present-day organisms that must have evolved early in the history of living things. We can hypothesise that as the newly-formed Earth cooled and the crust solidified, varieties of DNA evolved within self-made 'jackets' of protein and, somewhere about 4 000–3 500 million years ago, the first truly-independent, replicating, single-celled organisms appeared. Biologists generally believe that these early organisms were something like the bacterial cells we see today.

Some time later, single-celled organisms with a nucleus evolved, perhaps resembling the *protistans* that generations of schoolchildren dredge out of stagnant pools and examine under simple microscopes. A feature of many protistans is that they possess diverse means of moving about in their environment. An amoeba moves by altering the shape of its body (see Figure 3.17a, *overleaf*) as described earlier in the section on membranes, but many other protistans have various appendages which they can wave or vibrate and so push themselves along (Figures 3.17b and c, *overleaf*).

□ Why do you think the capacity for independent movement might have been an important stage in the evolution of life on Earth?

■ It meant that organisms could maintain themselves to some extent in *optimal* conditions. If the surrounding environment is hostile, they might be able to move to somewhere more hospitable.

Another important development in a hostile world is the ability to keep the conditions *within* the cell more conducive to life than the environment *outside* it. For single-celled organisms, the key to this vital property is the cell membrane, their interface with the outside world.

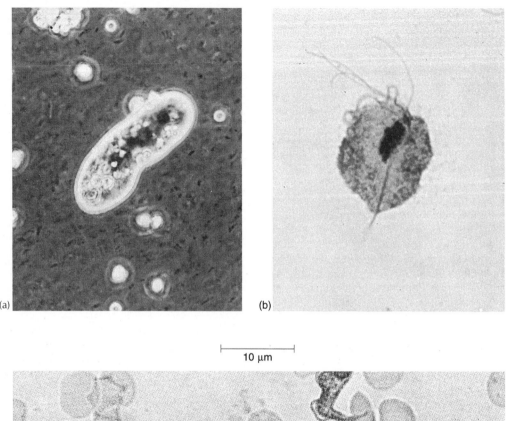

10 μm

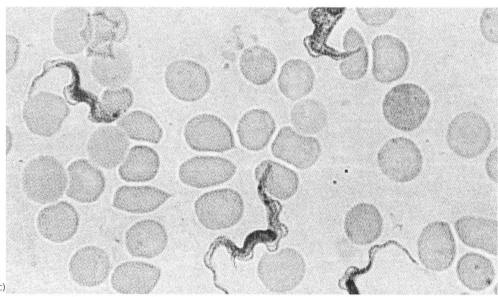

Figure 3.17 *Some protistans and how they move. (a)* Entamoeba hystolytica, *an amoeba that causes dysentery if it gets into the human digestive system; it moves by changing the shape of its outer membrane and 'flowing' over the surface beneath it. (b)* Trichomonas vaginalis, *a sexually-transmitted protistan which causes irritation in the reproductive tract; it moves by lashing four whip-like filaments called flagellae. (c) African trypanosomes move in human blood by 'thrashing' a long filament extending the length of the organism and projecting from one end; four trypanosomes are shown among red blood cells. Trypanosomes are transmitted by tsetse flies, and belong to several different species which cause sleeping sickness in humans and severe diseases of domestic cattle. (Sources: (a) Dr John Williams, London School of Hygiene and Tropical Medicine; (b) Dr J. P. Ackers, London School of Hygiene and Tropical Medicine; (c) Professor W. Peters, International Institute of Parasitology).* (Remember to finish reading page 55.)

Homeostasis: regulating the internal environment

As you have read, the cell membrane is a complex structure which has the capacity to control what passes in and out of the cell. As a result, the cell can, to a large extent, regulate its internal state. It can maintain such things as the concentration of essential nutrients and waste products in its cytoplasm with a degree of independence from the concentration of those substances *outside* the cell. This phenomenon of self-regulation is called **homeostasis** ('home-ee-oh-stay-sis'). Homeostasis literally means 'standing still' and is defined as the maintenance of a stable state close to the optimum conditions for maintaining life.

The principal process by which homeostasis is maintained is called **negative feedback**. Figure 3.18 illustrates in general terms how it works. An organism that can maintain homeostasis must be able to make a comparison between the *current* state of its 'internal world' and the desired *optimum* state, and then take action to reverse any drift away from that optimum. In order to achieve this, the organism has to have *sensors* that monitor the current state of the system and compare this with what the optimum state should be. Any difference between the two (the 'error') is then reduced; action is taken by *response mechanisms* that reverse the drift away from the optimum state. This process is called *negative* feedback

because the action taken reverses any change that has occurred in the system; that is, the error is negated.

A good analogy is the thermostat in a central heating system, which uses a negative feedback circuit to keep the temperature in the house close to the optimum set by the inhabitants. When the temperature falls below the desired level (the set point), the thermostat (sensor) switches on the heater (response mechanism); conversely, when the temperature rises too high, the thermostat switches the heater off.

☐ Look closely at the bottom of Figure 3.18 and notice that the arrows leaving the 'response mechanisms' box *cross over* each other. This is an essential feature of any negative feedback circuit diagram. Use the analogy of the central heating system to explain the function of this 'cross-over' in the circuit, starting from the moment when the temperature in the house falls below the set point.

■ The thermostat senses that the temperature is below the set point and switches the heating on; the house warms up, but the rising temperature will *overshoot* the set point because the thermostat can only detect 'too much' or 'too little' heat. The arrows cross over each other in the circuit diagram to show that the overshoot will trigger action to *reverse* it, in this example, by switching off the central heating. The temperature drifts downwards, overshoots the set point, and the sequence starts all over again.

Homeostasis is an essential process in self-maintenance, one of the two fundamental properties of living things that we identified in the first paragraph of this chapter. Even in a hostile external world, cells may be able to survive because they can keep their internal world stable. We will return to the subject of homeostasis a little later, when we focus on the maintenance of a stable internal state within large multicellular organisms such as ourselves.

The cell cycle and cell division

Another mechanism of self-maintenance, which *also* enables single-celled organisms and bacteria to reproduce, is the ability to split one cell into two, in other words, to make new cells.[11] New *somatic* (body) cells are formed by a process called the **cell cycle**. In essence, a cell enlarges and makes copies of everything it contains; it then divides to give two 'daughter' cells, each of which

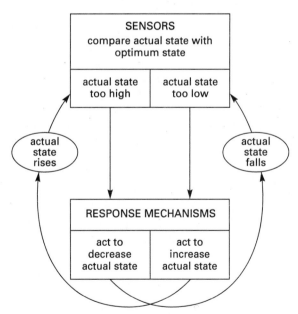

Figure 3.18 *Schematic diagram illustrating the basic principles of homeostasis, with particular emphasis on regulation via negative feedback.*

[11]Note that some protistans and bacteria can also reproduce by combining genetic material from different individuals, in a form of sexual reproduction.

receives a complete set of all the molecules and organelles that the 'parent' cell contained (see Figure 3.19). The new cells 'rest' for a time before the cycle starts again.

The triggers that initiate cell division are beyond the scope of this book, but they involve activation of certain genes, sections of DNA that instruct the manufacture of all the new components required to make two cells from one. An essential part of this replication process is the assembly of identical copies of all the DNA molecules in the cell, so that they can be 'shared out' between the daughter cells. This sharing out of two identical sets of DNA is a phase of the cell cycle known as **mitosis** (pronounced 'my-toe-sis'). The complete cell cycle involves a complex series of events divided into phases, as shown in Figure 3.20.

In the first phase of cell division, the DNA in the 'parent' cell *replicates*, that is, each original molecule of DNA acts as a template against which a new molecule of DNA is constructed (cell 1). These DNA molecules gradually compress (like a spring collapsing) and begin to be visible as a tangle of *chromosomes* when viewed

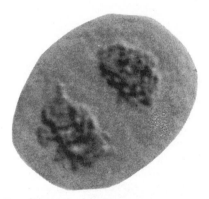

Figure 3.19 *Photograph of a plant cell in a late stage of cell division (the process is the same in animal cells but is particularly easy to see in plants). The cell contains two nuclei (the dark shapes), each of which has a copy of the DNA which the cell contained before it began to divide. A new cell membrane will soon form between the nuclei, dividing the original cell into two. (Photo: Open University)*

through a microscope (cells 2, 3 and 4); this is the start of mitosis. The cell now has two identical sets of chromosomes.

□ Can you remember how many chromosomes a human somatic cell usually has, and hence how many it would have at this phase of the cell cycle?

■ The normal chromosome number is 46, so there would be 92 chromosomes after DNA replication has occurred.

As mitosis proceeds, the chromosomes compress even further into short, sausage-shaped structures, which can be clearly distinguished from one another (cell 5). The chromosomes line up in the centre of the cell and then, quite suddenly, one copy of each chromosome migrates to opposite ends of the cell. The two identical sets of chromosomes are separated (cell 8) and a new membrane begins to form across the 'waist' of the cell, dividing it and its contents equally into two. The chromosomes gradually become invisible as the DNA molecules 'stretch out' again and mitosis comes to an end. The result is two daughter cells, each with exactly the same DNA as the original cell, and enough cytoplasm and organelles for normal cell metabolism to occur (cells 6 and 7; 9 and 10). The new cells go into a 'resting' phase until the time comes for them to divide in their turn: hence the term 'cell *cycle*'.

The part of the cell cycle known as mitosis normally takes between about 30 minutes and three hours, depending on the species of organism. Interestingly, the genes that were switched on or off in the parent cell remain in that state in the daughters: thus, a liver cell divides to produce more liver cells because the pattern of active and silent genes in the parent cell is preserved when the DNA replicates. Cell division involving mitosis enables one cell to become two, and two to become four, and so on; it is the process by which many single-celled organisms reproduce and increase their numbers, and it enabled larger organisms composed of many cells to evolve and grow, and to replace worn-out cells.

(a)

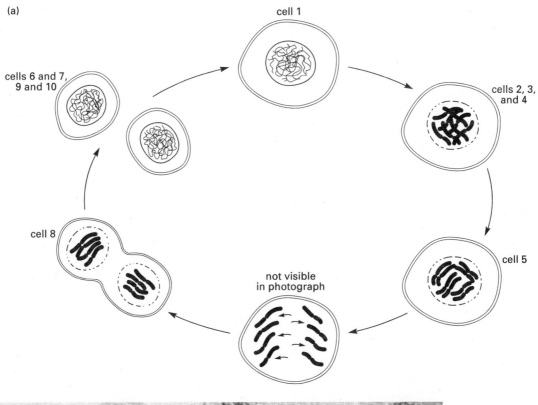

(b)

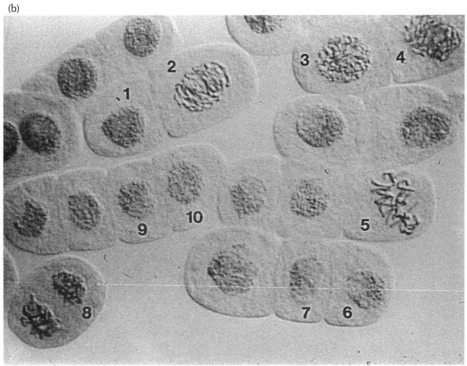

Figure 3.20 *The essential features of the cell cycle, illustrated (a) in diagrammatic form, numbered to identify corresponding cells in (b) a photograph of plant cells at various stages in the cell cycle. The phases are described in the text. (Photo: Open University)*

Towards larger organisms

We have only a hazy idea from the fossil record of what the evolutionary sequence might have been that resulted in the appearance on Earth of organisms consisting of many cells. The first multicellular organisms may have simply been clusters of cells that did not separate when a single-celled organism divided into two cells, and the daughters in their turn stayed together. Multicellularity provides a number of advantages, such as larger size and mutual protection against a variety of environmental threats. In a comparable way, many large animals live for all or part of their lives clustered together in flocks, herds and colonies, gaining safety in numbers and many other benefits that derive from sociality.

Specialisation of cells

The transition from simple multicellular organisms, that were essentially 'confederations' of identical cells, to more complex organisms such as humans, involved a crucial change in the properties of individual cells. From each cell being entirely self-sufficient and capable of *all* the processes necessary for self-maintenance and reproduction, cells became *specialised*, each carrying out only *some* of the functions required for the survival and reproduction of the whole organism.

Cells on the outside of the body evolved specialised features that formed a protective layer; within the body, different types of cells formed distinct *tissues* or *organs* with defined functions: some digest food, others collect and excrete waste products, and so on, as we showed early on in this chapter in Figure 3.3(b).[12] By analogy, individual members of a human society, or of a bee colony, each perform specialised tasks on behalf of the society or colony as a whole. Specialisation within different cell types occurs because (as mentioned earlier) each cell activates only a part of the genetic code, and hence

[12]A hierarchy of biological organisation, from atoms and molecules at one end of the spectrum, through increasingly complex levels of organisation (cells, tissues, organs, multicellular organisms) to interactions between species at the other end of the spectrum is illustrated in *Studying Health and Disease* (1994 edition), Chapter 9; see particularly Figure 9.1.

produces only those proteins involved in the specialised functions of that type of cell.

Transport and communication

As multicellular organisms evolved, they became larger. Above a certain size, cells within a multicellular organism face the problem that they are no longer close enough to the outside world to obtain all the nutrients they need, or to expel their waste, simply by *passive diffusion* across the cell membrane. Nutrients can pass into the body of the multicelled organism, diffusing from one cell to the next, but this is a slow process and above a distance of about 1 millimetre (1 mm) is inefficient.

An early stage in the evolution of multicellular organisms must have been the appearance of channels along which nutrients could be carried to the innermost cells and waste could be carried out. In many kinds of modern-day animals, these channels have evolved into blood vessels and the system includes a pumping organ, such as the human heart, which drives blood around the body. Figure 3.21 shows the basic layout of the human **cardiovascular system** ('cardio' is from the Greek word *kardia*, 'heart', and 'vascular' is from the Latin for vessel). The nutrients transported in the bloodstream are obtained from the breakdown of food by the *digestive system,* but we shall say no more about that here because it is discussed in Chapter 7.

If large, multicellular organisms, made up of cells of very different types, are to survive and reproduce, it is essential that their activities are coordinated effectively. The *homeostatic* control necessary for cells to function properly becomes a process that must occur, not just at the level of the individual cell as described earlier, but also at the level of the whole organism. Homeostasis at the organism level requires close coordination of the various fluids, cells, tissues and organs of the organism's body. Coordination of activities throughout a complex body requires effective *communication,* so that the requirements of cells in one part of the body can be recognised and responded to appropriately by cells elsewhere. Complex animals have a number of communication and control systems, of which the most important are the nervous system, the hormonal system and the immune system.

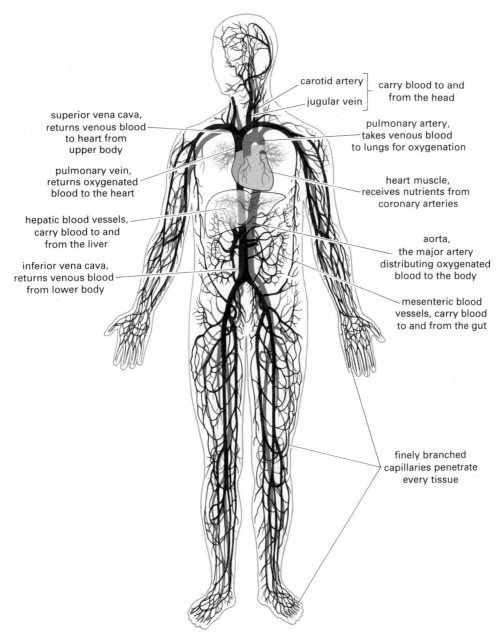

carotid artery ⎤ carry blood to and
jugular vein ⎦ from the head

superior vena cava,
returns venous blood
to heart from
upper body

pulmonary artery,
takes venous blood
to lungs for oxygenation

pulmonary vein,
returns oxygenated
blood to the heart

heart muscle,
receives nutrients from
coronary arteries

hepatic blood vessels,
carry blood to and
from the liver

aorta,
the major artery
distributing oxygenated
blood to the body

inferior vena cava,
returns venous blood
from lower body

mesenteric blood
vessels, carry blood
to and from the gut

finely branched
capillaries penetrate
every tissue

Figure 3.21 *The main features of the human cardiovascular system. The heart pumps blood to the body in the arteries (shown in red), and it returns to the heart from all parts of the body in the veins (black). The arteries and veins branch into an extensive network of fine vessels, called capillaries, which penetrate almost all parts of the body. The bloodstream acts as a transporter of oxygen, nutrients and dissolved waste, and of the specialised cells and molecules involved in defending against infection and in regulating growth, development and homeostasis. You are not expected to memorise the details of this diagram.*

The **nervous system** consists of specialised cells, called nerve cells or *neurons*, that are adapted to pass information one to another in the form of electrical impulses and chemical signals (these chemicals are collectively called neurotransmitters). To varying degrees, the nervous systems of animals include a *brain*, which is a large aggregation of neurons that controls the activity of the organism as a whole. An important function of the brain is to receive information about the outside world from sense organs, such as eyes, ears, the nose, etc. and to control the movements of the body through its environment (see Figure 3.22).

The **hormonal system** comprises a number of diverse and scattered groups of cells called *endocrine glands*, together with the hormones they synthesise and secrete into the bloodstream (for example, the pancreas secretes insulin, the ovaries secrete oestrogen). **Hormones** are signalling molecules that are carried around the body in the blood, and which influence the activity of 'target' cells elsewhere in the body.

☐ From your understanding of membrane structure, how do you expect a hormone to be able to 'select' the correct target cells with which it interacts?

■ By making a lock-and-key interaction with receptor molecules embedded in the surface membrane of the target cells. Cells that do not have the correct receptor cannot interact with that hormone.

Some hormones are chemically related to fats (these are the steroid hormones such as oestrogen and testosterone, involved in sexual development and reproduction); most are short chains of amino acids, some only a few amino acids long but others (like insulin) long enough to be called a protein. Certain hormones are intimately linked with the nervous system and some are secreted by the nervous system itself. (For example, the hormone prolactin is secreted by cells in the brain and causes the breasts of female mammals to secrete milk.)

Organisms can only survive if the many processes going on in the body operate within certain narrow limits. This 'whole organism' homeostasis is regulated by the coordinated activity of the nervous system and the hormonal system, together with the processes already described for regulating the internal world of every cell. Precise regulation is essential to life: humans, for example, become very sick and may die if their body temperature deviates by only a few degrees from the 'normal' temperature of around 37 °C.

☐ Look back at Figure 3.18. What response mechanisms are involved in temperature regulation in humans?

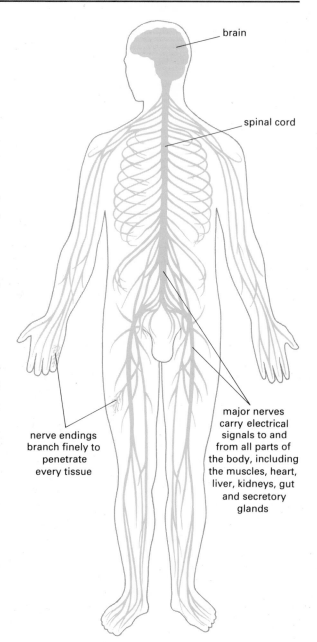

brain

spinal cord

major nerves carry electrical signals to and from all parts of the body, including the muscles, heart, liver, kidneys, gut and secretory glands

nerve endings branch finely to penetrate every tissue

Figure 3.22 *The main features of the human nervous system, conventionally distinguished into the* central *nervous system (the brain and spinal cord) and the* peripheral *nervous system (the nerves that penetrate almost every part of the body). Nerves generally consist of several different nerve fibres, which carry information in the form of electrical signals, either informing the brain and spinal cord about the state of the body, or bringing instructions from the brain and spinal cord to the muscles and organs. You are* not *expected to memorise the details of this diagram.*

■ You may have thought of sweating to lose heat by evaporation when we get too hot, or shivering to generate heat when we get cold. Other responses involve consciously-willed behaviour, such as removing or replacing clothing, and eating or drinking something cold or hot.

However, multicellularity has certain drawbacks. Large, multicellular organisms with homeostatically-controlled bodies provide wonderful places in which smaller organisms can survive and reproduce. At the very least, these 'passengers' use up precious resources that are needed by their host; at worst, they may be pathogenic and lead to their host's death. A vital aspect of homeostasis involves keeping the organism as free as possible from pathogens; in humans and many other animals, such control is achieved by the *immune system*. It operates in close association with the nervous system and with hormones to ensure, for example, that specialised defensive cells arrive as quickly as possible at places in the body where pathogens have entered. (The immune system is described in detail in Chapter 6.)

Reproduction in multicellular organisms

The evolution of sex was a very important development in the evolution of multicellular organisms. It is a feature that involves certain cells (the germline cells) becoming specialised for reproducing the organism, a capacity that is lost by all the other (somatic) cells. Most of the somatic cells in a complex organism can reproduce in one sense; skin cells can make more skin cells, for example, but they cannot make the special cells (eggs and sperm) from which whole new organisms develop. Whereas all somatic cells reproduce by mitosis, as described above, the production of eggs and sperms involves a quite different form of cell division, called *meiosis*. This is described in Chapter 4.

Whenever cells reproduce by mitosis, whether they be single-celled organisms or cells within multicellular organisms, there is a tendency for small changes, or mutations, to occur in the sequence of bases along their DNA. The rate at which such errors occur is increased by radiation and certain chemicals, as we mentioned earlier in this chapter. In a multicelled organism that lives a long time, and therefore undergoes millions of cell divisions, more of these errors will accumulate than in a short-lived one. This accumulation of mutations is responsible for many of the manifestations of ageing, a topic taken up in Chapter 8.

Adapting to change

The origin of multicellular organisms and their subsequent evolution into a huge diversity of forms involves the same process of natural selection that was described earlier in our story of life on Earth. Specialisation of cells to form organs with specific functions, homeostatic control, the immune system, and sexual reproduction are all features that make multicellular organisms better able to survive and reproduce. In the language of evolutionary biology, they are all **adaptations**. The story of the evolution of the huge diversity of organisms that inhabit the Earth today is largely one of new adaptations to particular environmental challenges. For example, the ancestors of living amphibians (frogs, newts and salamanders) evolved a set of adaptations that enabled them to make the transition from the purely aquatic life led by their fish ancestors to one that is lived partly on dry land. Feathers and wings are adaptations in birds that enable them to fly. Chapter 2 described a number of anatomical features, characteristic of humans, that evolved during our evolution as adaptations to our ancestral environment and way of life.

□ Can you recall what they were?

■ An upright posture and the ability to walk and run on two legs (bipedality) and a very large brain. These features are described as *adaptive* because they conferred a survival advantage on early humans in the transition to a savannah environment.

The evolution of organisms by natural selection is a process in which the phenomenon of competition plays a crucial role. The initial stages of the evolutionary process, as discussed earlier, can be regarded as involving competition between different versions of DNA. Those versions that could gather and use chemical compounds from the environment more rapidly would grow and reproduce faster than less effective versions. Competition, both within and between different species of living organisms, can be seen essentially as a continuation of the same process, since each individual represents a unique version of DNA, in competition with other versions.

This fundamental element of competition through reproduction raises a problem for any explanation of the evolution of complex organisms from simpler ones. How can one explain the fact that all the somatic cells in complex organisms have lost a fundamental property of living things, the ability to reproduce more organisms of that kind? Kidney cells can divide to make more kidney cells, skin cells can make more skin cells, and so on, but only the germline cells can divide to make the sperms and eggs from which all the different cell types of a whole new organism is made.

This problem is resolved when you remember that all the cells of an individual, whether they are kidney cells, nerve cells or skin cells, contain *the same version of DNA*. Thus all the cells in a complex organism, whatever their specialised functions, are more or less directly involved in the survival of the same version of DNA, and its transmission to the next generation. It is worth noting that cancer cells arise as a result of mutations; their genetic makeup is no longer the same as that of other cells in the body. They reproduce and multiply in a way that, ultimately, threatens the survival of the whole organism in which they grow.

Genotype and phenotype

Before we leave the story of life, it is necessary to make a few final points, and to introduce one more important term. As described above, DNA 'codes for proteins' and thus is responsible for the fact that organisms can produce the molecules that make up their structure, that conduct signals around the body, and which, in the case of enzymes, control the rate of chemical reactions within cells. For an organism to function normally, to be healthy and to be able to reproduce, its DNA must contain all the appropriate genes.

□ Can you remember the collective term given to all the genes that an organism contains?

■ The term is *genotype*. Each of us has a slightly different version of DNA and, hence, slightly different genes and a unique genotype (only identical twins have exactly the same genes and hence the same genotype).

Yet, even in identical twins there are distinguishing features, and you can imagine that a person raised under adverse conditions might develop rather differently than they would have done if raised in a healthy environment. The reason is that the *activity* of the genotype (the switching on and off of genes) can be influenced by the environment in which the organism grows and develops.

Biologists have a word meaning 'how the organism actually turned out': they describe the 'expressed' characteristics of the organism, its size, shape, metabolism, etc., as its **phenotype**. Each of us has a unique phenotype, partly because we have a unique genotype, but also because we have undergone a process of

development that is particular to each individual. The phenotype of an individual at a given point in its life results from a complex and continuous interaction between its genotype and its environment. You will learn a lot more about the relationship between genotype and phenotype in Chapter 4.

Although the genotype of an individual has to contain the 'correct' genes to produce a viable individual, it does not have to be the same as that of other individuals of the same species; there is considerable variation between the genotypes of individuals and any two mice or moose or humans with different genotypes can be equally *viable*. ('Viable' means 'able to survive'.) Each species has certain characteristic genes found in no other species, but some genes cross species boundaries; for example, humans have 98 per cent of our genes in common with chimpanzees. Against this background of uniformity, each individual in a species still possesses a unique genotype; each of us has some unique *variations* in our genes and some variations that are shared only with the closest members of our family. This fact is exemplified in the technique of *DNA fingerprinting*, a procedure used to determine unequivocally the parentage of individuals, which exploits the fact that specific variations in the genes possessed by an individual's mother or father can be detected in the DNA of their progeny. Genetic variation and inheritance are the subjects of Chapter 4.

Complexity and progress

We end this chapter on a cautious note. The language of evolutionary biology is full of adjectives, applied to organisms, that imply various kinds of value judgement. Humans are described as 'complex' and 'advanced', whereas bacteria or molluscs are 'simple' and 'primitive'. The use of such words stems from the fact that biological evolution is typically seen as a process that involves progress, with forms of life that are in some sense 'better' replacing existing forms. There is an important sense in which this view is appropriate and correct. From one generation to the next, those individuals of a given species that survive and reproduce more effectively than others are, by definition, described as being 'fitter'. Thus, over time, natural selection will insure that a species 'improves', in the sense that its individuals become better adapted to their environment.

This scenario assumes, however, that the environment is constant over time, which it is not. The environment is subject to continuous change, both long-term and short-term, and much of the evolutionary change in the form and physiology of organisms that results from natural selection is in response to environmental change. This phenomenon of a constantly shifting environment is central to an evolutionary concept called the Red Queen's hypothesis, after the Red Queen in Lewis Carroll's *Through the Looking Glass* who said, 'Now here, you see, it takes all the running you can do, to keep in the same place'. In other words, while natural selection is a process that tends to produce perfectly adapted organisms, a state of perfection is never achieved, because a continually-changing environment continually alters what 'perfectly adapted' means. This idea is important in the context of disease; as you will see in Chapter 5, organisms such as ourselves have to adapt continually to the rapid changes in pathogenic organisms that occur over evolutionary time.

Biological evolution involves not only the adaptation of *existing* species to a changing environment, but also the formation of *new* species. Sometimes new species replace existing species but, equally importantly, new species come to coexist alongside already established species. It can thus be misleading to regard all recently-evolved species as being in any sense *superior* to their ancestors. The important point is that they are *different*; they have evolved novel characteristics that enable them to exploit the *current* environment in different ways from existing species.

Evolution is not generally, therefore, a process in which new species replace older, less well-adapted ones, but one in which the number and variety of species, the diversity of life, tends to change over time. From the fossil record, it is clear that during evolution there has been a continual 'turnover' of species; at certain times there have been mass extinctions, when the number of species declined rapidly, and at other times there has been a rapid increase in the diversity of life-forms found on Earth.[13]

At any one time in evolutionary history, as at present, the Earth is inhabited by a large and diverse array of species, some of recent origin, others more ancient, some simple, some complex. The coexistence of complex and simple species is important in the context of disease, because most pathogens, particularly bacteria and viruses, are simple organisms that coexist with complex ones, such as humans. If evolution were a progressive process in which superior forms replaced inferior ones, one might reasonably expect that organisms would arise that are resistant to any kind of disease. That they have not is due to the fact that simple organisms hold certain advantages over more complex organisms, notably a very high reproductive rate. The evolutionary interaction between complex and simpler organisms, including pathogenic species, is examined in more detail in Chapter 5 of this book.

---

[13]Note that in geological timescales, 'rapid' means over a period of several hundred thousand years!

OBJECTIVES FOR CHAPTER 3

When you have studied this chapter, you should be able to:

3.1 Describe the basic features of a 'typical' animal cell, paying particular attention to the dynamic nature of cell metabolism and the crucial role of the cell membrane as the interface with the external world.

3.2 Give some examples of lock-and-key interactions between biological molecules and comment on their function in cell metabolism.

3.3 Describe the basic features of DNA structure, how it replicates during the cell cycle and is 'shared out' by mitosis; explain the significance of these features for the evolution of life on Earth.

3.4 Describe, in outline, how 'DNA makes RNA makes protein'.

3.5 Explain how a large multicellular organism, such as a human, can be composed of specialised cells of many different types, almost all of which contain exactly the same genes.

3.6 Illustrate the process of maintaining homeostasis by negative feedback, both at the level of a single cell and of a multicellular organism.

3.7 Describe the essential features of natural selection and mutation, and show how they may contribute to the evolution of diverse life-forms.

QUESTIONS FOR CHAPTER 3

Question 1 (*Objectives 3.1 and 3.2*)

Briefly describe the three mechanisms by which substances pass through cell membranes. Which of these mechanisms involves lock-and-key interactions?

Question 2 (*Objectives 3.3 and 3.4*)

How does the sequence of nucleotides in a length of DNA provide the 'genetic code' for the synthesis of a protein?

Question 3 (*Objective 3.5*)

What is the principal difference between the genetic material of an insulin-producing cell in the pancreas and a pigment cell in the skin of the same individual? Use the following terms in your answer: gene, genotype, gene product.

Question 4 (*Objective 3.6*)

Distinguish between the ways in which a single cell and a multicellular organism maintain homeostasis.

Question 5 (*Objective 3.6*)

Draw a rough sketch of a negative feedback circuit, using Figure 3.18 as a basis, showing how homeostasis of human body temperature is maintained.

Question 6 (*Objective 3.7*)

The theory of natural selection incorporates the idea of a 'struggle for existence'. Why is there a struggle for existence and why is inheritance of mutations an essential feature of the theory of evolution by natural selection?

4 Inheritance and variation

This chapter builds on the description in Chapter 3 of the structure of DNA and its replication during the cell cycle in the human body, and the process of nuclear division known as mitosis, which occurs during growth and repair as a body cell divides into two 'daughter' cells. The television programme 'Blood lines' on the structure, function and evolutionary significance of DNA, which was associated with Chapter 3, is also relevant here. The terms phenotype, genotype and gene were defined in Chapter 3 and are of central importance here.

The development of the human organism, from fertilised egg cell to mature adult, is not discussed here, but is a major theme in another book in this series, Birth to Old Age: Health in Transition.[1] In this chapter you will find other references to books in this series, in particular to World Health and Disease: Chapter 3 of that book describes global patterns of disease distribution and discusses what determines them, and Chapter 11 reviews the relationship between nutrition, infection and childhood growth.[2]

Introduction

This chapter explores the way in which genes and environments contribute to the development of the unique *phenotype* of individuals (that is, the sum total of all their characteristics), why individuals tend to resemble their parents, and how the enormous diversity of human phenotypes arises. Some of this variation is shown in Figure 1.1 (the frontispiece to this book). We trace the inheritance of certain characteristics, including

[1]*Birth to Old Age: Health in Transition* (Open University Press, 1985 and revised edition 1995).

[2]*World Health and Disease* (Open University Press, 1993).

susceptibility to certain diseases, which follow particular patterns. We begin with the individual and then move on to examine the family and finally whole populations. The frequencies of characteristics and diseases in different populations is discussed and we explain how and why these vary within and between populations. We begin by introducing the factors that contribute to the variation between individuals, namely genes and environments.

Inheritance and the individual

Our first task is to explore the nature of *genetically* determined differences between individuals. Though the focus is on the individual, in order to understand the inheritance of genes it is also necessary to look at events that occur within cells; so we jump between looking at the individual and focusing on particular cells, and we explore the relationship between the two.

A family photograph album

Imagine that you are sitting looking at a family photograph album in which there is a photograph of Sam when she was six months old. On the next page is Sam as a teenager and on the next as a mature woman of 21 years of age.

You could describe Sam's *visible* features or characteristics: whether she has curly or straight hair; whether her ears are 'unattached', that is, they are with lobes, or 'attached', without lobes (see Figure 4.1 *overleaf*); how tall she is; the colour of her skin and whether she tans easily in the sun. But what we can see is only a very small fraction of Sam's phenotype—the sum of all her characteristics. For example, we cannot see her blood group and blood pressure; and if we could look within individual cells, at the sequences of amino acids within the proteins (Chapter 3), we would find that some of them differ slightly from those of other individuals. A full description of Sam's phenotype, including her *morphology* (the shape and structure of her body), her speed of movement and coordination as well as her temperament, personality and the structure of proteins in her body, would show that, like you, she is quite unique. Our uniqueness is a consequence of the enormous amount of variation that exists between individuals.

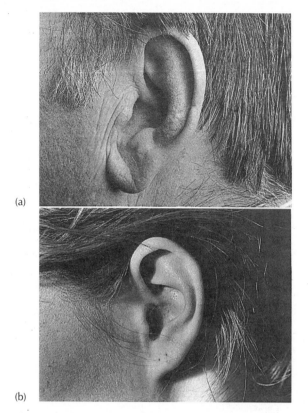

(a)

(b)

Figure 4.1 *Ear-lobes are either (a) free, unattached, or (b) attached. (Photos: Mike Levers)*

However, human babies usually resemble their parents, brothers and sisters, in particular ways. Why does Sam have some features in common with other individuals in her family and yet have strikingly different features that she shares with few other relatives? And how is her own unique combination of features, her individual pheno-type, brought about? A number of factors contribute, as you will see as this chapter unfolds.

Our first approach to the study of human variation comes from an understanding of the biological mechan-ism of reproduction. In order to understand why Sam or any other individual has her/his particular set of features, we need to look at the way in which living organisms reproduce themselves and what is transmitted from parent to offspring. Put another way we need to look at the *genes*, the units of genetic information that children *inherit* from their parents. Relatives are more likely to share genes than are unrelated people because they have an ancestor in common. The more closely related two people are to each other the more genes they have in common.

An important theme of this chapter is that individuals are the products of the *combined action* of their genes (the full complement of their genes is called the *genotype*) and their environments. Yet, some characteristics are influenced relatively more by genetic factors than by the environment, and for other characteristics the reverse is true. Later, we will examine examples of each situation, but first we consider how these two aspects, genes and environment, influence the development of the phenotype.

Chromosome pairs

Sam began life as a single cell which was formed from the combining of two different *gametes*, the collective term for egg cells and sperm cells (Figure 4.2). Each gamete has a *nucleus* which contains the DNA, the genetic material, and each fertilised cell contains the combined genetic material from sperm and egg. As you learned in Chapter 3, genes are sequences of DNA that are joined together in a linear order, as long strands called *chromosomes*. Like the gametes, most human somatic (body) cells have a nucleus in which the chromosomes are contained.

Laboratory techniques are available to aid in the preparation and staining of the chromosomes from a single cell, so that they are readily distinguished and can be photographed with the microscope (Figure 4.3). During *mitosis* (an important stage in somatic cell repli-cation, described in Chapter 3), the chromosomes become visible and their number, size and shape can be most easily studied. Every species has a particular num-ber of chromosomes, each with a characteristic size and

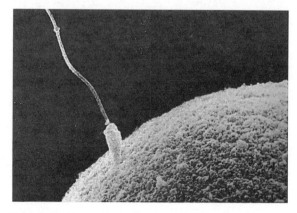

Figure 4.2 *Human gametes: a sperm and an egg (ovum), magnified approximately 4000 times, photographed with the aid of a scanning electron microscope. This sperm will penetrate the egg, resulting in the combining of genetic material from both gametes. (Source: Science Photo Library)*

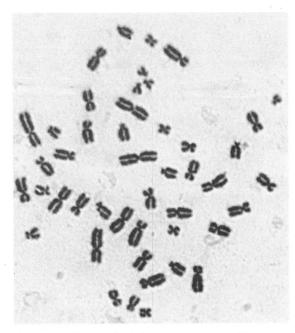

Figure 4.3 *Photograph of chromosomes prepared from a single white cell taken from human blood (photographed through a light microscope, magnified approximately 1 000 times). (Source: Department of Cancer Studies, The Medical School, University of Birmingham)*

shape. This characteristic number of chromosomes is found in the nucleus of every cell in the body, with the exception of mature red blood cells (which have no nucleus and no chromosomes) and the gametes. Humans have 46 chromosomes per somatic cell, and these have a similar genetic organisation to the 48 chromosomes of our closest living relatives, the chimpanzees.

The chromosomes of a single cell can be stained and photographed to reveal their distinct features. Once photographed, they can be cut out and lined up according to size. Figure 4.4 shows the chromosomes of a human female, arranged in this manner. This distinctive pattern is described as the human female **karyotype**, that is, the pattern of chromosomes that is unique to human females. (The same term, karyotype, is used for the standard chromosome set of an *individual,* as in 'human female karyotype', or of a *species*, as in 'human karyotype'.)

☐ What is the most striking feature of the human chromosomes shown in Figure 4.4?

■ The 46 chromosomes are present as 23 pairs of varying sizes; the members of each pair look the same.

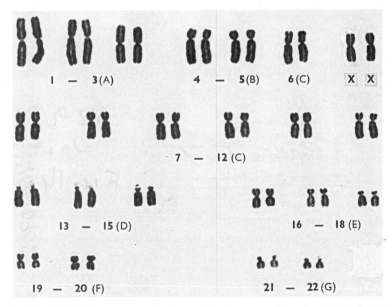

Figure 4.4 *Photograph of the stained chromosomes of a human female, arranged as a karyotype (photographed through a light microscope, magnified approximately 1 000 times). The pairs of chromosomes have been arranged in a conventional sequence and are numbered 1 to 22, with one pair of X chromosomes. (Photo: courtesy of Professor M. A. Ferguson-Smith, Department of Medical Genetics, Royal Hospital for Sick Children, Glasgow)*

The chromosomes in 22 of the pairs have been given a number; thus, there is a pair of chromosome 1, a pair of chromosome 2, etc. Members of a pair are said to be homologous, which in genetics means 'having a similar structure', thus there are 22 **homologous pairs** of chromosomes. Although the chromosomes of some homologous pairs are longer or shorter than others, it is still difficult to distinguish between several pairs of chromosomes on this criterion alone. For example, look at the pairs of chromosomes numbered 7 to 12 in Figure 4.4: if those chromosomes were mixed up it would be difficult to separate them into pairs again on the basis of visual appearance alone. This difficulty was overcome in the 1970s by the discovery of special staining techniques which produce distinctive patterns of bands on chromosomes. Such staining techniques have made it possible to define the differences between the members of one pair and those of another, as shown in Figure 4.5. This photograph of the chromosomes of a human male, arranged as a karyotype, could be from any cell in the body apart from sperm and mature red blood cells.

□ In Figure 4.5, what does the banding pattern of the homologous pairs of chromosomes numbered 7 to 12 reveal?

■ If you look closely, you can observe, first, that each chromosome appears to have an identical banding pattern with its partner and, second, that each pair can be distinguished from all other pairs.

The two observations that you have just made about chromosomes reveal important information about inheritance. We will look at the implications of each of these observations in turn.

The human female karyotype (shown in Figure 4.4) contains two chromosomes marked 'X'. In the human male karyotype (see Figure 4.5), one of the X chromosomes is replaced by a small chromosome called the Y chromosome. These **sex chromosomes** play an important role in sex determination: the sex chromosome constitution of females is XX, whereas that of males is XY. Apart from these sex chromosomes, both males and females contain similar sets of 22 homologous pairs of non-sex chromosomes.

We now know that each of the 24 *different* kinds of chromosomes that may occur in a human cell (that is, chromosomes 1 to 22, plus X and Y) carries different genes; each has particular genes arranged in a specific order along its length. However, both partners in an homologous pair of chromosomes, for example the pair

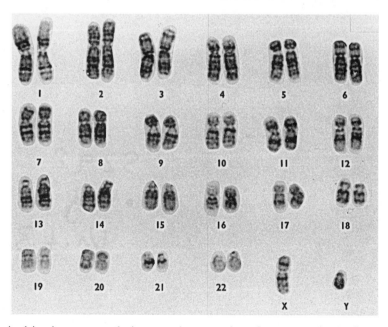

Figure 4.5 *Photograph of the chromosomes of a human male, arranged as a karyotype and stained to reveal their characteristic banding pattern (photographed through a light microscope, magnified approximately 1 000 times). (Photo: courtesy of Professor M. A. Ferguson-Smith, Department of Medical Genetics, Royal Hospital for Sick Children, Glasgow)*

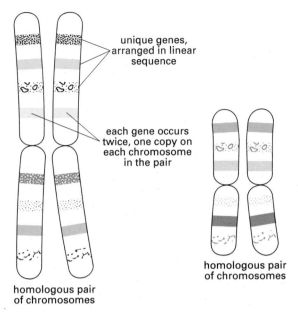

unique genes, arranged in linear sequence

each gene occurs twice, one copy on each chromosome in the pair

homologous pair of chromosomes

homologous pair of chromosomes

Figure 4.6 *Two homologous pairs of chromosomes; each pair has a different set of genes from those found on all the other homologous pairs. Two copies of each gene exist in the cell nucleus, one copy on each chromosome of a pair.*

of chromosome 1, carry the *same* genes in the *same* order (see Figure 4.6). This means that each gene present on the 22 non-sex chromosomes is present *twice* in the genotype, a feature that has important consequences for inheritance.

Figures 4.4 and 4.5 show clearly that the two sex chromosomes, the X and Y chromosomes, look quite different from each other; what you cannot see is that they carry quite different genes. Given the small size of the Y chromosome you may not be surprised to learn that it contains very few genes, the most important of which is the gene that carries instructional information for the development of testes rather than ovaries. Later in this chapter, we will look at the influence of the sex chromosomes on inheritance.

The formation of eggs and sperm

The presence of homologous pairs of chromosomes is particularly important for understanding reproduction and the passing on or *transmission* of genetic material from generation to generation. Observing the behaviour of chromosome pairs during the production of gametes provides a direct way of obtaining information about the inheritance of genes.

The process of gamete production involves a type of nuclear division which is different from mitosis and is

called **meiosis** (pronounced 'my-oh-sis'). Unlike mitosis, which occurs throughout the organism whenever growth by cell replication occurs, meiosis is confined to the egg-producing and sperm-producing cells in the *gonads*: ovaries in females and testes in males. Meiosis is a much more complex process than mitosis and is remarkably similar in all animal and plant species. The details of the process are not important here, but you should understand how differences between gametes can arise, since this variation has profound consequences for the phenotype of each individual.

The most striking way in which gametes differ from somatic cells in the body, and from the egg-producing or sperm-producing cells in the gonads from which they arise, is in the *number* of their chromosomes. The changes in chromosome number that take place during meiosis, gamete production and subsequent fertilisation of the egg by a sperm, are summarised in Figure 4.7. As a

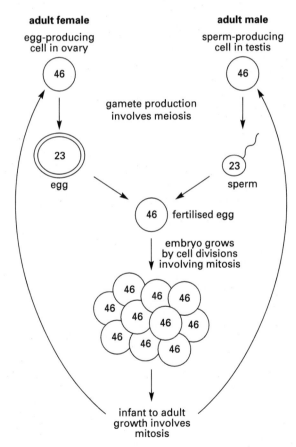

Figure 4.7 *Changes in chromosome number in the human life cycle.*

result of meiosis, each gamete contains only 23 chromosomes: one from each of the 22 homologous pairs of non-sex chromosomes, plus either an X or a Y chromosome. Not surprisingly meiosis is referred to as a *reduction division* since the usual number of chromosomes is reduced by half.

□ Look back at Figure 4.7. How many chromosomes will a fertilised egg contain and where did they originate?

■ 46 chromosomes in 23 pairs: one member of each pair came from the female parent in the egg and the other member of each pair came from the male parent in the sperm.

Thus fertilisation restores the full chromosome number. It also means that any individual inherits one of each pair of chromosomes from their father and one of each pair from their mother.

□ Why is reduction division (meiosis) such an important feature of reproduction?

■ If the chromosome number were not halved in the gametes prior to fertilisation, the fertilised egg would contain 92 chromosomes—twice the normal number in the parents' cells.

Fertilisation, which involves the combining of DNA from two different and unrelated individuals, is a powerful source of genetic variation. Growth and development follow, which among other events involve a staggeringly large number of cell divisions involving *mitosis,* in which the normal chromosome number is preserved (Chapter 3), to produce a fetus, baby, child and adult.[3] You, for example, consist of about 10 million million cells! Since the mature adult in turn usually produces gametes, some of which are fertilised, life constantly cycles, as shown in Figure 4.7.

Now look at Figure 4.8, which illustrates the production of gametes in each parent with reference to the sex chromosomes only; we have omitted all the other chromosomes to make the sex chromosomes easier to track. Each of the sperm-producing cells in the testes of the male contain both an X and a Y chromosome, whereas the equivalent cells in the ovaries of the female each contain XX. In the male, the X and Y chromosomes separate from each other during meiosis, the X

[3]Biological development is considered throughout *Birth to Old Age: Health in Transition.*

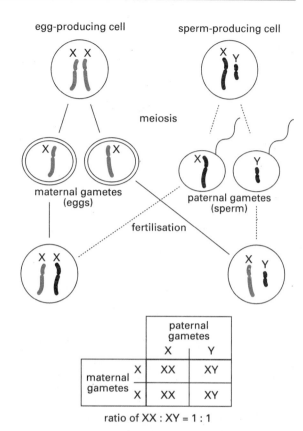

		paternal gametes	
		X	Y
maternal gametes	X	XX	XY
	X	XX	XY

ratio of XX : XY = 1 : 1

Figure 4.8 *Mating diagram showing the distribution of human sex chromosomes during gamete formation, the consequences for the possible sex of children, and the proportions of children of each sex.*

chromosome going to one sperm and the Y chromosome to another. Similarly, in the female, the two X chromosomes separate from one another, each one going to different egg cells.

□ On the basis of Figure 4.8, what is the ratio of X gametes to Y gametes produced by the male?

■ It is 1 : 1.

□ Since fertilisation of eggs by sperm is random, what is the expected proportion of female offspring?

■ It is a half, since half the sperm contain an X chromosome and so does every egg; therefore, 50 per cent of fertilised eggs will be XX.

Thus, for any individual (such as Sam), there is a 50 per cent chance of being a girl, or a boy. The process of meiosis, which governs the separation of X and Y chromosomes during gamete formation, not only accounts for the occurrence of XX (female) and XY (male) individuals, but is also responsible for the production of approximately equal numbers of the two sexes in any population.

Chromosome mixing during meiosis

The behaviour of chromosomes during meiosis is important for understanding how variation arises between gametes and in turn between individuals. Whereas cell division involving *mitosis* results in the production of cells that are genetically *identical* to the original cell and to each other (Chapter 3), *meiosis* results in the production of cells (sperms and eggs) that are genetically *different* from the original cell and from each other.

In fact, the behaviour of the sex chromosomes during meiosis is similar to that of all other pairs of chromosomes and it illustrates the pattern of inheritance of chromosomes from generation to generation. The members of each of the 22 homologous pairs of chromosomes in the gamete-producing cell also separate from each other during meiosis; one member from each chromosome pair enters each gamete. By the time cell division is complete, one chromosome of each pair is present in each of the resulting gametes, as shown in Figure 4.9. Thus each gamete contains:

- half the number of chromosomes, and
- one member of each pair of chromosomes.

Note that in Figure 4.9 the chromosomes we coloured red in the fertilised egg originated from the mother and the black ones came from the father. The fertilised egg contains half maternal chromosomes and half paternal chromosomes.

The fertilised egg in Figure 4.9 will develop into an individual which, in turn, will produce gametes. When this occurs, the members of each chromosome pair in the gamete-producing cells will separate and one of each pair will enter the resulting gametes. However, it is a matter of chance whether the red chromosome from a given pair enters a particular gamete, or whether the black one enters it. (Note: the red chromosomes originated from this individual's mother, and the black ones from the father.) Therefore, each gamete receives a *random assortment* of some red and some black chromosomes, but always one of each chromosome pair.

The more chromosome pairs there are in the gamete-producing cell, the greater the number of different combinations of red and black chromosomes are possible in the resulting gametes. A gamete-producing cell with only two pairs of chromosomes could produce a total of four different possible combinations of red and

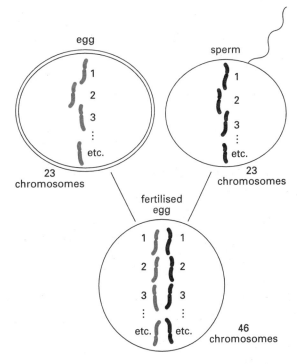

Figure 4.9 *The chromosome content of male and female gametes and the resulting fertilised egg (only four chromosomes are shown in each gamete, and four pairs in the fertilised egg). The fertilised egg contains half maternal (red) and half paternal (black) chromosomes.*

black chromosomes in the gametes; with 10 pairs of chromosomes there are 1 024 possible different combinations, and with 23 pairs of chromosomes (the number in human cells) a staggering total of 8 388 608 different combinations of red and black chromosomes can be produced!

This 'reassortment' of chromosomes during gamete formation produces various combinations of maternal and paternal chromosomes, but it does not break up the normal set of genes on individual chromosomes. However, a process known as *crossing over* does. Crossing over is the physical exchange of genetic material between the two chromosomes in an homologous pair, following breakage and rejoining as shown in Figure 4.10 (*overleaf*). This process, which occurs during meiosis, brings about a considerable rearrangement of genetic material in the original parental chromosomes.

Thus far, we have shown how and why the process of sexual reproduction is an important source of *variation* between individuals. During gamete production, genes *within* a chromosome are rearranged by crossing over, and red and black chromosomes are assorted into different combinations by meiosis. Further mixing of chromosomes occurs when gametes from two different individuals combine at fertilisation.

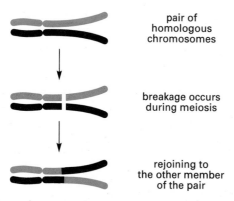

pair of homologous chromosomes

breakage occurs during meiosis

rejoining to the other member of the pair

Figure 4.10 *The process of crossing over between the two chromosomes in an homologous pair, which breaks up and rearranges the combination of genes on individual chromosomes.* (Remember to turn back to finish reading page 73.)

Environment

We turn now to the influence of the environment on the development of the phenotype from the time of fertilisation to adult maturity and into old age. Environmental factors are another very important source of variation between individuals.

You are already familiar with the general meaning of 'environment', but what do we mean by it in the context of the development of the phenotype? In fact, when considering the development of the phenotype, **environment** has the very broadest meaning, ranging from the cytoplasm surrounding the nucleus within a cell, to a specific biological environment such as the uterus, to the Earth's climate and contact with pathogens, and the whole of human culture. It includes any factor, *other than the genes,* that influences the development of the phenotype. The phenotype, which changes during the lifetime of an individual, is continuously affected by many aspects of that individual's changing environment.

□ Given this very broad definition, can you give some examples of environmental factors that affect physical or mental growth and development?

■ You may have thought of some of the following (there are many others): diet, education, lifestyle, number of children in the family, level of income, amount of pollution.

Some of these factors may influence the phenotype only at one particular stage of development; for example biological environments are particularly important during fetal development (as discussed briefly below). On the other hand, diet affects the phenotype throughout an individual's lifetime.[4]

Intra-uterine environment

As discussed elsewhere in this series, the *nutritional* environment inside the uterus has been implicated in possible long-term effects on the susceptibility of adults to a range of diseases in later life, including heart disease and diabetes.[5] Such dietary effects are controversial and difficult to prove because of the long time-scale involved, but there is no doubt that certain chemical or infectious agents entering the intra-uterine environment can have serious adverse effects on the developing fetus in a matter of weeks or months.

Some agents are not harmful to the mother yet can damage the developing fetus. The majority of malformation-producing agents (such as the drug thalidomide, prescribed in the 1960s to combat morning sickness) are especially damaging in the early stages of pregnancy, when the embryonic limbs and major organs are taking shape. Another example is the rubella virus: if contracted in the first three months of pregnancy this may result in serious eye, ear and cardiovascular (heart and blood vessel) malformations in the fetus, while the mother experiences only mild symptoms of German measles. In contrast, the harmful effects of excessive alcohol consumption by the mother are not restricted to a sensitive period in early pregnancy, but extend through the entire nine months. Excessive alcohol consumption (greater than 80 grams *per day,* i.e. a full bottle of wine or about 5 pints of beer) during pregnancy is the current major cause of mental retardation in newborn babies.

[4]See *World Health and Disease,* Chapter 11, for a discussion of nutrition and health; later in the present book (Chapter 7) we return to the subject of human digestion and dietary change.

[5]The 'programming' hypothesis is discussed in *Studying Health and Disease,* Chapter 10, which includes an audiotape on this subject for Open University students; it is mentioned again in *World Health and Disease,* Chapter 11.

Distinguishing between genotype and phenotype

The development of the phenotype of an individual is not a simple straightforward process, but rather is the result of the *dynamic interaction* of the genes with the environment. How much are characteristics determined by the genes and how much are they influenced by the environment? This question is difficult (if not impossible) to answer, because a person's phenotype is a product of growth and development brought about by a certain genotype in a *succession* of environments. The phenotype at a given moment is determined not only by the environment that prevails at that moment, but also by the succession of environments experienced during its lifetime. Every person is the product of their genotype *and* their life experiences.

Over the last forty years or so, there has been heated debate among biologists as to the relative contribution of the genotype (sometimes referred to as *nature*) and the environment (*nurture*) to the development of characteristics. From this so-called **nature–nurture debate** there has emerged a reasonable consensus for the view that the two are generally inseparable. This *interactionist* view is epitomised by the words of the eminent biologist and expert in animal behaviour, D. O. Hebb who, writing in 1953 about attempts to differentiate between instinct (nature) and learning (nurture) in the development of behaviour, suggested that such attempts are

> ...exactly like asking how much of the area of a field is due to its length, and how much to its width. (Hebb, 1953, p. 44)

Nevertheless, some attempts have been made to partition the causes of variation for some characteristics. The difficulty of this task is illustrated by the example of human birth weight which, although it might be considered a characteristic of the *baby*, is also affected by a number of genetic and environmental factors *outside* the baby.

> □ Can you suggest some genetic and environmental factors that might affect human birth weight?

> ■ You might have thought of some of the following: fetal genotype, maternal genotype, maternal environment including socio–economic factors, and the environment inside the uterus when the fetus was developing there (the intra-uterine environment).

This example illustrates the complexity of the interactions between the genotype and environment. Studies on identical twins can shed some light on this interaction. Identical twins are *genetically* identical and can represent a sort of 'natural' experiment to test whether two individuals who are genetically identical may develop differently. Clearly, if genes are paramount in determining a characteristic, then that characteristic will be similar in identical twins who are reared *apart* (i.e. in different environments). But suppose, for example, that one identical twin contracts a serious infection such as polio and the other does not; the former may become physically disabled and the latter may not. Clearly, their difference in physical form is then due to environmental factors.

However, it is very rare to find identical twins who were separated early in life, so the information on humans is limited; we will consider some examples later in this chapter. It is much easier to carry out studies of how the same genotype may react to different environments in plants. In the case of grasses, for example, it is possible to split one individual into a number of genetically identical pieces, grow them in different environments and observe the phenotypic differences between them. The results of one such experiment are shown in Figure 4.11 (*overleaf*). You can see from this drawing how wide the range of phenotypes, all with the same genotype, can be. Experiments such as this show that the phenotype is the result of the *interaction* between gene action and the particular environment.

This interaction is as important in humans as it is in other organisms. *The genotype sets the boundaries within which the phenotype develops in different environments.* For example, however perfect the diet that promotes the growth of a particular individual, there is a maximum height above which he or she cannot grow that is determined by their genotype. On the other hand, the potential height may never be reached because of an inadequate diet and/or the extent of childhood diseases the individual has suffered.[6]

We can put these ideas into a broader context by considering a different example, tuberculosis.

> □ If every individual in a family of two parents and four children has a similar characteristic, such as tuberculosis, would you conclude that the condition was bound to be genetic in origin (that is, a result of family members sharing similar genes)?

> ■ No. If a condition is *familial*, which means that it runs in families, one may *suspect* a genetic origin, but there could be something about the environment that they all share which leads them all to succumb to the same disease.

---

[6]The relationship between nutrition, infection and growth in height among children is discussed in *World Health and Disease*, Chapter 11.

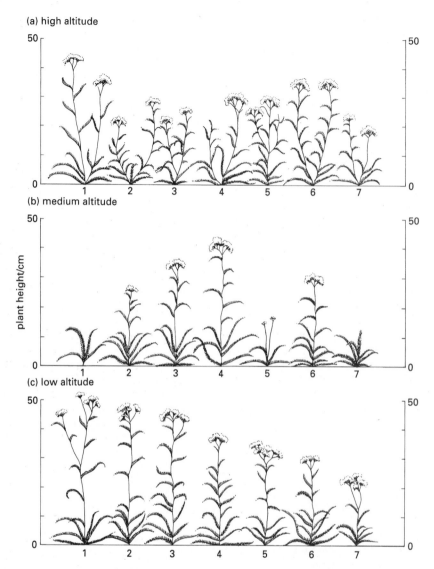

Figure 4.11 *Responses of seven different* Achillea *(yarrow) plants to environments of different altitude. Cuttings from each of the seven plants were grown at (a) high altitude, 3 040 metres above sea-level, (b) medium altitude, 1 400 metres, and (c) low altitude, 30 metres. Numbers identify plants from the same parent. (Source: S298 Course Team, 1987,* The Process of Heredity, *Unit 1, Figure 1, p. 4, redrawn from Suzuki, Griffiths and Lewontin, 1981, p. 18)* (Remember to turn back to finish reading page 75.)

To be sure that a characteristic is inherited, it is necessary to look at the occurrence of the characteristic in more distant relatives, including grandparents. This is our next task: to explore the patterns of inheritance and the extent to which different characteristics recur in different members of the same family.

The family

We now turn to an examination of *specific* characteristics, such as hair texture, size of ear lobes, blood group and adult height, in order to explore patterns of inheritance in family members and how these patterns contribute to the production of variation between individuals.

Phenotype, as well as meaning the sum total of *all* characteristics, has another more-restricted shade of meaning; it is also used by geneticists as a 'shorthand' way of referring to the expression of a *particular* characteristic. So instead of talking of the 'characteristic of brown hair', geneticists frequently talk of the 'brown hair phenotype', as in 'all the members of a brown-haired family share the brown hair phenotype'.

Why has Sam or any individual a particular characteristic? To understand the reasons we need to broaden our interest to look at other members of Sam's family. A family history can show that a particular phenotype is genetically influenced and can clarify the pattern of inheritance from generation to generation. It can also show why children in a family share some characteristics, but differ from each other in other ways.

Another word of warning about the terminology sometimes used to describe the *relationship* between genes and the phenotype is appropriate here. Biologists often use a shorthand such as 'the gene for brown hair' or 'the brown hair gene' (and we shall do this in this book). This expression suggests a direct causal relationship between a particular gene and the production of brown hair. But this may be an over-simplification because the gene involved in making hair brown may *primarily* be involved in pigment formation throughout the body, not just hair colour.

Patterns of single-gene inheritance: dominant and recessive characteristics

A single human chromosome carries many genes, each with its own function and each with its own specific location on a particular chromosome. Here we focus on the behaviour of *single* genes during gamete production and fertilisation, by tracing the patterns of **single-gene inheritance**.

Each gene in the genotype can exist in one or more *alternative* forms called **alleles**. Each allele is associated with an alternative phenotype. We will illustrate the vital importance of alternative alleles for the pattern of single-gene inheritance by considering a specific example, which gives rise to a disease called *multiple lipoma*. Individuals with this disease have non-malignant (non-cancerous) fatty tumours, usually occurring beneath the skin. Multiple lipoma is probably the most common form of tumour in adults and is not normally harmful to health. Each person has one of two alternative phenotypes: each of us is either affected, with tumours, or unaffected, free of tumours, as a consequence of inheriting a particular allele (form) of a single gene, the multiple-lipoma gene. These alternative phenotypes are part of *normal variation*, just as some individuals have blue eyes and others have brown, or some have attached ear lobes and others unattached or free lobes. The existence of alternative alleles of the same gene is a powerful source of variation.

The example of multiple lipoma is helpful in explaining the relationship between the alternative alleles of a single gene and the phenotypes associated with each allele. It is conventional in genetics to represent each allele by a letter (either capital or lower case), printed in *italics.* In this example, we will use the letter *L* for the allele associated with the presence of lipomas, and *l* for the allele associated with the absence of lipomas. You already know that in any individual, there are *two* copies of each gene present in every somatic cell (we will look at the gametes shortly), one inherited from the mother and one from the father, each on one chromosome of a homologous pair (if you are unsure, look back at Figure 4.6). Now that we have introduced the term 'allele' to mean 'alternative forms of a gene', we can re-state the previous sentence in more precise genetic language: in any individual, there are two *alleles* of each gene present. In the case of multiple lipoma, individuals could be *LL, ll* or *Ll*.

An individual with two copies of the *L* allele (one copy on each chromosome of a homologous pair) is said to have the *LL* genotype; such individuals will develop multiple lipomas. A person with two copies of the *l* allele has the *ll* genotype and will be free of tumours. (Note that here we are using 'genotype' in its restricted sense to mean the inherited alleles of a *particular* gene, rather than in the comprehensive sense used up to now to refer to the sum total of all the genes of an individual.) We can follow what happens to the *LL* and *ll* alleles, first during meiosis when gametes are produced, and second at fertilisation when gametes combine (Figure 4.12).

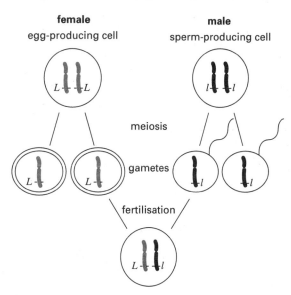

Figure 4.12 *Mating diagram between a female with the genotype LL and a male with the genotype ll, illustrating the behaviour of these alleles during gamete formation and fertilisation. (Only the chromosomes containing the multiple-lipoma gene are shown here.)*

The two alleles of the multiple-lipoma gene are located on a pair of homologous chromosomes, one allele on each member of the pair, as shown in the egg-producing and sperm-producing cells at the top of Figure 4.12. It is important to note that because members of a homologous pair of chromosomes separate during gamete formation (as shown earlier in Figure 4.9), the alleles they contain *also* separate.

☐ How many alleles of the multiple-lipoma gene are present in each gamete?

■ Only one allele in each gamete.

☐ What alleles do the gametes contain?

■ In this example, the female's gametes all contain *L*, whereas the male's gametes all contain *l*.

☐ What are the possible genotypes of the children of this couple with respect to the multiple-lipoma gene?

■ They would all be *Ll*.

Notice that not only do *all* the progeny have the *same* genotype, *Ll*, but that it is different from either parent. We need some way to distinguish between situations in which the two alleles of a particular gene are the *same* (as they are in each of the parents in this example, *LL* or *ll*), and where the two alleles are *different* (for example, *Ll*, as in the children in this example). Geneticists use the following terms, which will recur many times in this chapter and elsewhere in this book, so it is well worth learning them now: where the two alleles are the *same*, the alleles are said to be **homozygous** (pronounced 'hom-oh-zy-gus') and the individuals are referred to as **homozygotes** ('hom-oh-zy-goats') for that particular gene; where the two alleles are *different* they are said to be **heterozygous** ('het-er-oh-zy-gus') and the individuals are referred to as **heterozygotes** for that particular gene. In our example, the offspring shown in Figure 4.12 are heterozygotes with respect to the multiple-lipoma gene; their parents are both homozygotes, the mother is *LL* and the father is *ll*.

But what is the *phenotype* of offspring with the heterozygous genotype *Ll*? One of their alleles (*L*) is associated with the presence of tumours, but the other (*l*) is not. In fact, they have multiple lipoma like their mother. The characteristic which is *expressed* in the heterozygote individual is said to be the **dominant characteristic** because it masks the effect of the *l* allele. The characteristic which is *not* expressed in the heterozygote is said to be the **recessive characteristic**. In this case, absence of lipomas is *recessive to* (or masked by) the dominant characteristic, which is presence of lipomas. It is noteworthy that there is no 'blending' of the two different alleles in the heterozygote to produce an intermediate condition, and the children (*Ll*) have the same phenotype (presence of tumours) as one of the homozygous parents (*LL*).[7]

Strictly speaking, it is the phenotype (such as presence or absence of lipomas) rather than the allele that is dominant or recessive; however, alleles are classified as dominant or recessive on the basis of their associated phenotype and the terms 'dominant allele' and 'recessive allele' are widely, if loosely, used by geneticists. By the same convention, phenotypes such as multiple lipoma which require the inheritance of only *one* defective allele, are often referred to as **dominant disorders**.

Characteristics due to dominant alleles, such as multiple lipoma, show a particular pattern of transmission from generation to generation. The important point to note is that by knowing the pattern of inheritance of alleles, predictions about future generations can be made. If the genotypes of the parents are known (for example, *LL* and *ll*), the possible genotypes of the children can be predicted, and so can the chance or probability of each child inheriting a particular genotype. Alternatively, it is possible to work out the genotype of some members of the family solely from observation of their phenotypes with respect to certain characteristics. Thus, since the male's phenotype in our example is *absence* of multiple lipoma, we can conclude that he must have the genotype *ll*, because if he had even one *L* allele he would have developed tumours. Such information is less important for characteristics such as non-malignant tumours, but it is crucially important for parents, paediatricians and genetic counsellors when potentially-fatal disease genes are under consideration, a point which is elaborated in Chapter 9 of this book.

[7]Note the convention that the allele for the *dominant* characteristic is represented by a capital letter (*L* in this example), and the *recessive* characteristic by a lower-case letter (*l*).

Sex-linked characteristics: colour-blindness

Genes on the X chromosome have to be considered as a special case under the general heading of single-gene inheritance. This is because females have two X chromosomes and males only one X and one Y chromosome. Although the Y chromosome carries very few genes, the X chromosome carries many genes which have a pattern of inheritance described as **sex-linked** (or *X-linked*) inheritance. The genes associated with colour vision are carried on the X chromosome and demonstrate this pattern of inheritance.

Consider red colour-blindness which is a *recessive* characteristic, that is, it is masked by a single allele for normal colour vision. In this example, we will represent the normal colour-vision allele by *C*, and the recessive colour-blindness allele by *c*. A mating diagram between a *heterozygous* female (*Cc*) who has normal colour vision, and a male with normal colour vision is given in Figure 4.13. She will produce two types of gametes, half with the normal allele, *C*, and half with the colour-blindness allele, *c*.

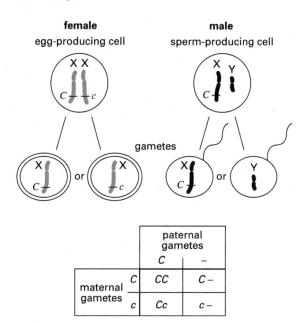

<table>
<tr><td></td><td></td><td colspan="2">paternal gametes</td></tr>
<tr><td></td><td></td><td>C</td><td>–</td></tr>
<tr><td rowspan="2">maternal gametes</td><td>C</td><td>CC</td><td>C–</td></tr>
<tr><td>c</td><td>Cc</td><td>c–</td></tr>
</table>

Figure 4.13 *Mating diagram illustrating the behaviour of alleles on the X chromosome associated with normal colour vision (C) and with red colour-blindness (c) during gamete formation and fertilisation. These alleles are missing from the Y chromosome.*

☐ What are the possible phenotypes of the children of the couple in Figure 4.13, for both sex and red colour-blindness?

■ Half the children would be female and half would be male. All the daughters would have normal colour-vision and so would *half* the sons, but the other half would be red colour-blind.

☐ Why would these males be red colour-blind even though this phenotype is recessive?

■ They would be red colour-blind because their genotype is *c*–; there is no dominant (normal colour vision) *C* allele present to mask the single recessive *c* allele. Males only have one allele of this gene.

Consequently the incidence of sex-linked characteristics is much higher in males than in females, because daughters would have to inherit *two* copies of the red colour-blindness *c* allele (one from each parent) before they expressed the abnormal phenotype. The pattern of inheritance of sex-linked characteristics is never from father to sons.

Multiple alleles: blood groups

So far, characteristics with just two alternative phenotypes have been described. However, some genes have more than two alternative alleles. One well-known example is that of the so-called **ABO blood groups**, where at least three alternative alleles (*A*, *B*, and *O*) of the *ABO* gene exist. A person's blood group partly depends on which of these alleles they inherit. This information is vital for blood transfusion. Blood cannot be transfused between one person and another without first checking the blood groups of both the recipient and the donor. It is safe to transfuse blood from an individual of one group into another individual of the *same* group; but when blood is transfused between individuals with *different* blood groups, strict rules of compatibility must be followed. Breaking these rules may result in serious harm or even the death of the person receiving the transfusion.

☐ Three alternative alleles of the *ABO* gene exist, but how many of them are present in any one individual?

■ Only two, one on each member of a pair of homologous chromosomes.

An individual may be *homozygous* for any one of the three possible alleles (that is, *A A* or *B B* or *O O*) or *heterozygous* for any possible combination (*A B* or *A O* or *B O*). To determine the phenotype (that is, the blood group) arising from these genotypes, you need to know that both the alleles *A* and *B* are dominant to *O* (or put another way, *O* is recessive to both *A* and *B*).

☐ What is the blood group of individuals with the following genotypes: *A O*, *B O*, and *O O*?

■ Blood group A, B and O, respectively.

The relationship between *A* and *B* when present together in an individual is such that one allele is *not* dominant to the other; in such a case the alleles are said to be **codominant.** The consequence is that the individual has the blood group AB.

The existence of many alternative alleles, or **multiple alleles**, of the same gene is quite common; a great variety of characteristics are known to be associated with multiple alleles and others are sure to be found in the future. Although the pattern of inheritance seems more complicated for multiple alleles than for those with just two alternatives, the same rules are obeyed: only *two* of the many possible alleles of a gene are present in each individual, these are separated and reduced to one during gamete production, and two are restored at fertilisation.

Multiple alleles are an important source of variation. To emphasise the amount of variation that exists within the human species we will consider one protein in detail, **haemoglobin**, the most widely studied of all our body constituents. Haemoglobin, which is present in red blood cells, transfers oxygen from the lungs to all the cells in the body. This complex protein is made up of a sequence of amino acids which is the same in most people. However, nearly 500 variant forms of hameoglobin have been found, each coded for by a different allele, which have arisen due to *mutation*, the change of one DNA message into another (as described in Chapter 3).[8] When you consider that there are about 100 000 genes coding for proteins in humans and that many of these exist as multiple alleles, you can begin to get a measure of the variation that exists within our species.

The patterns of inheritance of alternative phenotypes (such as presence or absence of lipomas) associated with single-gene inheritance, are found not only in humans but in all organisms with sexual reproduction. Understanding the patterns of inheritance for recessive, dominant, sex-linked and codominant alleles helps us to learn more about *normal variation* between individuals and why particular characteristics tend to run in families. These patterns are even more important when the inheritance of genetic diseases is considered, a subject we turn to later in this chapter.

Multifactorial inheritance: adult height

Patterns of single-gene inheritance associated with the *presence* or *absence* of a characteristic, such as the presence or absence of multiple lipoma or A, B or O blood group, were considered above. But the inheritance of many characteristics does not follow this pattern: characteristics such as height, blood pressure, susceptibility to infectious diseases, rate of growth, or skin pigmentation, do not fall into two or three clearly-defined alternative phenotypes (for example, height does not occur as either 'tall' or 'short'), but instead show *continuous variation*, each category of which differs from the next in the range by only a small measurable amount.

Such phenotypic characteristics are therefore *quantitative* rather than *qualitative* in nature and are usually distributed continuously in the population, in the manner shown in Figure 4.14. This pattern is called a **normal distribution** curve: the majority of individuals fall within the middle of the range, with few people at the two extremes. If this represented (for example) the range and distribution of the height of adult Englishmen, then the majority of individuals fall around the national average height, with few very tall or very short men.

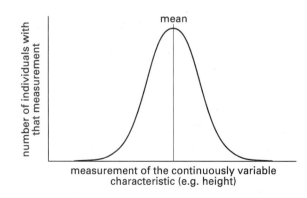

Figure 4.14 *A normal distribution curve.*

---

[8]A television programme 'Blood lines', for Open University students, focuses on mutations in the haemoglobin gene.

Table 4.1 Average intra-pair difference for four multifactorial characteristics between the two individuals in pairs of identical and non-identical twins, reared in similar and in different environments

Multifactorial characteristics	Average intra-pair difference		
	Identical twins reared together	Identical twins reared apart	Non-identical twins reared together
height/cm	1.7	1.8	4.4
weight/kg	1.9	4.5	4.5
head length/mm	2.9	2.2	6.2
head width/mm	2.8	2.9	4.2

Source: Stern, C. (1973) *Principles of Human Genetics*, 3rd edn, W. H. Freeman, San Francisco, Table 78, p. 661 (after Newman, H. H., Freeman, F. N. and Holzinger, K. J., 1937, *Twins: a Study of Heredity and Environment*, University of Chicago Press, Chicago, p. 369)

Quantitative phenotypic characteristics such as height are thought to reflect the *cumulative* effect of *several different* genes, each of which has a small individual impact on the phenotype. The *multiple genes* associated with a quantitative characteristic (such as height) are scattered throughout the chromosomes; this is in contrast to the *single-gene* effects we discussed earlier, which are due to alternative forms (alleles) of the *same* gene. In addition, environmental factors play a particularly large part in the development of the phenotype of quantitative characteristics, such as height, which is why they are often referred to as **multifactorial characteristics**, since many genetic and environmental factors are involved.

As we pointed out earlier in this chapter, studying identical twins is one way of estimating the *relative influence* of environmental and genetic factors on variations between individuals for multifactorial characteristics such as height. Identical twins reared together are compared with those in which members of each twin pair are separated at birth and raised in different households. Each twin-pair is genetically identical since both individuals are formed from a single fertilised egg, which splits early in development to form two distinct embryos with identical genes.[9] Thus, identical twins separated at birth permit studies of the effect of different environments on the same genes. Non-identical twins, on the other hand, are genetically different, since they develop from two different eggs, each fertilised by different sperm. Studies on non-identical twins reared *together* permit studies of the effect of different genotypes in a similar environment.

Table 4.1 compares the phenotypes of four multifactorial characteristics in identical twins when raised in the same household and when reared apart, and in non-identical twins when reared in the same household.

Identical twins reared together (first column of figures) show differences in all four characteristics between the two individuals in each pair of twins (intra-pair differences); for example, on average there is a difference of 1.7 cm between the heights of the two individuals in each pair of twins. This is an effect of the environment during pregnancy and after birth, which gives rise to small phenotypic differences in spite of the twins having identical genotypes and being reared together. By themselves, the results from identical twins reared together are not very informative; they become significant, however, when comparisons are made between them and the corresponding findings for the other two groups of twins. Comparing the first and the last columns of figures shows that the average differences between the individuals in each pair are larger for all four characteristics in *non-identical* twins reared together than in *identical* twins reared together. The middle column in the table contains the important average intra-pair differences for identical twins reared apart. It is important to note that in this study the home environments were not strikingly different.

□ What do the results in Table 4.1 suggest about the genetic influence on weight compared with that on height, head width and head length?

■ The results indicate that a greater genetic influence exists for height and head dimensions than for weight; the latter is more subject to environmental influences. (If you are unsure about this, notice that height and head dimensions are similar for identical twins, regardless of whether they were reared together or apart, but their weights are strongly affected by their environment.)

[9] The development of the human embryo from a single fertilised egg cell is described in *Birth to Old Age: Health in Transition* (Open University Press, revised edition 1995).

So even within the group of multifactorial characteristics, the amount of influence exerted by the environment or by the genes varies according to the particular characteristic.

More can be learnt about genetic and environmental influences on multifactorial characteristics by broadening the view to compare populations who live in different parts of the world. There are enormous differences in both the rate of growth and the ultimate height of children belonging to different countries of the world. Are these differences related (at least partly) to differences in their genes? To answer this question we can, for example, estimate the growth rate between the age of onset of puberty and achievement of ultimate adult height, and compare people in the Far East with those in Western Europe. Studies reported by J. M. Tanner (1992), have shown that people with good nourishment in the Far East, such as the Japanese, have puberty about a year earlier than Western Europeans and end up about six centimetres shorter.

□ Assuming that environmental conditions were ideal in both populations, what do these data suggest about genetic influences on growth rate and ultimate height?

■ They suggest that there are genetic differences between different populations for these characteristics.

So even among children who are well nourished there are clear indications that genes influence growth and height differently in different countries. But there are a number of environmental factors that lead to enormous differences in the size of children within and between populations.

□ What environmental factors might contribute to these differences?

■ Many are due to differences between rich and poor, urban and rural dwellers, children subject to periodic or chronic undernutrition, and children subject to periodic bouts of disease.

As living conditions improve, the growth of children speeds up and adult height increases. In the industrialised nations, these trends towards taller individuals reaching their adult height at earlier ages are now slowing down and in some cases height and growth rate have almost stabilised, at least in the children of the well-off. Differences in growth between rich and poor are still present in practically all countries; only in Norway and Sweden have they been eliminated (these trends are reviewed in

Brundtland *et al.*, 1980, and Lindgren, 1976). Because similar environmental factors affect growth and health, one of the best monitors of the health of a nation is the growth of its children. Continuous surveillance of childhood growth is carried out in a number of countries, including the United Kingdom; this has practical value in monitoring the health of individuals and *indirectly* surveying the living conditions of populations.

You saw above that in the case of characteristics caused by an allele of a *single* gene (such as the allele that causes multiple lipoma), inheritance of the characteristic follows a distinctive pattern from generation to generation. But for multifactorial characteristics, such as height, there is no distinctive pattern of inheritance. Since many disorders are multifactorial, this information is crucially significant when trying to make predictions about the likelihood of genetic relatives inheriting or manifesting such disorders, as discussed later in this chapter.

Other families in the same town

Life for a minority of families in the same town as Sam's is not so straightforward as it is in her case, because one member of the family was born with a serious genetic disorder. So far this chapter has been primarily concerned with the inheritance of *normal variation* and how this follows particular patterns according to whether the phenotype is dominant, recessive, sex-linked, codominant or multifactorial. Here we move on to look at *disease phenotypes* which are considered to be outside the usual range. However, the alleles and genes involved follow identical patterns of inheritance as non-disease alleles, so the rules or laws already described also apply to their inheritance.

Human diseases can be classified in a number of ways. Here we consider disease on a spectrum, from the *environmentally* determined conditions such as those due to nutritional factors (for example, rickets), and those caused by *infectious agents* (for example, polio and tuberculosis), to the *genetically* determined diseases or abnormalities (for example, sickle-cell disease and Tay–Sachs disease).[10] In both these last two examples the individuals are ill because they were born with a defective gene. About 5 000 **genetic diseases** have been identified as being due to defective genes. One in 30 children in the United Kingdom has a genetic disorder, and these account for about one-third of all hospital admissions of young children.

[10]Sickle-cell disease and Tay–Sachs disease are introduced in *World Health and Disease*, Chapters 3 and 9.

Some genetic diseases occur when the individual inherits only one copy (allele) of a single defective gene ('dominant disorders'); others require *both* alleles of the gene to be defective ('recessive disorders'); and some genetic diseases are sex-linked. There are many common disorders in which *both* environmental and genetic factors play a part; these include developmental disorders (such as spina bifida), and diseases of later adult life (such as coronary heart disease).

Here we consider three examples of the inheritance of diseases. The first is the biggest killer of adults in Western societies, coronary heart disease which, in a minority of cases, is related to a genetic disorder called familial hypercholesterolaemia (pronounced 'high-purr-kol-esterol-eemiyah'). Then we turn to cystic fibrosis and phenylketonuria ('fee-nile-kee-toe-new-rea'), two genetic disorders that are manifested in childhood.

Familial hypercholesterolaemia: a dominant disorder

Although some human diseases are inherited as the result of a single defective gene, by far the most common *non-infectious* diseases of adult life, for example diabetes, schizophrenia, cancers and coronary heart disease, are not caused by a single defective gene. In addition, many *congenital malformations* (malformations that are present at birth but do not necessarily have a genetic basis), such as cleft lip and palate and congenital heart defects, are not inherited as single-gene characteristics. All these conditions are multifactorial in origin, the role of the environment is relatively large and the underlying causes may be heterogeneous and complex.[11]

As we said earlier, multifactorial disorders do not follow distinctive patterns of inheritance from generation to generation, so it is difficult to make predictions about the frequency with which individuals are likely to be affected within a family. However, these disorders do recur within a family more frequently than expected from their incidence in the population as a whole, and the risk of a child being affected is higher when more than one family member is affected.

A number of adverse *risk factors* that play a part in the development of the disease phenotype, some genetic and some environmental, have been associated with *coronary heart disease* (CHD).

☐ Which environmental factors do you think may play a causative role in CHD?

■ You may have thought of (among others) lack of exercise, a high fat diet, smoking, stress or poverty.

A full discussion of the risk factors involved in CHD occurs in another book in this series, which emphasises the complex interaction between environmental factors and a person's genes.[12] Here we focus on the genetic aspects. Although the cause of CHD is multifactorial, one specific single-gene defect, called *familial hypercholesterolaemia,* has been identified in a minority of cases of the disease. It is a *dominant* disorder (that is, inheritance of only one defective allele of the relevant gene is necessary to produce the disorder), which has a relatively high incidence in certain geographic areas; for example, 1 in 500 people in populations of European or Japanese descent have a defective allele of this gene.

Familial hypercholesterolaemia is important not only because it is common, but because the elegant investigation by Michael Brown and Joseph Goldstein (awarded the Nobel prize for medicine in 1985; for a review, see Goldstein and Brown, 1989), clearly illustrates the dynamic interface between medicine and genetics. Their investigations clarified how the cells in the body take in fat and, in the process, they identified a major cause of CHD.

Consider the imaginary case of Chris. He is 33 years old and has familial hypercholesterolaemia, which is characterised by elevated blood cholesterol (a type of fat, which is mainly produced by the liver, but a small percentage comes from the diet). This means that Chris has a genetic predisposition to developing premature CHD. Since the characteristic phenotype of familial hypercholesterolaemia cannot readily be seen, how does Chris know he has it? There is a family history of heart disease that is known to extend back over a number of previous generations and, of utmost significance, an older brother died from CHD at the age of 40. Consequently, all surviving first-degree relatives (parents, siblings and offspring) were given a blood cholesterol test, which detected Chris's abnormally high cholesterol.

Fortunately for Chris, the disease can be treated because the underlying abnormality in the function of his cells is understood. Normal cells obtain the cholesterol they need to manufacture membranes and other cellular components (see Figure 3.7 in Chapter 3) by uptake from

[11]Neural-tube defects (NTDs) are discussed in *Studying Health and Disease,* Chapter 8; the debate about the possible role of dietary factors in the causation of NTDs is summarised in a collection of articles and correspondence taken from medical journals, which appears in *Health and Disease: A Reader* (the 1994 edition has a larger collection than the 1984 edition).

[12]*Dilemmas in Health Care,* Chapter 10.

the blood, a process which relies on receptors for cholesterol in the surface membrane of the cell. Brown and Goldstein showed that individuals with familial hypercholesterolaemia have defective cholesterol receptors, with the result that their cells take up reduced quantities of cholesterol from the blood.

With any single-gene disorder it is useful to know whether it is dominantly or recessively inherited since the number of children likely to be affected is different in these two situations. To learn about the genetics of a single-gene disorder, **pedigree charts** can be constructed, describing the incidence of the characteristic within a family over a number of generations. The extent to which the characteristic recurs in different members of the same family may provide clues about its possible mode of genetic transmission. Figure 4.15 gives the pedigree chart for four generations: I, II, III and IV of Chris's family. Individuals who manifest the characteristic, in this case familial hypercholesterolaemia, are shaded. By studying Figure 4.15 you can see that male and female 1 and 2 respectively had three children: 3, 5, and 6, the first of whom was affected.

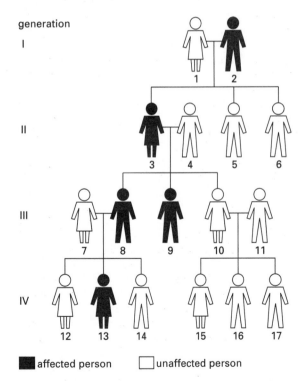

generation

□ Chris's mother is number 3 in the pedigree; she married number 4. How many children and of what sex did they have?

■ Two male children (numbers 8 and 9) and one female (number 10).

□ How many of these children were affected?

■ Two (numbers 8 and 9), Chris and his older brother.

Often, it is possible to deduce from such family trees whether a disorder is the result of the presence of recessive or dominant alleles. Notice in this pedigree that every affected person has an affected parent, who also had an affected parent, and so on. This feature is characteristic of *dominant* inheritance. The reason for this is that each child has a 50 per cent (or a half) chance of inheriting the affected parent's abnormal allele. Chris, for example, must have inherited one copy of the disease allele (which we will call *FH*) from his mother; his father must be *homo*zygous for the normal or non-disease allele (i.e. he has two normal alleles of the gene, *fh fh*).

□ In the pedigree shown in Figure 4.15, would phenotypically normal family members transmit the disease allele to their children?

■ No; *both* their alleles for the gene would have to be normal because the disease allele is dominant.

Some other disorders that have the same pattern of inheritance as familial hypercholesterolaemia because they are due to dominant single-gene effects are Huntington's disease (a degenerative disease of the nervous system) and achondroplasia ('ay-kondroh-play-zeeah', short-limbed dwarfism).

Cystic fibrosis and phenylketonuria: recessive disorders

Recessive disorders are those in which *two* defective alleles of a certain gene must be inherited before the disease phenotype is expressed. Put another way, in a recessive disorder, the presence of *one* normal allele masks the effect of one abnormal allele and the person is unaffected. The most common single-gene recessive disorder in populations of European descent is *cystic fibrosis*, with as many as 1 child in 2 000 affected. Affected children have chronic lung disease and problems with their digestive system. A less common recessive

■ affected person   □ unaffected person

Figure 4.15 *Chris's family pedigree of familial hypercholesterolaemia, tracked across four generations. Chris is number 9.*

genetic disorder is *phenylketonuria* or PKU, which occurs with a frequency of 1 in 15 000 people in populations of European descent. Development is delayed in PKU-affected children, who may also show behavioural disturbances. Significantly, both cystic fibrosis and PKU have a lower frequency in non-European populations, a point to which we return later in this chapter.

In contrast to dominant genetic disorders (like familial hypercholesterolaemia), in which affected persons are usually *heterozygotes*, recessive disorders are expressed only in *homozygotes*, who must have inherited *two* defective alleles, one from *each* parent. A pedigree illustrating the inheritance of PKU is shown in Figure 4.16. Both parents of the affected children are heterozygotes and are said to be **carriers** because they each have one disease allele; the parent does not express the disease phenotype because the defect is recessive and so is masked by the presence of the normal allele. When two carriers become sexual partners, the chance of having an affected (homozygous) child is a quarter, that is, one in four of their children will (on average) be affected.

□ What is the most striking difference between the pedigree chart in Figure 4.16 and the one shown earlier in Figure 4.15 for a dominant genetic disorder?

■ Far fewer individuals are affected by the recessive disorder than by the dominant disorder.

Notice in the pedigree chart in Figure 4.16, that it is possible for the recessive disease allele to be handed down for generations without ever combining with another PKU allele at fertilisation to produce a homozygous person who is affected by the disorder. In fact we all carry disease alleles for a number of recessive disorders that would be severely damaging, if not lethal, if we had two such alleles (that is, if we were homozygotes with respect to any of those genes).

The chance of two carriers mating is increased if their parents are genetic relatives, since the probability of

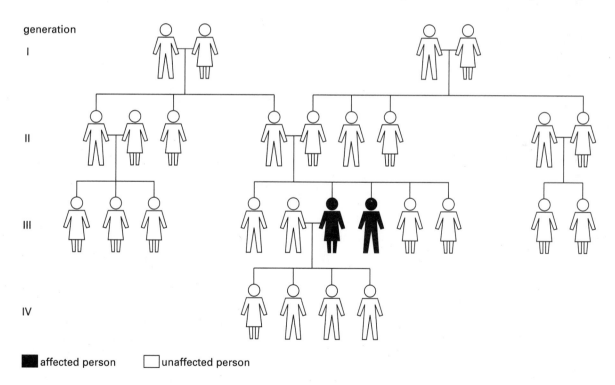

■ affected person   □ unaffected person

Figure 4.16 *Typical pedigree of a recessive genetic disorder, in this case phenylketonuria.*

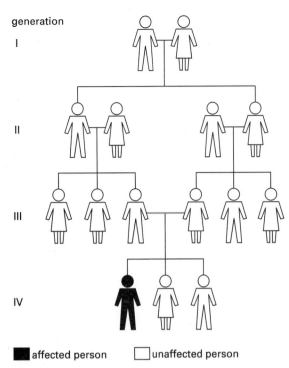

generation

I

II

III

IV

■ affected person   □ unaffected person

Figure 4.17 *Pedigree for a recessive genetic disorder which, in this case, involves genetically-related partners (linked by a red bar).*

them carrying the same recessive allele is higher than for the population as a whole (Figure 4.17).

□ How are the parents of the affected child in Figure 4.17 genetically related to each other?

■ One of each of their parents are brother and sister, which means they are first cousins.

The tendency for rare disorders to appear with unusual frequency in the offspring of cousins was recognised long before the underlying genetic principle was understood, and it led to the prohibition of cousin marriages in many societies. Recessive disorders have a higher incidence today in societies where cousin marriages remain common.

This discussion of genetic diseases has shown the importance of focusing attention at the level of the family and the use of pedigree charts to illustrate the patterns of inheritance of disease alleles. We turn next to focus on the *biochemical* level of a genetic disease. In Chapter 3 you learned that the *products* of genes are *proteins* whose structure is specified by the DNA code contained in the gene. Here we compare the normal functioning protein with the product of a disease allele.

The biochemical basis of disease: phenylketonuria

The primary aim for medical science in trying to understand any disease is to determine the link between the cause of the disease and its symptoms. Here we explore the mechanism by which an abnormal *gene product* is related to the medical phenotype, i.e. the signs and symptoms, of the person who has it. Epidemiological studies can be very revealing, but useful insights, particularly for single-gene abnormalities, can come from a biological approach. Biomedical research has led not only to a greater understanding of the normal function of genes and the nature of disease defects but also, in some instances, it has informed the development of effective treatments (we return to treatments in Chapter 9 of this book).

Relationship of the abnormal gene to the clinical features of PKU

Although for many genetic disorders the relationship between the abnormal gene and the clinical features is still not clearly understood, for some diseases treatment is available because a great deal is known about the abnormal gene product. PKU was the first disease for which treatment in the form of dietary restriction was successfully used. We have chosen to focus on this disease again because it demonstrates a general principle of genetic disorders, the loss or deficient function of the protein product encoded by the abnormal gene. However, it is important to remember that there are many different types of proteins in cells, each type having different functions (Chapter 3), so we must take care in drawing general conclusions about the changed function resulting from disease alleles on the basis of this one example.

The biochemical and genetic origins of PKU were discovered by a Norwegian physician, A. Følling, in 1934. It was the first demonstration of a genetic defect causing mental retardation. He showed that babies who failed to make a certain enzyme became mentally retarded when they grew up. The normal enzyme breaks down phenylalanine to tyrosine (both of which are amino acids, the building blocks of proteins). In children with PKU, phenylalanine cannot be broken down so it accumulates in the body (Figure 4.18) and, since tyrosine is not produced, there is a deficiency of tyrosine. We now know that the enzyme is the product of a particular gene. Children with PKU inherit two abnormal alleles of this gene, which do not have the correct sequence of nucleotides and hence cannot produce the correct enzyme.

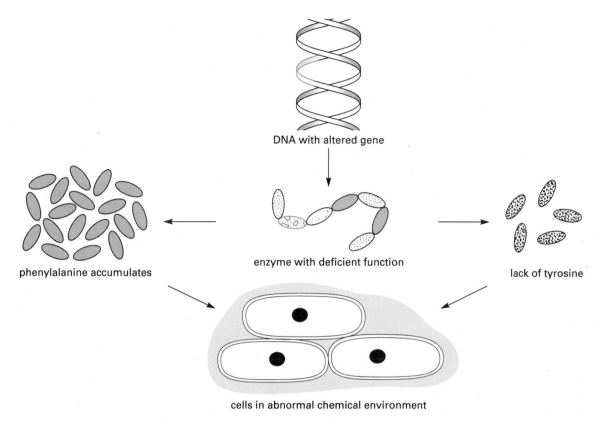

DNA with altered gene

phenylalanine accumulates

enzyme with deficient function

lack of tyrosine

cells in abnormal chemical environment

Figure 4.18 *A schematic representation of the biochemical consequences of the deficient gene product (enzyme) associated with phenylketonuria (PKU). (Note: nothing in this diagram has been drawn to scale!)*

☐ Since both phenylalanine and tyrosine are constituents of a normal diet, in what way could mental retardation be prevented in babies born with the PKU alleles?

■ By restricting the intake of phenylalanine in the diet and ensuring a sufficient intake of tyrosine.

Such treatment renders most affected children free of symptoms. Thus, changing the *environment* leads to a change in the phenotype. This example illustrates an important principle: care is needed when talking about the *cause* of genetic diseases since, as with normal variation, the environment is also important in determining the final phenotype.

The clinical features associated with PKU are quite diverse. Children with the disease show a developmental delay, first apparent in infancy, which is accompanied by seizures, hyperactivity and behavioural disturbances. They also tend to have blond hair and skin pigmentation is absent. At first sight, such diverse features appear to be entirely unrelated, but studies on the function of the enzyme coded for by the PKU allele have revealed how these different clinical symptoms are connected. The absence of the functional enzyme in individuals with PKU affects the synthesis of *myelin* in the brain. Myelin is a component of the protective fatty sheath that surrounds nerves and it is essential for their normal activity. The deficiency in myelin may be responsible for the mental retardation and behavioural changes. Tyrosine is required for pigment formation, so its deficiency accounts for the fair complexion and blond hair.

PKU shows how the function of one gene influences the development of the phenotype of the individual in a number of ways. But are all individuals with the disease affected in the same way; do they share the same clinical features? In fact, the disease phenotype can vary considerably between individuals, as we now explain.

Variations in the disease phenotype

One reason for the disease phenotype differing between individuals is because the action of the disease gene is affected by the rest of the genotype. A clear example is the case of children with PKU, for whom most of the symptoms of the disease can be prevented by a carefully controlled restriction of phenylalanine in their diet, together with the addition of sufficient tyrosine.

There is extreme variability from individual to individual in the amount of phenylalanine and tyrosine per kilogram of body mass required to prevent biochemical disturbances and intellectual impairment. The variability is due to the different degrees to which individuals use *other* enzymes for changing phenylalanine into other substances, and the level of *tolerance* for abnormal concentrations of phenylalanine that different individuals have. Thus, different individuals have different responses to the diet; each child with PKU has a different *overall* genotype and therefore responds in a distinctive manner to changes in diet, despite the fact that all such children have the same genetic deficiency.

PKU is a striking example of how each genotype interacts differently with the environment. But it also illustrates another important point; the effect of a single allele cannot be considered in isolation from the rest of the genotype. What a person inherits is *not* a set of independent characteristics, but a vast number of genes, the products of which *interact* both with other gene products and with the environment to produce the individual's unique phenotype.

You have seen that genetic diseases are associated with phenotypes which are considered to be outside the normal range. But how did disease alleles and normal alternative alleles of a gene (such as *A*, *B* and *O* of the ABO blood group) arise in the first place? Are disease alleles different in some important way from normal alleles? We turn next to the mechanisms by which the large amount of genetic variation that exists in the human population arises.

The process of genetic change: mutation

Genetic differences are due to *mutation*, the introduction of 'genetic errors' that result in *permanent* changes in the DNA (mutation and its effect on the sequence of nucleotides in DNA was introduced in Chapter 3). Mutation is the raw material of evolutionary change and the accumulation of genetic changes over time has contributed to the evolution of different species, including humans, and their separation from other primates. Different kinds of mutation can occur in the DNA: sometimes nucleotides are lost, occasionally extra nucleotides are inserted into a gene, or a nucleotide may be changed into a different one or relocated elsewhere in the DNA.

Most mutations occur as minor changes involving only one or a few nucleotides of DNA. Nevertheless, a small change in the nucleotides may lead to a profound change in the gene product (the protein). Some mutations may have little effect on the phenotype, and a few may even be beneficial; others are harmful and some give rise to genetic disease alleles. In the case of genetic disease alleles, such as the one associated with PKU, the protein produced as a result of the abnormal allele has altered properties because its structure is different from that of the normal protein. These points are summarised in Figure 4.19.

☐ Is the origin of genetic diseases significantly different from the process that produces alternative alleles of normal genes?

■ No, mutation underlies both.

In fact an important concept of medical genetics is that genetic diseases are only the most obvious, and often the most extreme, manifestations of genetic change, superimposed on a background of entirely normal variation, all of it generated by random mutations.

Gene mutations can arise spontaneously as errors during the normal process of DNA replication in any cell. But only mutations in the cells that give rise to the *gametes* can be perpetuated from one generation to the next. Some of the defective alleles transmitted in the gametes are descended from mutations that happened many generations ago, which have been copied and passed on from parent to offspring; others are new errors that arose very recently as new gametes were formed. Indeed, there is a high probability that each of us has received a newly-mutated gene from one of our parents. Fortunately, most of these new mutations are recessive and so remain hidden, since they do not affect the structure of a protein nor the form or function of the person who inherits the mutation.

The *rate* at which mutation occurs can be increased by external agents, such as ultraviolet light, X-rays, temperature and noxious chemicals. Interestingly, the male survivors both of the Hiroshima bomb and of the accident at Chernobyl nuclear power station did not suffer an increase in the number of mutations in the DNA of their sperm cells. (We discuss the effect of industrial chemicals on human DNA in Chapter 10 of this book.)

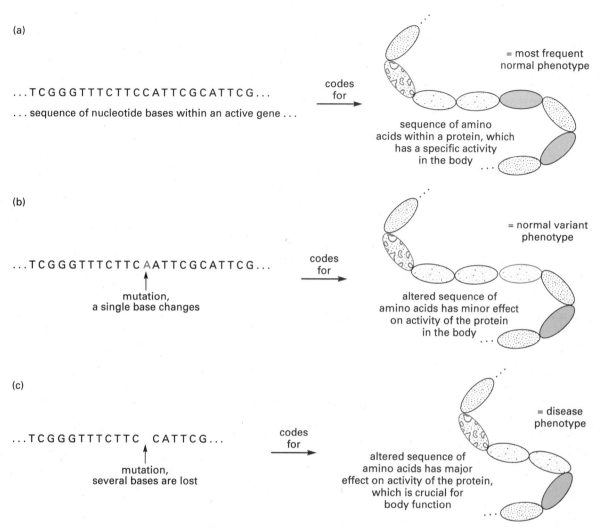

Figure 4.19 *A general outline of how mutations lead to changed phenotypes. (a) The normal nucleotide sequence codes for an active protein found in the most frequent normal phenotype; (b) a mutation gives rise to a variant protein without changing its activity significantly, leading to a normal variant phenotype; (c) a mutation has a damaging effect on the activity of the protein, giving rise to a disease phenotype. Note: a single base change, as in (b), could result in a disease phenotype if the protein activity is altered, as is the case in sickle-cell disease; similarly, the loss of several bases, as in (c), could result in another normal variant phenotype if the activity of the protein remained unaffected by the change in amino acid sequence.*

Mutation is a constant process and continues to occur in the cells of our bodies as we age. Depending on the nature of the mutation, its location in the DNA, and the tissue affected by the gene product, a mutation may possibly lead to a cancer (as Chapter 8 describes). As age increases, so does the number of mutations in the cells, which is one reason why cancer is mainly a disease of older people. Mutations also increase with age in eggs and sperm. The most widely known example of the effect of age on the number of mutations is Down's syndrome. The incidence of Down's syndrome increases with the age of the mother, as shown in Figure 4.20 (*overleaf*).

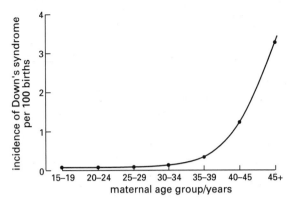

Figure 4.20 *The incidence of Down's syndrome births and maternal age. (Source: Jones, S. et al. (eds) (1992)* The Cambridge Encyclopedia of Human Evolution, *Cambridge University Press, un-numbered Figure, p. 275, acknowledged as 'after Penrose, L. S. and Smith, G. F. (1966)* Down's Anomaly, *Churchill Livingstone')*

The mutation associated with Down's syndrome involves a whole chromosome, not just a few nucleotides. A typical karyotype of a person with Down's syndrome is shown in Figure 4.21.

□ How does this karyotype differ from normal (look back at Figures 4.4 and 4.5)?

■ There is an extra chromosome 21, giving a total of 47 instead of 46 chromosomes.

This kind of mutation is called a **chromosomal mutation.** Such mutations may involve either changes in chromosome *number* (the loss or gain of a chromosome), or changes in chromosome *structure*, such as the loss of a piece of chromosome.

Children with Down's syndrome have a slight slant to their eyes, a small round head, short stature, broad hands and feet, an unusual crease extending across the palm of the hand, a loving nature and a varying degree of mental retardation. How the additional chromosome produces these features is unknown, but the *origin* of the extra chromosome is understood.

One gamete, usually the egg, carries an extra copy of chromosome 21; fertilisation by a normal sperm leads to an embryo with three copies instead of two. But why should an egg cell carry an extra chromosome? We know that something goes wrong during *meiosis*, the reduction division which produces gametes with half the usual number of chromosomes; the two copies of chromosome 21 fail to separate into two different gametes.

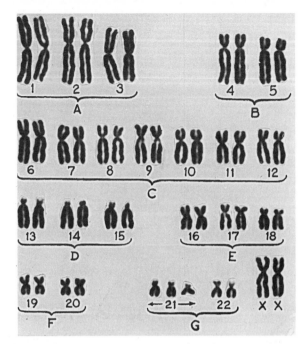

Figure 4.21 *Karyotype of a person with Down's syndrome.*

Why should an extra chromosome occur more frequently in the eggs of older women? A major clue lies in the process of meiosis, which is particularly lengthy in females. In human males, meiosis takes only a few hours and the production of mature new sperm cells is completed in about three weeks; the process does not begin until puberty and is repeated throughout adult life. In females, meiosis begins in the *embryo* but is arrested at an early stage and is not completed in individual eggs until a time between the onset of sexual maturity and the menopause. This means that in the eggs of older females the process of meiosis lasts over 40 years. It appears that, as the duration of meiosis increases, the chance of chromosome separation going wrong also increases.

Chromosomal mutations are rarely perpetuated, either because the affected individual has a short life span, or because he or she is infertile. About three quarters of fertilised eggs that would develop into a child with Down's syndrome spontaneously abort and many live-born Down's children die soon after birth. Those who survive to adulthood are usually infertile.

Even though some mutations are harmful, useful ones survive and, over the course of evolution, the steady influx of new alternative alleles has led to a high degree of variability and individuality.

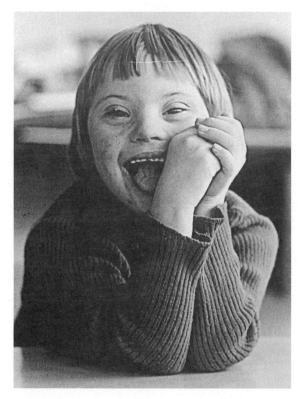

A child with Down's syndrome. (Source: MENCAP National Centre)

A world census

So far we have confined our discussion to the inheritance of genes within families, but in order to understand the 'genetic health' of nations and the distribution of genetic diseases, we need to look at the frequencies of genes within countries and larger groups. This is because the genotype of individuals, including people with genetic diseases, is a reflection of the population to which they belong. The genotype of individuals is not only affected by immediate members of their family, but also by the genotype of the general population that has married into that family. The focus of the last part of this chapter is on **population genetics**, the study of factors influencing the distribution and frequencies of genes in populations. Here we are using the term **population** in its biological sense, meaning a group of individuals among whom mating occurs, or occurs more often than with members of other populations.

Differences between populations

In order to understand the present-day genetic structure of human populations we need to look at our evolutionary history (as described in Chapter 2). About 10 000 years ago the number of human inhabitants of the Earth was at least 1 500 times smaller than it is now; since population density was low, 'breeding' populations would have been relatively isolated from each other. There is evidence to suggest that major genetic differences between such populations must have evolved before population growth increased the contact between them.

Earlier in this chapter the idea of genetic differences affecting height and growth rate between populations was introduced (recall the discussion of multifactorial inheritance). In fact, there are some striking geographical patterns for genes controlling visible characteristics. Human populations in different parts of the world became adapted to the physical environment in various ways, height being only one of them. Body form and proportions are in the main under genetic control. Most tropical people have slim bodies and long limbs; their large surface area helps them to lose heat, in contrast to the squat heat-conserving shape of the Eskimos (Inuit) and other Arctic peoples. Indians living in the high altitudes of the Andes evolved big chests which enabled them to extract oxygen more easily from the thin air, and Northern Asians evolved pads of fat around their eyes which narrow the aperture and protect the eyes, both against the cold and the sun glaring off the snow. The striking geographic patterns of genes controlling visible characteristics such as these have their equivalents in the distribution of genetic diseases.

However, the fact that the distribution of certain alleles (for example for body form or eye-shape) varies between different populations has often led to the mistaken assumption that humans can be divided into distinct 'races' on the basis of their genes. In colloquial speech, the term 'race' as applied to humans usually refers to a set of visible characteristics such as skin colour, hair texture and body shape, as well as cultural features, which are associated with people whose ancestors came from a particular part of the Earth—such as Africa, Europe or Asia. But to a biologist, *race* means a group in which the frequency of particular alleles differs in distinctive ways from the frequency found in other groups. When the allele frequencies of human genes are actually measured between different populations, no such distinctive pattern emerges. A minority of alleles certainly differ in frequency (which is why some skin is black and others white), but no distinctive pattern of alleles across a range of human genes can be found to correspond to the 'races' commonly distinguished on the basis of appearance and culture.

In genetic terms, there is only *one* human race and it is extremely diverse. In fact, over 90 per cent of the total genetic diversity world-wide is found *within* the perceived 'races', rather than between them. The differences between the alleles of two individuals from different perceived 'races' (such as a European and an African) are, on average, no greater than the differences between any two Europeans or between any two Africans.

The mistaken idea that distinct human 'races' exist was promoted by geneticists in the early part of this century, and demolished by their successors in the 1970s and 1980s, who mapped the frequency of certain alleles across the world's populations. Each population (that is, an interbreeding group) is said to have a **gene pool**. This is defined as all the alleles ever found in that population; put another way, it is the total genetic variation existing among the people in that population. Of course, populations overlap and interbreeding occurs at the margins of population groups (increasingly as transportation of people around the world rises), but some variations in the frequency of certain alleles can be found in the gene pools of different populations. Remember that these variations affect a minority of human genes and show no consistent relationship with so-called 'races'. People living in a remote region of a country may have a higher frequency of a particular allele than their countrymen and women living some miles distant, yet the two populations are indistinguishable in terms of their appearance and culture. For example, there is a much-studied village in central Portugal where a genetically-determined blood disorder is common, but the same disorder is rare among other Portuguese.

How did these genetic variations between different populations arise? Investigation of this question has largely been carried out by focusing on the frequency with which disease-causing alleles are distributed in different gene pools, but the processes involved must be the same for alleles that influence physical characteristics such as height, body shape and skin colour. Three processes have been identified, which together explain why the frequencies of certain alleles vary in different parts of the world: they are mutation rate, chance or random processes, and natural selection. We consider each of these in turn.

Mutation rate

Although mutations occur at random, the **mutation rate** (their frequency, i.e. the chance of a change happening in the DNA), falls within a range between 1 and 12 mutations per gene in every 100 000 gametes. Once a mutation has occurred in a gamete, then it is transmitted to all the cells in the individual formed from that gamete (after fertilisation), because the mutant allele is *copied* when DNA replicates before each cell division, in just the same way as the normal alleles are copied.

The incidence of certain genetic diseases depends *solely* on the mutation rate because, in such diseases, the mutation results in a severe genetic abnormality which prevents the person from having children. Mutations that produce a *dominant* disease allele often prevent reproduction and so are not transmitted to the next generation. Since the disease allele is not transmitted, it can only occur in a population as a newly-arisen mutation. Thus, the incidence of the disease reflects the rate at which new mutations of the affected gene arise. This also applies to chromosomal mutations. For example, the incidence of chromosomal mutations involving a whole chromosome (as in Down's syndrome) is about 6 per 1 000 newborn babies and about 250 per 1 000 miscarriages. As we noted earlier, these chromosomal mutations are not passed on since children who survive are usually infertile.

The mutation rate is less significant for *recessive* diseases because the mutant alleles have accumulated in the population from previous generations. The number of carriers (heterozygotes) is far more significant in determining the incidence of the disease. Recall that recessive alleles can be transmitted invisibly from generation to generation by carriers, their presence being masked by the dominant allele. Consider the following data for PKU, which can be determined from the known incidence of the disease in the white population of the USA, estimated to be 200 million people in 1976 when these figures were quoted by Lerner and Libby (p. 238):

> number of carriers of newly-arisen PKU mutations in 10 million gametes = 400

> number of carriers with inherited PKU mutations = 2 500 000

These data clearly demonstrate the importance of carriers of mutations descended from previous generations, relative to the number of newly-arisen mutant alleles, in determining the frequency of the disease. The risk that any carrier will have an affected child depends partly on the *carrier frequency* (proportion of heterozygotes) in the general population; the higher the frequency, the greater the chance that a carrier will mate with another carrier and produce an affected child.

Chance or random processes

Surnames illustrate the process of chance events in genetic inheritance rather well. You can think of surnames as being analogous to genes in that they are passed on from generation to generation, but only through one parent. In social systems like those in most of Europe, where surnames pass from father to son, a particular surname will be lost from the population if it is shared by only a few families and none of them has a son. This is less likely to happen if many children are produced and they remain within the same isolated population. In remote Italian villages in the Parma Valley with 200 to 300 inhabitants for example, there are on average only 12 surnames per village. Often half the village have the same surname, and in some cases the surname is found in no other village.

The analogy between surnames and genes can be readily illustrated. Human populations that are geographically close to each other, or who have recently evolved from a common ancestor, usually share some of the same alleles. There is, however, an important exception to this, which occurs when a population lives in relative *isolation* from other populations. A rare genetic mutation may arise in such an isolated population as a chance event, but can be absent in a related but geographically separate population. The inhabitants of the island of New Guinea provide a remarkable example of this. Until relatively recently, isolated populations lived in separate valleys unaware of each others' existence. These populations had their own distinctive genetic abnormalities, such as premature ageing in one valley, delayed puberty in another, and one population had the highest known incidence of profoundly deaf individuals in the world. Such effects suggest that a different ancestral disease mutation became prevalent in each isolated population.

Groups may be isolated not only for geographic reasons, but because they hold strong religious beliefs, as in the case of the Old Order Amish, an American religious sect which split into three isolated communities in Pennsylvania, Ohio and Indiana. Even today, rare recessive diseases exist with an increased frequency, each one in a different community, clearly illustrating the strong interrelationship of social structure and genetic structure. The Amish in Pennsylvania is a small genetically-isolated population with large families and with a high frequency of marriages between relatives, leading to unusual disease frequencies. A form of dwarfism (Ellis–van Creveld disorder) is present at a high frequency in the Pennsylvania Amish, but is absent in the Amish in Ohio and Indiana.

□ Can you deduce when in time the mutation leading to this disorder arose?

■ It must have arisen after the three groups of Amish separated from each other, or have been present in one of the founders of the Pennsylvanian group.

There is one important systematic difference in the incidence of recessive diseases between industrialised countries and more traditional populations in other parts of the world. In general, in the populations of industrialised countries, recessive diseases are much rarer than in parts of the Third World because the proportion of marriages between genetic relatives (for example first cousins) has gone down sharply during the past century.

Natural selection in action: sickle-cell disease and malaria

So far, we have considered two of the three processes that affect the frequency of alleles in different parts of the world: mutation rate and chance processes. We now consider the third, natural selection. The process of natural selection (described in Chapter 3) is one of the driving forces of genetic change; harmful mutations are 'weeded out' whereas mutations that increase the ability of individuals to survive and reproduce are favoured by selection. Is there any evidence of selection working today? There are a number of examples, but by far the best understood is that of sickle-cell disease and the haemoglobin gene.

As you learnt earlier, more is known about haemoglobin and its variants than any other human protein. Remember that haemoglobin is present in red blood cells and has the crucial function of carrying oxygen from the lungs to all the cells of the body. One of the variants of this molecule, called *haemoglobin S* or sickle-cell haemoglobin, is common only in regions of the world where there is (or once was) a high prevalence of malaria.

Haemoglobin S is the protein product of an allele conventionally represented by the letters Hb^S. Individuals with two copies of this allele ($Hb^S Hb^S$) have *sickle-cell disease*, a severe disease in which the red blood cells take on a sickled shape instead of being round.[13] These cells block capillaries and produce a variety of symptoms from anaemia to heart failure. Individuals with this genotype often die before they reproduce and so do not pass on the mutant allele. Despite this, the mutant allele persists in certain parts of the world at a high frequency. For

[13]Sickle-cell disease is introduced in *World Health and Disease*, Chapter 3; Figure 3.4 in that book shows photographs of normal and sickled red blood cells.

(a) distribution of malaria

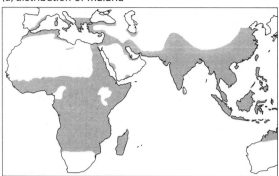

(b) frequency of sickle-cell allele

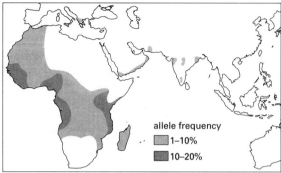

allele frequency
1–10%
10–20%

Figure 4.22 *Distribution (a) of malaria and (b) of the* Hb^S *allele; shading denotes the percentage of the population that has this allele. (Source: Jones, S. et al. (eds) (1992) The Cambridge Encyclopedia of Human Evolution,* Cambridge University Press, *un-numbered Figure, p. 16, based on Strickberger, M. W. (1990)* Evolution, *Jones and Bartlett, Figures 21–23)*

example, in Africa south of the Sahara and north of the Zambezi river, Hb^S is so common that in some groups five per cent of newborn babies are homozygous and thus suffer from sickle-cell disease.

Why then is the Hb^S allele so common? You might have expected that natural selection would lead to its gradual disappearance, since it clearly reduces the reproductive potential of people with sickle-cell disease. The answer lies in the remarkable advantage gained by *heterozygotes*, who carry one copy of Hb^S and one normal haemoglobin allele, Hb^A. They have some resistance to the organism that causes malaria. Let us look at the evidence for this explanation.

Figure 4.22(a) shows the distribution of malaria in Africa and southern Asia. Compare this with Figure 4.22(b), which shows the distribution of the Hb^S allele in the same part of the world.

□ What relationship is there between the two distributions?

■ They overlap. The regions with a high frequency of the Hb^S allele, and hence of sickle-cell disease, coincide with areas of the world where malaria is rife. In areas where malaria is less common, such as the Sahara and southern Africa, the Hb^S allele is also less common.

The parasite responsible for one form of malaria (a protistan called *Plasmodium*) spends part of its life cycle in the red blood cells of mammals, including humans, where it multiplies.[14] The red blood cells of normal homozygotes ($Hb^A Hb^A$) are susceptible to this parasite and consequently they, like sickle-cell homozygotes ($Hb^S Hb^S$), produce fewer children than heterozygotes ($Hb^A Hb^S$), who have some resistance to malaria. Heterozygotes with only one Hb^S allele have *sickle-cell trait*, an intermediate phenotype with respect to the red blood cells since some are the normal round shape and some are sickle-shaped. The sickled shape confers some protection against the debilitating effects of malaria since the parasite is killed inside the collapsed sickle-cells. Thus, heterozygotes tend to have more surviving children than either of the two homozygote genotypes and some of these children will inherit the Hb^S allele. Another way of saying this is that natural selection acts to retain the Hb^S allele in the population because it confers some advantage in areas of the world where malaria is rife. A summary of the phenotypes associated with each genotype of the Hb^A and Hb^S alleles is given in Table 4.2.

[14]A photograph of the malarial parasite inside a red blood cell appears in *Studying Health and Disease*, Figure 9.1; the parasite's life cycle is shown in *World Health and Disease*, Figure 3.3.

Table 4.2 Genotypes and phenotypes of the Hb^A and Hb^S alleles

Genotype	Phenotype
$Hb^A Hb^A$	normal homozygotes: at risk of dying from malaria
$Hb^S Hb^S$	sickle-cell homozygotes: at risk of dying from sickle-cell disease
$Hb^A Hb^S$	sickle-cell trait heterozygotes: some resistance to malaria, some symptoms of anaemia

For a final piece of evidence that the Hb^S allele confers some resistance to malaria, we can look at a population genetically-related to those shown in Figure 4.22a, which became geographically separate in a part of the world where malaria is absent. 15 million black Africans were transported to the Americas as slaves in the eighteenth century, taking the sickle-cell disease allele with them.

☐ If sickle-cell disease confers an advantage only in those regions of the world where malaria is rife, would you expect the frequency of the mutant Hb^S allele to have decreased, increased or stayed the same in the present-day black population of the USA?

■ Since sickle-cell homozygotes ($Hb^S Hb^S$) rarely leave descendants and heterozygotes ($Hb^A Hb^S$) would no longer be at an advantage compared with normal homozygotes ($Hb^A Hb^A$), the frequency of the mutant Hb^S allele would be expected to decrease in the population.

In fact, the frequency of heterozygotes in US blacks has decreased to 1 in 500 of the population, compared with 1 in 25 in parts of present-day equatorial Africa.

The example of sickle-cell disease shows clearly how the environment affects the distribution of a genetic disease. The transmission of the malarial parasite to human hosts depends in part on a suitable climate and habitats for mosquitoes to breed. It also illustrates the influence of culture on the change of gene frequency, since the introduction of agricultural practices to Africa involved the clearing of forests, which improved the environment for the mosquito. These insects, which carry the malarial parasite and transmit it to humans, increased

in number. So the increased probability of malarial infection depends in part on agricultural practices among different African populations.[15]

Although natural selection, acting through the climate and disease, is responsible for many geographical changes in gene frequency, it is important to remember that such patterns can also arise at random. Differences in gene frequencies between populations and ethnic groups means that, in order to determine the *current* risk of being affected by a disease allele, it often matters whether a family has its origins in (for example) the United Kingdom, Italy or Japan. Given the changes in movement of people round the world, particularly in the last 5 000 years, how are gene frequencies being affected? This is the topic with which we conclude this chapter.

Present trends and future prospects

With the advent of global travel and in the process of world conquest, human populations have undergone a basic change in their relations with one another. Our long heritage of cultural diversity is being blurred, leading to the gradual 'homogenisation' of language and culture. What might the effect of these cultural changes be on the genes carried within and between populations? The genes found in most present-day populations show evidence of their origins in the relatively isolated populations of the past. For example, Welsh-speaking Welsh have a higher frequency of certain alleles than English-speaking Welsh, and vice versa, but as the two cultures mix, so will their genes.

☐ How do you think the exchange of people between formerly separate populations might affect the frequency of recessive genetic disorders?

■ They will decline in incidence, because the chance of a carrier of the recessive allele mating with another carrier will go down.

Recessive genetic disorders are usually associated with particular populations (for example, cystic fibrosis is

[15]Malaria persists for a complex set of reasons outlined in *World Health and Disease*, Chapter 3. The difficulties encountered by the many campaigns to eradicate malaria are discussed in *Caring for Health: History and Diversity* (Open University Press, revised edition 1993), Chapter 8.

highest in white Americans and Europeans, but rare in black African peoples, whereas sickle-cell disease shows the opposite distribution). Increasing rates of intermarriage between people from different population groups will tend to reduce the incidence of any recessive genetic disorders that either population experiences.

Conversely, improvements in social, economic and medical provision tend to *reduce* the impact of natural selection on disadvantageous genes. In the past, natural selection acted against the passing on of genes that increased a young person's susceptibility to infectious disease, or contributed (at least in part) to certain congenital abnormalities, low birth weight and so forth. In the 1990s, an increasing proportion of human babies survive to reproduce in their turn, passing on to future generations genes which might not, in the past, have been passed on.

However, disease-causing organisms themselves evolve in unpredictable ways, and it is difficult to determine whether new infectious diseases might influence the selection of particular alleles in human populations in the future. This is emphasised by the evolution of one relatively new disease, AIDS. Suppose that in some imaginary future, a few individuals in areas of high

infection, such as parts of Africa, were found to be resistant to HIV (the virus that causes AIDS) as the result of a new allele arising by mutation.

☐ What do you predict would happen to the frequency in the population of this imaginary allele?

■ If an allele that confers resistance to HIV infection ever arose, it could be expected to *increase* in the population as more children would be born to people who had that allele, and more of the children who inherited it would survive to reproduce in their turn. (This is the opposite case to that described earlier for the Hb^s allele, which is *decreasing* in the USA as selection pressure favouring its transmission declines in the absence of malaria.)

In Chapter 6, we will return to the subject of infectious diseases and genetic resistance to infection and, at various points later in this book, we will continue to speculate about the future course of human evolution. It may be closely bound up with the evolution of other species; in Chapter 5 we turn to the relationship between humans and other organisms and examine their impact on our health and disease.

OBJECTIVES FOR CHAPTER 4

When you have studied this chapter, you should be able to:

4.1 Use examples to illustrate the difference between: genotype and phenotype; dominant and recessive characteristics; homozygotes and heterozygotes; and sex-linked and non-sex-linked characteristics.

4.2 Explain why each individual is phenotypically unique, with reference to: the behaviour of chromosomes during meiosis and at fertilisation, single-gene and multifactorial inheritance, the contribution of mutations and the influence of the environment.

4.3 Using phenylketonuria (PKU) as an example, explain (a) how the diverse clinical features of an affected individual are related to a single deficient gene product, and (b) how the overall genotype and the environment can influence the expression of this disorder.

4.4 Describe the mechanisms that influence the distribution and frequencies of genes in populations, and discuss how this knowledge explains the patterns of genetic diseases (with reference to particular examples) in the world today.

QUESTIONS FOR CHAPTER 4

Question 1 (*Objectives 4.1 and 4.2*)

Match one of the *situations* described in (a) to (e) with one of the *explanations* 1–5 given in the list below.

Situations

(a) Parents of normal stature have a child with the dominant disorder *achondroplasia* (short-limbed dwarfism).

(b) A study was conducted on twins in which at least one member of each twin-pair had club-foot at birth. All these twin-pairs had a similar home environment. In 32 per cent of the *identical* twins in the study, *both* twins in the pair had club-foot; of the remaining 68 per cent of identical twins, only one twin in each pair was affected. In 3 per cent of the *non-identical* twins in the study, *both* had club-foot; of the remaining 97 per cent of non-identical twins, only one twin in each pair was affected.

(c) A child is born with the recessive disorder *atrophy of the retina,* in which the back of the eye degenerates, but neither parents have the disease.

(d) A woman is heterozygous for two genes, one associated with PKU, which is on chromosome pair number 12, and the other gene associated with cystic fibrosis which is on chromosome pair 7. She transmits the defective allele for PKU and the normal allele for cystic fibrosis to her daughter.

(e) A woman has two sons, both of whom have *haemophilia,* a disease in which the blood fails to clot, and four unaffected daughters. Neither she nor the children's father have the disease, but *her* father had haemophilia.

Explanations

1   A new mutation occurred during gamete formation in one parent.

2   Assortment of chromosomes during meiosis accounts for this situation.

3   This situation is best understood as a multifactorial characteristic with both genetic and environmental influences.

4   The affected individual is homozygous for two recessive alleles of the gene.

5   This situation is characteristic of a sex-linked recessive disorder.

Question 2 (*Objective 4.1*)

What is the sex of the person whose karyotype is shown in Figure 4.21?

Question 3 (*Objective 4.2*)

Normal individuals have an enzyme that repairs damage in the DNA of skin cells brought about by exposure to ultraviolet light. Individuals with *xeroderma pigmentosa* are unable to repair such damage because of a defective enzyme and consequently they develop skin cancers. How could the development of skin cancers be prevented?

Question 4 (*Objective 4.2*)

What are the possible genotypes of the gametes of a person who is heterozygous for the gene that causes cystic fibrosis?

Question 5 (*Objective 4.3*)

Using PKU as an example, describe the diverse clinical features of this disease and explain how these are related to a deficiency in the product of the defective gene.

Question 6 (*Objective 4.4*)

Explain the distribution of each of the following diseases: (a) porphyra, (b) thalassaemia, and (c) neurofibromatosis, each of which is described below.

(a) The dominant genetic disorder *porphyria* is rare in most parts of the world but is relatively common in South Africa. The gene normally has little effect, but its carriers have a severe, and sometimes fatal, reaction to barbiturate drugs. About 30 000 Afrikaners carry the disease allele today, which we know they all inherited from a couple from Holland who arrived in South Africa in the 1690s.

(b) *Thalassaemia* (featured in the TV programme 'Blood lines') is a recessive genetic disease, prevalent in Mediterranean countries, the Indian sub-continent, Malaysia and the Far East and in parts of Central and West Africa. Affected individuals have anaemia and other associated blood problems. The disease is associated with loss of part of the haemoglobin molecule. Its distribution overlaps part of the area where malaria is currently or was once prevalent.

(c) The dominant disorder *neurofibromatosis* affects the nervous system and is associated with the risk of malignant tumours. It occurs at high frequency in certain families, but these families have no known previous history of the disease.

5 *Living with other species*

This chapter discusses the relationship between humans and those organisms, called pathogens, that cause the infectious group of human diseases. It builds on an understanding of the story of human evolution presented in Chapter 2 and of the theory of biological evolution, which was discussed in Chapter 3. From Chapter 2, we assume a knowledge of the origin of a number of infectious diseases caused by pathogenic organisms that humans have acquired from other animals; from Chapter 3 we assume some understanding of the concepts of natural selection, adaptation and fitness.

Introduction

This chapter is about relationships between pathogenic organisms and their human hosts. *Pathogen* is the term we are using in this book to refer to any organism, large or small, that causes disease by infecting or infesting another organism. When you fall ill with an infectious disease caused by a pathogen, such as the measles virus, you probably regard it as an unfortunate, random event, like falling off a ladder. In fact, your misfortune is part of a pattern, and a manifestation of a complex relationship that exists between us, as members of the human species, and whichever organism has caused the disease that has afflicted you. This relationship has a history and an origin, as outlined in Chapter 2. The pathogenic organism may have been affecting humans for many thousands of years or may be comparatively new. Infectious diseases can kill and, if we are to survive and reproduce, we must respond to every infection by inactivating the organism that causes it, or by becoming less adversely affected by it.

The history of *host–pathogen relationships* is like a very prolonged war, made up of countless, often-repeated battles fought out within individuals in the form of illnesses that end in the incapacitation or death either of the pathogen or of the host. The outcome of each little battle changes, by an infinitesimal amount, the relationship between pathogen and host *at the species level* and determines whether, over evolutionary time, the disease becomes more or less common and harmful to humans. (Note the use of 'military metaphors' in this account, a common form of expression in discussions of infectious disease, which is considered further in Chapter 6.)

The phrase 'at the species level' defines what this chapter is about. Here we are concerned with the ways in which species (rather than individuals) are affected by diseases and how, over evolutionary time, the host species and the pathogen species respond to one another. For example, the bacterium that causes tuberculosis, TB (*Mycobacterium tuberculosis*), infects and kills many thousands of people every year and thus affects our numbers as a species. It has been a more potent threat to species survival in the past than it is today, but TB is again on the increase in the 1990s.[1] Falling ill with TB is also a personal experience as well as a threat to the species; the nature of the interaction between an individual *person* and a pathogen such as the TB bacterium is discussed in Chapter 6.

The chapter begins by looking in very general terms at the ways in which species interact with one another in nature. We discuss the biological importance of pathogenic organisms, their diversity, classification and effects on their hosts, giving most attention to those pathogens that affect humans. In the middle of the chapter, we examine the interaction between infectious diseases and the life history of the host. The life of humans, and of other hosts, consists of a series of stages, in which birth, reproduction and death are the three crucial biological events. What impact does infectious disease have on the normal progression from one stage to the next?

The chapter then looks in more detail at the idea that hosts are engaged in a protracted, evolutionary 'war' with their pathogens; we expose the limitations of this

---

[1]The history of tuberculosis (TB) is described in *Medical Knowledge: Doubt and Certainty* (1994 edition), Chapter 4.

militaristic analogy and describe some of the different outcomes that can result during host–pathogen evolution. Host–pathogen relationships change over evolutionary time but rarely come to a definite, stable conclusion; we consider the intrinsic instability of this relationship and show how it is influenced by environmental changes. A brief overview of how diseases are thought to have influenced the course of evolution of humans and of other species brings the chapter almost to a close, as we consider how pathogens are implicated in some fundamental aspects of human biology, such as the fact that we reproduce sexually, that we choose our mating partners and that we tend to live socially. Finally, we emphasise the importance of micro-organisms in maintaining the survival of the rich diversity of life-forms on Earth.

Interactions between species: a general framework

□ Can you recall the definition of a species from Chapter 2?

■ A species is a group of organisms that most closely resemble one another and that, typically, can mate with one another in their natural habitat and produce fertile offspring.

The current concern for the future of the Earth and its living inhabitants has given a sharp emphasis to the question 'How many species are there?'. It is estimated that the Earth currently contains some 30 million species, of which only about 1.5 million have been named and described by biologists. It may well surprise you that, despite all their efforts, biologists are apparently so woefully ignorant. A major problem is that biological knowledge is very fragmentary and biased. Most of the Earth's approximately 4 000 mammal and 9 000 bird species have been described, but much less is known about the majority of insects, which account for more than half of the world's species. Knowing about the Earth's species is not simply an academic exercise. The Oxford evolutionary biologist, Robert M. May wrote in 1992:

> More immediately, utilitarian reasons for counting and cataloguing species are also noteworthy. A considerable fraction of modern medicines has been developed from biological compounds found in plants. Society would be well advised to keep looking at other shelves in the larder rather than destroying them. Many nutritious fruits and root crops remain largely unexploited; cultivating them could expand and improve the global food supply. (May, R. M., 1992, p. 19)

Species of organisms are not only very numerous; they are also very diverse. They exist in a vast range of sizes and have a rich variety of life styles. To cope with this diversity, biologists need to classify organisms, to arrange them in sensible groupings of manageable size. There are many ways to classify organisms, just as there are several ways of organising books in a library. They could be categorised, for example, by size, by colour, by method of movement, by habitat, and so on (we shall attempt to classify pathogens in some of these ways in a moment). At this early stage in the chapter, however, we shall classify organisms according to the major ways in which they *interact* with one another.

Two simple examples can help to clarify important differences in types of interaction. When a cow browses on a plant, it destroys much of the plant's previous growth and perhaps its flowers, preventing it from reproducing. In this interaction, between a *herbivore* (plant-eating animal) and its food, the cow gains food that it needs to sustain its own survival, growth and reproduction, while the plant loses tissue and reproductive potential; this relationship is one of *exploitation*. When a bee visits the flowers of a plant, it gains food in the form of nectar. This modest loss to the plant is greatly offset, however, by the fact that the bee takes pollen from the flowers and pollinates other plants elsewhere, promoting the plant's reproduction; the relationship is one of *reciprocal benefit*. Table 5.1 (*overleaf*) lists a number of kinds of relationship between organisms according to whether the participants appear to gain (+) or lose (–) from the relationship or whether it has a neutral effect (0) on their survival and reproduction.

□ In which of the categories of interaction in Table 5.1 would you place the association between humans and the bacteria that live in our guts and which help us to digest our food?

■ Because both species benefit from the association, it is an example of *mutualism*.

While much of the emphasis of this chapter is on organisms that cause human disease, it is important to remember that humans have other kinds of relationship, sometimes positively beneficial, with other organisms. Many help us to lead healthy, disease-free lives. The last four interactions in Table 5.1 can be grouped under the single heading **symbiosis**, meaning 'living together' in intimate and prolonged association. (Note that in some older biology texts symbiosis is used in the same sense as 'mutualism' in Table 5.1, but in modern biology it is used, as here, in a more general sense.)

Table 5.1 A classification of interactions between species

Interaction	Consequences for species A and B		Comments
	A	B	
competition	0	–	competition for one or more essential resources (e.g. food, space) in which A excludes B: competitive exclusion
	or		
	–	–	competition in which A and B compete for resource(s) but neither excludes the other: coexistence
predation	+	–	carnivorous animals: A typically kills B
	+	–	herbivorous animals: A typically browses on but does not kill B
symbiosis parasitism	+	–	A is a parasite on or in B, its host; A derives benefit at a cost to B
commensalism	+	0	A derives benefit by living on or with B, but at no cost to B
mutualism	+	+	A and B live in close association and both derive a benefit
neutralism	0	0	A and B live in close association but neither derives a benefit or incurs a cost

In the context of health and disease, however, the type of interaction described as **parasitism** in Table 5.1 is of the greatest relevance, because it covers the various relationships that exist between large animals, including humans and their livestock, and simpler pathogenic organisms that actually or potentially cause disease.

The nature of human pathogens

To a biologist, all pathogenic species, from microscopic bacteria and viruses to large tapeworms, are properly described as **parasites**, a term defined in Table 5.1 as any organism that derives benefit from living in or on another organism (the host), at a cost to the host. The cost may be anything from using small amounts of the host's food supply to causing a fatal illness. However, in everyday language, the word 'parasite' tends to refer only to *animals* and the single-celled *protistans* that cause significant irritation or illness; the common meaning of parasite generally *excludes* bacteria and viruses. To avoid confusion, we shall make it plain whenever we use the term parasite exactly what kinds of organisms we are referring to.

☐ Compile a short list of parasitic animals or protistans that you have directly encountered or heard about (some were mentioned in Chapters 2 and 3).

■ The list is potentially enormous. If you own a cat or a dog, you have probably had to treat it for worms

in its gut, or for fleas, ticks and lice in its fur. Many of us have had to comb headlice out of children's hair, or combat them with special shampoo. At some time in your life, a small amount of your blood has surely been sucked out of your body by a mosquito. Protistans cause malaria, sleeping sickness, some diarrhoeal diseases and some genital tract infections (among others).

Parasitic animals and protistans come in a wide range of sizes and shapes, from tapeworms several metres long to the tiniest of creatures visible only with powerful microscopes. Humans who live in an affluent modern society generally fail to appreciate the biological importance of these parasites because they are so rarely encountered in everyday life. In fact, on a world-wide scale, they are a major cause of human sickness and many millions of people are killed each year by parasitic animals and protistans, as Table 5.2 shows.[2] (You are not expected to memorise this Table.)

☐ According to Table 5.2, approximately how many cases of infection with parasitic animals and protistans did the WHO estimate existed in 1989?

[2]The percentages of deaths caused by infectious and parasitic diseases in industrialised countries and the Third World are compared in *World Health and Disease*, Chapter 3, Figure 3.1.

Table 5.2 The numbers of people infected world-wide in 1989 with the commonest diseases caused by parasitic animals and protistans

Medical name of disease	Common name of disease	Infected people (millions)
dracunculiasis	guinea worm	10
Intestinal infections		
amoebiasis	amoebic dysentery	400
ancylostomiasis	hookworm	900
ascariasis	roundworm	1 000
giardiasis	giardia	200
strongyloidiasis	threadworm	30
trichuriasis	whipworm	500
leishmaniasis	kala azar	12
lymphatic filariasis	elephantiasis	90
malaria	malaria	150–200
onchocerciasis	river blindness	18
schistosomiasis	bilharzia	200
trypanosomiasis		
(African)	sleeping sickness	0.04
(South American)	Chagas disease	13–15

Source: World Health Organisation (WHO) estimates for 1989, quoted in Dobson, A. (1992) Chapter 10.4 in Jones, S. *et al.* (eds) *The Cambridge Encyclopedia of Human Evolution*, Cambridge University Press, pp. 418–9.

■ Over three and a half billion cases. Even allowing for the fact that a high proportion of cases can be attributed to individuals who were infected with several different parasites at the same time (each parasitic infection counting as a 'case'), the prevalence of diseases caused by these organisms is immediately apparent.

Parasitic animals and protistans are also a major cause of mortality and of reduced reproductive success among non-human animals and plants; a major preoccupation of agriculture is to control parasites that can wipe out crops and livestock.

There are many different kinds of animal and protistan parasites and they are extremely diverse. Figure 5.1 (*overleaf*) summarises the type and location of the principal parasites that can be found in and on a human host. These range from single-celled organisms resembling an amoeba to quite large, complex creatures like tapeworms and ticks.

One important general distinction is between **endoparasites**, those that live within the body of their host, usually within a specific organ, and **ectoparasites**, those that live attached to the outer surface of the host, like leeches, fleas and lice. As well as animals and

protistans that live inside cells and organs, the term 'endoparasites' includes a huge variety of bacteria and viruses. Ectoparasites commonly suck blood from their host and, in themselves, are often little more than an irritant. In some instances, however, they carry endoparasites and provide the means of transmission (they are the *vectors*) by which endoparasites get from one host to another. For example, the malarial parasite (*Plasmodium* species) is transmitted by several species of mosquitoes.

A feature of many endo- and ectoparasites is that they are, to a greater or lesser degree, highly specific to particular species of host. For example, as described in Chapter 2, species of *Toxocara* are nematode worms which are specific parasites of dogs and cats.

☐ Both species of *Toxocara* can infect humans and can cause severe symptoms. What is this phenomenon called?

■ Cross-infection (discussed in Chapter 2).

It follows from the great number and diversity of parasites of all kinds (in the widest biological sense of the term), and from their specificity in certain hosts, that there must be many more species of parasite in the world than there are of hosts. It is estimated that 25 per cent of all insect

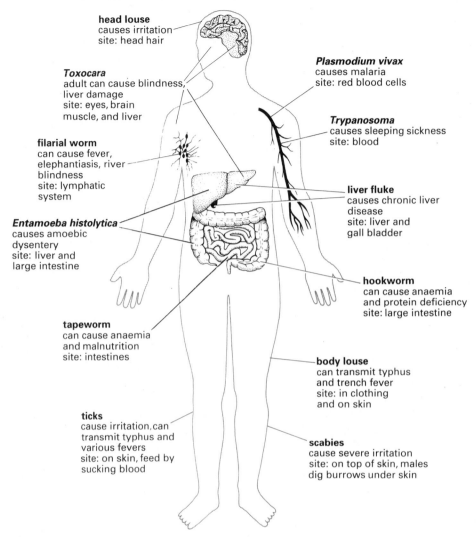

head louse
causes irritation
site: head hair

Toxocara
adult can cause blindness,
liver damage
site: eyes, brain
muscle, and liver

filarial worm
can cause fever,
elephantiasis, river
blindness
site: lymphatic
system

Entamoeba histolytica
causes amoebic
dysentery
site: liver and
large intestine

tapeworm
can cause anaemia
and malnutrition
site: intestines

ticks
cause irritation, can
transmit typhus and
various fevers
site: on skin, feed by
sucking blood

Plasmodium vivax
causes malaria
site: red blood cells

Trypanosoma
causes sleeping sickness
site: blood

liver fluke
causes chronic liver
disease
site: liver and
gall bladder

hookworm
can cause anaemia
and protein deficiency
site: large intestine

body louse
can transmit typhus
and trench fever
site: in clothing
and on skin

scabies
cause severe irritation
site: on top of skin, males
dig burrows under skin

Figure 5.1 *The diversity of animal and protistan parasites that infect and infest humans.* (Compiled by Sarah Keer-Keer, not previously published) (Remember to turn back to finish reading page 101.)

species (which account for more than half the world's species) are parasites of *other insects*, laying their eggs inside the eggs or juvenile stages of other insect species.

> So, naturalists observe, a flea
> Hath smaller fleas that on him prey;
> And these have smaller fleas to bite 'em,
> And so proceed *ad infinitum*.
> (Jonathan Swift: 'On poetry', 1733)

This maxim is most clearly demonstrated by a group of viruses known as *bacteriophages,* which infect bacteria.

Parasitic animals and protistans are at the larger end of the scale of pathogens that cause disease in humans; they range from metre-long tapeworms to viruses that are only visible with the electron microscope (Figure 5.2). Size is another way of classifying the enormous diversity of human pathogens; put simply, the big ones are termed *macroparasites* and the tiny ones are termed *microparasites.*

Macroparasites are relatively large, multi-celled *invertebrate* animals ('invertebrate' means without a backbone), which mainly belong to two groups: the

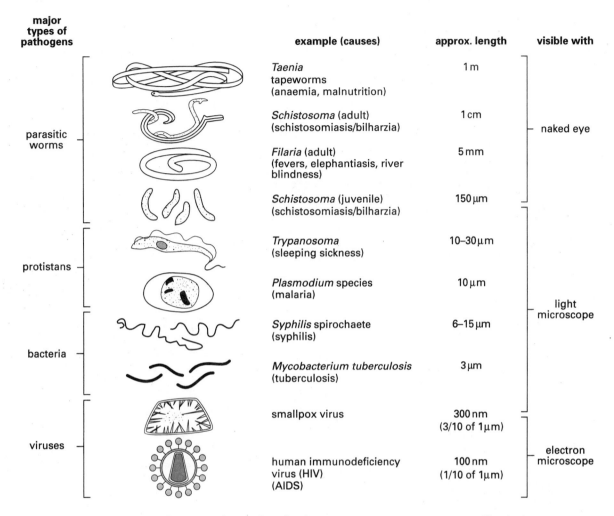

major types of pathogens		example (causes)	approx. length	visible with
parasitic worms		*Taenia* tapeworms (anaemia, malnutrition)	1 m	naked eye
		Schistosoma (adult) (schistosomiasis/bilharzia)	1 cm	
		Filaria (adult) (fevers, elephantiasis, river blindness)	5 mm	
		Schistosoma (juvenile) (schistosomiasis/bilharzia)	150 μm	
protistans		*Trypanosoma* (sleeping sickness)	10–30 μm	light microscope
		Plasmodium species (malaria)	10 μm	
bacteria		*Syphilis* spirochaete (syphilis)	6–15 μm	
		Mycobacterium tuberculosis (tuberculosis)	3 μm	
viruses		smallpox virus	300 nm (3/10 of 1μm)	electron microscope
		human immunodeficiency virus (HIV) (AIDS)	100 nm (1/10 of 1μm)	

Figure 5.2 *Comparative sizes of various pathogens that affect humans. (1 μm (1 micrometre) = one-millionth of a metre; 1 nm (1 nanometre) = one-thousand-millionth of a metre.) (Compiled by Sarah Keer-Keer, not previously published in this form)*

flatworms include flukes, tapeworms and nematode worms; the arthropods (a large group of jointed-limbed invertebrates) include lice, fleas and ticks (Figure 5.3, *overleaf*).

Macroparasites present a major problem in many parts of the world because they infect very large numbers of people (as Table 5.1 showed), and they have particular properties that make them very difficult to eradicate.

Immune responses to macroparasites are typically not fully effective, as you will see in Chapter 6. Macroparasite infections tend, therefore, to be persistent; individuals can become reinfected and, consequently, people tend to carry such parasites for the greater part of their lives. They cause a diverse array of diseases that are typically chronic in form, causing long-term morbidity rather than mortality.

Some macroparasites have complex life cycles involving two or more host species; this complexity prolongs the time it takes to produce the next generation. Typically the eggs are laid in one host, but they mature in another. Tapeworms (Figure 5.4), for example, reproduce sexually in the human gut; their eggs are passed out in the host's faeces and are later eaten by, and develop in, other large mammals, such as pigs or cattle (described in Chapter 2).

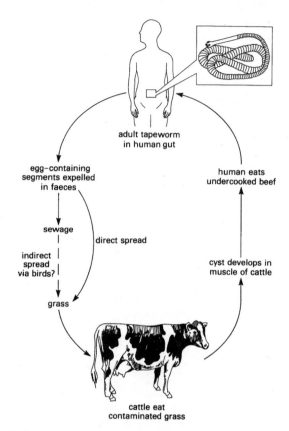

Figure 5.4 *Life cycle of the tapeworm* Taenia saginata.

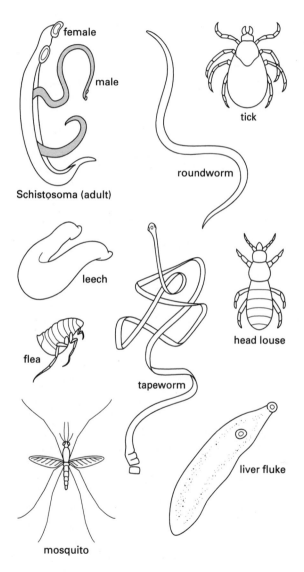

Figure 5.3 *A selection of macroparasites of humans. These animals have not been drawn to scale; simply admire their diversity!* (*Drawings by Tim Halliday*) (Remember to turn back to finish reading page 103.)

Microparasites, as their name implies, are very small organisms visible only through a microscope; they are generally endoparasitic, that is, they live in their host's cells and organs. Typically the entire life cycle is completed in a single host. They include viruses and a wide variety of organisms, such as bacteria and protistans (single-celled organisms), many of which are pathogenic. Transmission from host to host may be through a variety of mechanisms, including the following:

1   Simple transmission from host to host through the external environment, for example, in airborne water droplets, e.g. the viruses that cause the common cold and influenza can be transmitted by sneezing.

2   Transmission from host to host through intimate contact involving exchange of body fluids, e.g. sexually-transmitted bacteria, viruses and protistans.

3   No direct transmission between hosts, but infection occurs by contact of a new host with intermediate stages of the parasite in the external environment; e.g. the anthrax and tetanus bacteria can be transmitted in soil.

4   Transmission by vectors or intermediate hosts in which development and reproduction of the microparasite may or may not occur, e.g. the malarial parasite is transmitted by mosquitoes, typhus is transmitted by lice, and the worms that cause schistosomiasis (bilharzia) are transmitted by snails.[3]

The extraordinary variety of the organisms that infect and infest people around the world helps to explain their great importance for human survival.

The impact of infectious diseases on human survival

A major effect of many infectious diseases is that they reduce the survival of their human hosts, either by killing people directly, or by debilitating them so that they become more susceptible to other infections, or by limiting their capacity to work and hence acquire the means of subsistence. Figure 5.5 shows the general shape of *survival curves* for humans living in a prosperous, industrial society and in a poor, developing country in recent times. The difference between the two is largely attributable to the impact of infectious diseases, exacerbated by malnutrition, in the developing world.

□ What aspects of survival are similar in the two populations shown in Figure 5.5, and what aspects are different?

■ The maximum survival in the two populations is very similar, at 90 and 85 years. The main difference lies in the survival rate during the first five years of life. This is much lower in the developing country's population, with the result that a much smaller proportion of those born survive to reproductive age.

Differences such as these between developed and developing countries are generally much less marked today than they were 20 years ago. The important point about the general shape of the curves in Figure 5.5 is that they show that, from one part of the world to another, or from one period of human history to another, infectious diseases can have a varying effect on the *age structure* of the human population.[4]

[3]The life cycles of the malarial parasite and of the worms that cause schistosomiasis (bilharzia) are illustrated in *World Health and Disease*, Chapter 3.

[4]Population age structure is discussed in *Studying Health and Disease* (1994 edition), Chapter 7, and in *World Health and Disease*, Chapter 2.

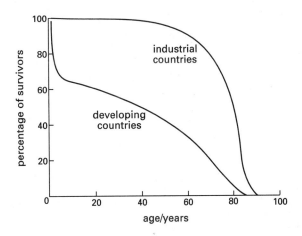

Figure 5.5   *Survival curves showing the percentage of individuals living to a given age in a prosperous industrial country and in a poor developing country. (Source: Begon, M., Harper, J. L. and Townsend, C. R., 1990,* Ecology: Individuals, Populations and Communities, *2nd edn, Blackwell Scientific Publications, Oxford, Figure 12.19(b), p. 418; adapted from Bradley, D. J., 1977, in* Origins of Pest, Parasite, Disease and Weed Problems, *ed. Cherrett, J. M. and Sagar, G. P., Blackwell Scientific Publications, Oxford.)*

Parasites may adversely affect the reproductive success of their host in a variety of ways. Some kill their host before it reaches reproductive age, while others allow the host to survive but cause infertility; some reduce the host's life expectancy or cause reproduction to be delayed to later in the host's life, so that it produces fewer offspring. However, the survival of the pathogen species depends on an adequate population of hosts surviving long enough for the pathogen to reproduce and be transmitted to new hosts. This brings us to the central aspects of existence!

Life, sex, death and disease

Viewed from an evolutionary perspective, in the life of an individual organism there are two fundamental events, reproduction and death. These reflect the two components of biological *fitness*, survival and reproductive success, survival being (in essence) the delaying of death.

□ Can you recall, from Chapter 3, what the word 'fitness' means in a biological context?

■ It is a measure of the lifetime reproductive success of an individual, usually expressed in relative terms. For example, an individual that leaves six surviving offspring who themselves survive to reproduce has twice the fitness of one that produces and raises three.

Life histories

The pattern and timing of reproduction and death during the lifespan of an organism are called its **life history**, and *life-history theory* seeks to explain how the very different life histories of different species have evolved by natural selection. It examines such questions as why individuals of some species are short-lived, while those of others are long-lived; why some species reproduce only once in their lives and others do it several times. In answering such questions, life-history theory seeks to address the general hypothesis that different kinds of life history are *adaptations* to particular features of the environment of the species under consideration.

Of major concern in the study of life histories is the reproductive 'schedule' which is characteristic of a species. Some species breed early in life, others delay breeding until they are relatively old. Some produce several young at each breeding episode, others a few or only one. In comparison with other animals, humans are late breeders, breed several times and produce a small number of young at each breeding episode.

Most animals and plants die soon after breeding or, put another way, continue to breed until they die. The timing of death in a given species depends a lot on whether or not there is parental care of the young. Some species of salmon, which do not care for their young, die immediately after spawning, but in many other fishes and in most mammals and birds a protracted period of post-natal feeding and care is essential for the survival of the young. Death of the parents does not occur, except by disease or predation, until the rearing of their offspring has been completed. A very unusual feature of the human life cycle is that women have a protracted period of post-reproductive life that continues long after all the children have become independent (a point we return to in Chapter 8 when we consider human ageing). In this chapter, we are concerned with the question of why organisms die when they do; indeed, why do they die at all?

A superficial interpretation of the theory of natural selection suggests that the fittest organisms would be those with the highest *fecundity*, i.e. those that produce the greatest number of surviving progeny in the shortest possible time; in the words of Oscar Wilde, 'nothing succeeds like excess'. We might expect evolution, therefore, to have produced a 'super-organism' that shows all the life-history features that confer high fitness.

□ What might these features be?

■ Such an organism would reproduce soon after birth, producing large numbers of progeny, and would continue to do so throughout an extremely long life. It would out-compete any competitor, would be highly efficient at finding food, would ward off all predators, and be resistant to all diseases.

Such super-organisms do not exist, and nor could they, for a number of reasons, of which we shall consider two.

Consider, first, the specific question 'Why do organisms die?'. The evolution of death is an interesting problem, about which there are several theories. One such theory argues that natural selection cannot prevent death because it cannot eliminate certain kinds of *genes*. Genes that cause death *before* an individual has reproduced are, obviously, not passed on to progeny and so are eliminated by natural selection whenever they arise by mutation. However, genes that cause death *after* reproduction has begun are passed on to the progeny and thus persist in the gene pool of the species. (The term 'gene pool' refers to all the genes carried by all the individuals of a population or a species, as defined in Chapter 4.) Put another way, the capacity of natural selection to eliminate harmful genes becomes weaker as an organism progresses through the reproductive phase of its life. According to this argument, death is an inevitable *consequence* of natural selection, but it is not an *adaptation*, that is, a characteristic that has been favoured by natural selection.

The second, more general, reason why super-organisms cannot evolve invokes the concept of *trade-offs* between one component of a life history and another. Trade-offs arise because the resources organisms need in order to survive and reproduce, such as food, water and energy, are often in limited supply, at least for part of an organism's life cycle. This shortage arises largely because individuals, of the same and of different species, are sometimes in competition with one another for such resources. Given a finite supply of resources that they have managed to acquire, organisms have to make what amount to life-history 'decisions'. A major decision is how much of their available resources should be allocated to bodily survival and growth (*somatic* effort) and how much to reproduction (*reproductive* effort). An individual that puts everything it has into reproduction may not have enough left to survive to another breeding episode, whereas one that limits its reproductive output at its first breeding episode may have enough left to survive and then breed again.

☐ Humans typically have one child at a time, though twins and triplets occur occasionally. What trade-offs do you think might be involved that prevent twins becoming the norm for humans?

■ There are at least two possible trade-offs to be considered. First, space in the womb and nutritive resources for the developing fetus or fetuses are limited, leading to twins typically being born prematurely and each being smaller than single babies. The apparent two-fold advantage of producing twins may be offset by their post-natal survival chances being reduced as a result of their smaller size. Second, babies have to be fed by their mother. The effort of feeding twins may cause a delay before the next breeding episode can be undertaken. Thus, the reproductive success of a woman having one baby at a time at short intervals may be greater than that of a woman having pairs of twins at longer intervals.

As a result of many trade-offs such as these, various aspects of the life history of organisms tend to be associated with one another. So, for example, animals that breed only once tend to have a large number of young during their single breeding episode and to be short-lived, whereas those (like ourselves) that breed several times tend to produce a small number of progeny per breeding episode and to be long-lived.

Small animals usually breed early in life and die young; large animals are older when they first breed and tend to live long, although there are exceptions to these general rules. As a general rule, small, short-lived, fast-breeding animals and plants, pursue what is often called a 'boom and bust' life history, and are found in environments that are unpredictable or unstable, and in those habitats where there are a large number of competing species. Large, long-lived, slow-breeding species are more typical of environments that are stable over long periods and in which the level of competition between species is relatively low. Like all generalisations in biology, however, there are many exceptions to this general rule.

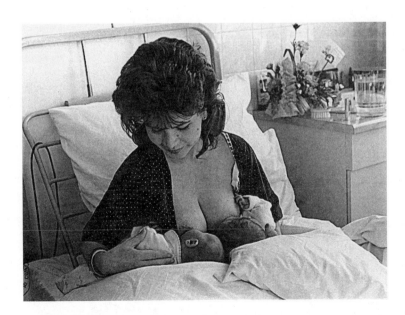

The reproductive success of a woman having one baby at a time at short intervals may be greater than that of a woman having pairs of twins at longer intervals. In industrialised countries the advantage of single births is very small. (Photo: Mike Levers)

Vulnerable stages in the life history

Many diseases and other causes of death typically occur most often at particular stages in the life history of a certain species. For example, young individuals are particularly vulnerable to infectious disease; hence the low survival of humans up to five years in developing countries (as shown in the survival curve in Figure 5.5). There are two major reasons for this pattern.

First, young individuals have not had the opportunity to develop **immunity** to common pathogens. Many infectious diseases, such as measles and whooping cough, can affect individuals at any age but, typically, are 'diseases of childhood'. This is because once an individual has recovered from the first episode of infection, he or she is never susceptible to that pathogen again. The person is said to be *immune* to that type of pathogen. (The mechanisms by which this occurs are discussed in Chapter 6.) Some young individuals who have not yet developed immunity succumb to an infection and die. Second, early life is a period of rapid growth requiring abundant food that, in a harsh, unpredictable environment, may not be available. In many species, including our own, high mortality early in life is due partly due to malnutrition leading to increased vulnerability to infection.[5]

Once the early growth stage is completed, the survival curve for most species declines much less rapidly. The next vulnerable stage in the life history is during reproduction. This exposes animals to disease risks peculiar to reproduction, in the form of sexually transmitted diseases (STDs). An interesting feature of STDs such as syphilis and gonorrhoea is that individuals do not develop immunity to them and can be reinfected again and again. STDs typically do not kill their hosts immediately but may have a debilitating effect leading to premature death. Very little is known about STDs in other animals and so it is not clear whether the effects that they have on humans are typical of animals generally. STDs are known for some plants; they are carried from flower to flower by pollinating insects.

Reproduction is also typically very stressful for animals, particularly for females, though often also for males. In red deer (*Cervus elephas*), for example, the autumnal mating period, or rut, involves intense fighting among stags which leaves some of them injured or so weakened that they are unable to survive the winter. Females may be so weakened by feeding their calves that they are unable to breed in the following year.

[5]See *World Health and Disease*, Chapter 11.

☐ Patterns such as these have echoes in human lives. Can you suggest some parallels?

■ As described in Chapter 2, birth in humans is more stressful than it is in the majority of primates. Some male violence against other males is undoubtedly linked to sexual competition.

Finally, old age is a period of increasing susceptibility to infectious disease and therefore reduced expectation of survival. In old age, the immune system generally becomes less and less capable of coping with infections, as you will see in Chapter 6.

We turn now to the question of how these life-history relationships between humans and their pathogens may have evolved

The evolution of host–pathogen relationships

As described in Chapter 3, bacteria may have been among the first organisms to evolve on Earth. We can speculate that they lived suspended in a slurry of mud and water containing a variety of chemical compounds, which provided the raw materials to support their survival, growth and reproduction. Much later in evolution, a few of the descendants of these early life-forms had new environments to invade, which offered a much more hospitable habitat than the 'primeval soup'. This new environment was inside the cells and organs of multi-celled animals and plants, a protected place, full of nutrients. In such a favourable environment, micro-organisms are able to reproduce at a very high rate.

A bacterium that infects a human may generate several dozen generations within a single day. For example, the time that it takes for a common inhabitant of the large intestines of mammals, the bacterium *Escherichia coli* (known as *E. coli* for short), to complete the process of reproduction is 20 minutes under optimal conditions. Put another way, the **generation time** of *E. coli* is just 20 minutes. Many pathogenic bacteria can reproduce just as quickly. (*E. coli* sometimes occurs in pathogenic forms and can cause severe outbreaks of diarrhoea.) If hosts are not to be swiftly overwhelmed in the face of the massive reproductive potential of pathogens, they must have effective defenses in the form of an *immune system*.

The differential between the very short generation time of a microscopic pathogen and the relatively long generation time of its host has profound implications for the evolution of the relationship between them. During the course of its host's life, a pathogen living within it can

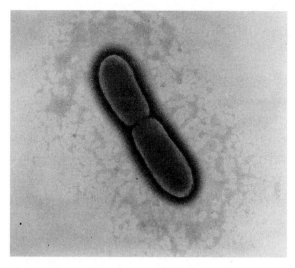

The bacterium Escherichia coli *takes only 20 minutes to grow and divide into two bacterial cells, as in this photograph taken with an electron microscope (magnified 40 000 times). (Photo: Heather Davies)*

complete many hundreds or thousands of generations and may therefore actually *evolve,* becoming better and better adapted to life in its host and acquiring ever-improving counter-defenses against the defenses of its host.

> ☐ What are the two main processes underlying the ability of an organism to evolve and adapt (become fitter) in a given environment, as described in Chapters 3 and 4?

> ■ They are *mutation,* random changes in the sequence of nucleotides in the organism's DNA, which are passed on to its offspring in the gametes, and *natural selection,* which ensures that advantageous genes gradually spread throughout a population over many generations.

Under pressure from the reproductive advantage of micro-organisms, the immune systems of larger animals have evolved enormous flexibility, which gives the host some chance to counter any new varieties of pathogen that evolve. In recent times, these 'natural' defences have been reinforced by artificially-produced chemicals, which (in some cases) have changed the balance of survival in favour of the host species. For example, in the middle years of the twentieth century, the incidence of malaria world-wide was greatly reduced through the use of drugs to combat the malarial parasite itself and of insecticides that killed the mosquitoes which transmitted

it to humans. However, both the rapidly-reproducing parasite and its mosquito vector have evolved resistance to these compounds; this is one reason why malaria is returning to areas until recently declared free of infection.

The consequences of the great differential between pathogen and host reproductive rates are of great concern to an evolutionary biologist. Viewed from this perspective, there are three important facets of host–pathogen relationships.

1   The association is often very intimate. Pathogens typically possess a number of adaptations that enable them to maintain a position in or on their host and to resist all the host's efforts to remove them. For example, different species of mammals have fleas and lice with grasping limbs specifically adapted to clasp the hair of their host species (Chapter 2). Thus cat fleas cannot maintain a secure grip on human hair. Pathogenic organisms of all kinds are adapted to resist the defensive responses of their host's immune system (as you will see in Chapter 6).

2   The pathogen is largely or wholly dependent on its host for the resources that it requires for survival, growth and reproduction. A major problem for pathogens is that, to reproduce, they, at some stage in their life cycle, must get to a new host before their current host dies. In many macroparasites, dispersal is effected by means of one or more vector species.

3   The activities of the pathogen, to varying degrees, reduce the fitness of the host by reducing its survival and/or reducing its reproductive success. In extreme instances a pathogen may kill its host.

The harm caused by pathogens to their hosts is very variable, both within and between species. Within a host species, there are typically individuals that are totally unaffected by a particular pathogen, others that have slight infestations that cause little or no impact on their fitness, and some that are seriously debilitated or killed. Between species, there is a spectrum of effects from organisms that are generally benign, such as most types of gut bacteria (e.g. *E. coli*), to those that are generally lethal, such as the human immunodeficiency virus (HIV).

Such is the specificity and intimacy of the relationship between pathogens and their hosts, that it is clear that each has become adapted in many ways to the other, an example of what is called **coevolution.** Coevolution refers to specific, reciprocal adaptations between two or a few species, that have evolved through prolonged, intricate interaction between those species. Coevolution between hosts and pathogens, one or both of which has a harmful effect on the other, is often likened to the human arms race, because any adaptation by one side that increases its effectiveness tends to lead to counter-adaptations by the other side. This analogy is a poor one, however, because, in the natural world, coevolution commonly leads to adaptations by each organism that reduce, rather than increase, its harmful effects on the other.

Pathogens vary in the degree to which they harm their hosts, a property called **virulence**. The virulence of a particular pathogen is measured as the percentage of infections that lead to death. Among human pathogens, that which causes cholera can have a virulence of 15 per cent (i.e. 15 per cent of infected people die), that causing dysentery 6 per cent. These two were among the most virulent of human pathogens until the advent of HIV, which has a virulence close to 100 per cent.

Any new mutation arising in the host, which causes it to be more resistant to a pathogen, or mutations in the pathogen causing it to be more virulent, has the effect of altering the relationship between them. This leads to evolutionary changes in the other 'partner' in that relationship. If the pathogen becomes more virulent, the host must evolve greater resistance or die out; if the host evolves a more effective immune response, the pathogen evolves counter-measures. For this reason, host–pathogen relationships are evolutionarily *unstable* and are subject to change over time, favouring one partner or the other at different times.

This instability becomes particularly apparent when a disease is passed from its usual host to a new host. For example, plague, which has devastated human populations many times during recorded history, is contracted from rats and other rodents, in some of which it is a far less lethal disease.

□ What is the term that is used for such diseases?

■ They are called zoonoses (Chapter 2).

Other examples of diseases that are more harmful to humans than to their natural hosts are rabies (which originated in foxes), yellow fever (which originated in monkeys) and brucellosis (which originated in cattle). These and other examples suggest that host–pathogen relationships tend to evolve towards a situation in which *both* organisms can coexist without the host being affected as severely as it once was. Is this due to evolutionary changes in the host, the parasite or both?

Coevolution in action: myxomatosis

The history of myxomatosis provides some answers to this question. The *Myxoma* virus is indigenous to South America and rabbits there are prone to the disease, which produces fibrous lesions on the skin, but do not usually die from it. The virus was unknown in other parts of the world until it was deliberately introduced into Australia in 1950 in an attempt to control the rabbit population, which threatened the livelihood of sheep farmers. Rabbits had themselves been introduced to Australia from Europe in the nineteenth century and had undergone a population explosion.

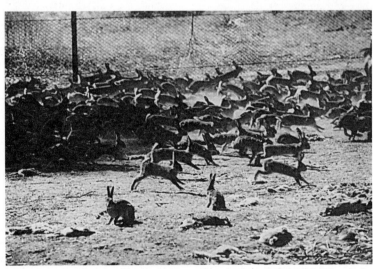

Faced with abundant food and few natural predators, rabbits introduced into Australia from Europe in the late nineteenth century underwent a population explosion which, by the mid-twentieth century, was devastating farm land. (Photo courtesy of Dr Roger Trout)

Carried by mosquitoes, the newly-introduced *Myxoma* virus caused an epidemic that killed 99.8 per cent of all rabbits; a second epidemic killed 90 per cent of the generation that resulted from those that survived the first. A third epidemic, however, killed only 50 per cent of the remaining rabbits. This rapid decline in the virulence of myxomatosis was due both to the rabbits evolving resistance to the virus, and to the virus evolving reduced virulence.

☐ Why do you suppose that reduced virulence might be *adaptive* for the *Myxoma* virus (i.e. improve its chances of surviving long enough to reproduce)?

■ A pathogen that does not kill its host has greater opportunity itself to survive, reproduce and infect new hosts than one that kills its host quickly. At the point when it had reduced the host population by 99.8 per cent, the *Myxoma* virus must itself have been at some risk of becoming extinct.

Transmission routes and the evolution of virulence

It appears to be a feature of some host–pathogen relationships that, during evolution, they have changed from being one of true parasitism towards one of commensalism (recall Table 5.1). It has been widely assumed that there is a general trend during evolution for pathogens to become less virulent, but this view is erroneous. There are other directions in which pathogens may evolve.

An alternative adaptive solution to the pathogen's problem of getting from one host to another is to evolve the ability to survive for a long period outside the host. For example, the bacillus (a rod-shaped bacterium) that causes anthrax, a highly virulent disease, can survive in soil, in a dormant state, for many years. The small island of Gruinard off the coast of Scotland was uninhabitable for more than 40 years after it was used for testing the anthrax bacillus as a biological weapon in World War II. A pathogen with the ability to survive outside its host, and which can thus survive if its host has become rare, does not need to adapt to the problem posed by a reduced host population by evolving decreased virulence. By contrast, a pathogen that cannot survive independently for long (like *Myxoma*) can adapt to a shortage of hosts by evolving reduced virulence.

The mode of transmission between hosts may be a key factor in the evolution of virulence. Parasites that are carried by vectors tend to be more virulent than those that are passed directly from host to host; if their hosts become rare, they can survive for some time within the vector.

Where evolution *does* appear to have led to decreased virulence is in pathogens that are passed directly from host to host, by direct contact or through the air, such as the rhinoviruses that cause the common cold (Chapter 2). If such pathogens were to make their hosts very ill so that they had to 'go to bed' and thus engage in much less social contact, the transmission of the pathogen to new hosts would be greatly reduced. Rhinoviruses and other pathogens that are transmitted directly tend to have low virulence. There are exceptions, however, to this generalisation; anthrax is one and HIV (the human immunodeficiency virus) is another.

☐ HIV remains dormant in the body for several years without causing any symptoms. How might this be an adaptive feature of this virus?

■ The long period of dormancy allows more opportunities for it to be passed from person to person than would be the case for a pathogen that debilitates or kills its host soon after infection.

Medical and social intervention can influence the evolution of a pathogen's virulence, in either direction. For example, the increasing availability of purified water in parts of India in the 1950s and 1960s led to an evolutionary change in the water-borne cholera pathogen, *Vibrio cholerae*. This bacterium exists in two forms: the original form has a virulence of up to 15 per cent, but there is a less virulent 'El Tor' form of the bacterium, with a virulence of 2 per cent. As the water purification schemes progressed, the proportion of El Tor forms of cholera in India rose, but the original, more virulent form still persists in Bangladesh where water purification schemes have been delayed by natural disasters such as flooding, and lack of finance.

☐ Can you explain this phenomenon?

■ Water purification tilted the balance of survival against the more virulent bacteria, but the El Tor form increased in the population because its lower virulence allowed more opportunities for transmission between infectious individuals who (usually) did not die.

Conversely, there is evidence that attempts in hospitals in the USA to counter outbreaks of pathogenic *E. coli* with disinfectants have led to the evolution of more virulent strains. The virulence of *E. coli* ranges from 0 to 25 per cent. (See Ewald, 1993, in the Further Reading list at the end of this book for a more detailed discussion of these and other examples.)

Host–pathogen dynamics

Another common feature of host–pathogen interactions is that pathogens are distributed in the population such that the number of pathogens per host individual does not show a *normal distribution*, that is, one in which a majority of host individuals carry an average number of pathogens.[6] This is difficult to demonstrate with bacteria and viruses, but can easily be shown for visible ectoparasites such as the head louse.

□ Look at Figure 5.6. How are head lice distributed among individual people?

■ Their distribution is highly 'clumped', such that most individuals carry no lice, some carry a few, and only a small proportion are heavily infested.

There are a number of possible reasons for this distribution pattern, each of which may apply more or less in different cases. It may, for example, reflect the fact that it is difficult for pathogens to disperse from one host to another, with the result that infections only affect a restricted number of individuals living in a confined area. Another common factor is that pathogens may reproduce prolifically only in individual hosts that are already weakened by other factors such as starvation or another kind of infection. A third possibility is that a large proportion of the host population is resistant to the pathogen.

The dynamic properties of an infection by a pathogen, that is, the way the impact of the infection on the host changes over time, can be described and analysed by reference to certain properties of the host population. Every individual in the host population must belong to one of the following four categories, which are represented in Figure 5.7:

(i) *Susceptibles*: individuals who are capable of being infected, but have not been infected by the pathogen.

(ii) *Latents*: individuals who are currently infected with the pathogen, but do not show symptoms of infection. Individuals with latent infections may or may not be *infectious*, i.e. capable of passing the pathogen on to susceptibles. Some latents are not infectious because the pathogen has not yet produced infective stages; others are infectious even though symptomless.

(iii) *Symptomatic infected*: individuals who are currently infected with the pathogen, show symptoms of infection and are usually capable of passing the pathogen on to susceptibles.

[6]For an example of a normal distribution curve, look back at Figure 4.14 in Chapter 4.

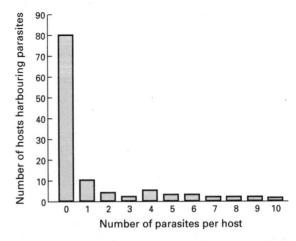

Figure 5.6 *The distribution across a population of people of the head louse* Pediculus humanis capitis. *(Adapted from Begon, M., Harper, L. J. and Townsend, C. R., 1990,* Ecology, *2nd edn, Blackwell Scientific Publications, Oxford, p. 407, Figure 12.13(b))*

(iv) *Immunes*: individuals that have previously been infected with the pathogen, have recovered from their symptoms and are now immune to that pathogen. Immunes may or may not still be carriers of an infection; if they are they can pass it on to susceptibles, as in the celebrated case of Typhoid Mary. She was a domestic cook named Mary Mallon, who worked in the USA at the turn of the century. In a ten-year period she is believed to have infected 54 people with typhoid, three of whom died. She always denied that she was the source of the infection.

Any one host individual may pass through all of categories (i) to (iv) during the course of its life, or may die at any stage (Figure 5.7a). If the individuals in the host population are adult, all can reproduce and replace members of the population that die. Deaths occur in all four categories, but only those in category (iii) can be the direct result of the disease caused by the pathogen. As discussed above, it is generally not adaptive for pathogens to kill their hosts early in the course of an infection.

□ If you were to draw a diagram like Figure 5.7 for HIV, a relatively new infection in the United Kingdom with a very high fatality rate, what would the relative proportions of the various segments look like, and why?

■ It should look something like Figure 5.8. HIV is of relatively recent origin, so in most Western populations the susceptibles segment is still very large; however, in some Third World cities it is much smaller than shown here, because a high proportion of the population are infected with HIV. The majority of infected individuals are in category (ii), the latents, who show no symptoms of HIV-related illness (the long period of dormancy of this virus was mentioned earlier), but *all* of these are believed to be infectious. The proportion of infected people who belong to category (iii), symptomatic infected, is small because of the high rate of fatality within a short time of symptoms developing. No one falls into category (iv) because, to date, no one is known to have developed immunity to HIV.[7]

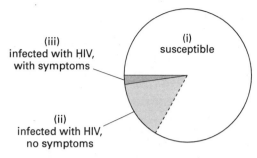

Figure 5.8 *The relative proportions of susceptible, latent (symptomless) and symptomatic individuals in a theoretical population, with respect to HIV, the human immunodeficiency virus. The proportions shown here vary enormously from one population to another, but the absence of immunes is common to all. Everyone with a latent HIV infection is believed to be infectious to susceptible individuals.*

The rate at which the number of hosts infected by a given parasite increases depends on a number of features of the parasite itself and on certain properties of the host population. For example, if the host population contains a high proportion of immunes and a low proportion of susceptibles, then the rate at which the parasite spreads is likely to fall. If the rate falls below that at which each parasite produces one surviving offspring in the next generation, the disease will become extinct.

☐ Under what circumstances do you suppose that these conditions would arise?

■ In the late stages of an epidemic, when most members of the host population have been infected by the parasite and, if they have not died, have become immune to it.

Thus, diseases to which humans can develop immunity tend to occur erratically, with epidemics separated by periods in which their impact is slight or negligible. By contrast, sexually-transmitted diseases, to which hosts do not become immune, persist in human populations at a more constant frequency. Immunisation programmes, by

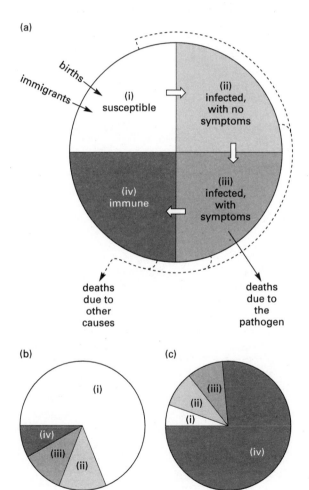

Figure 5.7 *(a) During the course of an infectious outbreak, an individual in the host population may pass through all of categories (i) to (iv), which are defined in the text. For most infectious diseases, the relative proportions of the four categories in the population of a host species are different in (b) an early stage of an epidemic, compared with (c) a late stage.*

[7]HIV and AIDS are discussed in another book in this series, *Experiencing and Explaining Disease* (Open University Press, revised edition 1995), and in a supplement for Open University students in 1994.

increasing the proportion of immune individuals in a population, greatly reduce the impact of a parasite and can sometimes eliminate it altogether. Such was the case with smallpox, which the World Health Organisation declared had been eradicated world-wide in 1980.

Latency, infectious periods and host density

If a pathogen has a long latent period and/or infectious period, as in the case of HIV, the transmission of the pathogen to relatively few new hosts in a widely dispersed population will adequately maintain its survival in the population.

> □ Can you explain why this is so?

> ■ The longer a pathogen has a hold on an individual, the more time there is to come into contact with potential new hosts, even if these are few and far between, so the greater is its chance of being transmitted to susceptibles.

In contrast, measles is a disease with a relatively short latent period (6–9 days) and an even shorter infectious period (6–7 days). Host density becomes a critical factor in the survival of such a pathogen. It has been calculated that measles can only persist in densely-populated human settlements of at least 300 000 to 400 000 people. Such large concentrations of people have existed for less than 2 000 years, suggesting that the measles virus has been a common and prevalent pathogen among humans for less than 100 generations, although it probably occurred sporadically for a long time before that. Two additional factors that affect the need for a high density of susceptible hosts are: individuals readily become immune to measles, and the measles virus is not readily transmitted from person to person, being very short-lived in the external environment.

> □ By contrast, a relatively *low* density of susceptible hosts is required to maintain sexually-transmitted infections in human populations. Can you suggest why?

> ■ There are three reasons. First, the mode of transmission, sexual contact, is affected very little by population density (humans manage to mate with one another whether they are living far apart or close together in dense aggregations). Second, transmission is very efficient, because the pathogen does not need to survive in the outside world at all. Third, immunity to most STDs is very weak (as mentioned earlier), so virtually everyone in the population who is not already infected is susceptible.

Macroparasites, such as flukes and tapeworms, tend to have very long latent and infectious periods; most species have a life expectancy of more than one year in the adult stage and produce eggs for most of their adult life. The nematode worm *Onchocerca volvulus*, which causes river blindness, lives for eight to ten years in humans. Because of their very long infectious periods, these macroparasites tend to be very persistent, and are prevalent even in very small and highly dispersed human populations.

Instability in host–pathogen relationships

Over long periods, in terms of tens or hundreds of years, the balance of relative advantage between a pathogen and its host changes; as a result, certain pathogenic diseases have had a greater impact on human populations at some times in history than at others. These fluctuations have many underlying causes, but two arise from the biology of the host species. Hosts have two distinct forms of defence against infectious disease, *resistance* and *immunity*, which must be considered on different time-scales.

Immunity was defined earlier, and is a property of an *individual*. It develops during the life of that individual and is not passed on to its progeny. **Resistance** is a property of a *species*, or of a *population*; it evolves by natural selection and is passed on from generation to generation. Resistance is largely a consequence of genes that contribute to a fast and effective immune response to common pathogens. Over many generations, natural selection favours those individuals that are most resistant to the common pathogens in that environment; resistant individuals have greater reproductive success than more adversely affected members of the population, and so the genes that contribute to the resistance have a greater chance of being passed on. Over time, genes that confer some resistance to infection spread through the host population.

The coevolution of host resistance and pathogen virulence

The example of myxomatosis, described above, is one in which greater resistance has evolved in the host, rabbits. This effect, combined with the evolution of decreased virulence in the virus, typically leads to a relatively stable state in which pathogen and host coexist, with only a relatively small proportion of the host population being adversely affected by the pathogen. This situation is not truly stable, however, because at any time a mutation may occur in the pathogen population, producing a more virulent form.

☐ What effect do you think this might have, over time, on the relationship between the pathogen and the host?

■ The more virulent form of the virus will spread through the host population, killing the least resistant individuals. Since only the most resistant survive to pass on their genes ('survival of the fittest'), this favours the gradual evolution of greater resistance in the host population as a whole. Eventually a stable state of coexistence between host and pathogen is restored, until the next significant mutation occurs in either.

The instability of host–pathogen relationships is of profound importance for medical and social intervention to reduce the incidence of infectious diseases. The fact that pathogens are continually evolving means that the 'war' against them may never be won. An example is provided by TB, which is discussed extensively in another book in this series.[8]

The bacterium *Mycobacterium tuberculosis* kills about three million people each year throughout the world and, in parts of some developing countries, infects about 95 per cent of the population. In the aftermath of World War II, TB was almost eliminated from most developed countries by improved nutrition and housing across the whole population, coupled with the use of drugs, vaccination and isolation of infected people. However, TB is now increasing in most countries of the world. There are a number of reasons for this increase, including the spread of another pathogen, HIV. People with a very poor immune response (whether due to HIV or some other cause such as chronic malnutrition) are more likely to develop infectious diseases, including TB.

A change in the TB bacterium itself has contributed to its increased prevalence. Strains of the TB bacterium that are resistant to all drugs have evolved in recent years, known as multi-drug resistant (MDR) strains. The evolution of drug-resistant strains has occurred in many different types of pathogenic bacteria, and in *Plasmodium*, the malarial parasite, a fact which has contributed to its increase in parts of the world where malaria had been eradicated. The existence of drug-resistant strains of bacteria provides the basis for the fact that, if you are prescribed antibiotics to treat an infection, you are strongly exhorted to 'finish the bottle', that is, to continue taking the antibiotic after your symptoms have been alleviated.

[8]*Medical Knowledge: Doubt and Certainty* (revised edition, 1994), Chapter 4.

☐ Can you explain the rationale for this instruction, based on your knowledge of natural selection and the discussion (above) of the evolution of resistance?

■ Among the population of bacteria infecting a person, there will typically be much variation between individual bacteria in their degree of resistance to a given antibiotic. The first few doses of the drug will kill the least resistant bacteria, leading to a rapid alleviation of the symptoms, but more resistant bacteria will remain alive. These may eventually be killed by subsequent doses of antibiotic. People who do not finish a course of antibiotics risk a renewed bout of the disease, caused by a population increase among the more resistant bacteria that have not been killed at the beginning of the course of treatment. Such people are also carriers of those resistant bacteria, which can be passed on to others. Over time, with repeated but inadequate prescription of a common antibiotic, strains of bacteria can evolve which are completely resistant to it.

Cyclic outbreaks of infection

Diseases to which hosts develop immunity, such as measles, typically show cyclic outbreaks (Figure 5.9) because, during each outbreak, a large proportion of the host population becomes immune.

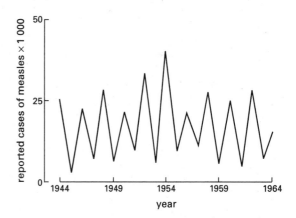

Figure 5.9 *Reported cases of measles in New York City from 1944 to 1964. (Source: Begon, M., Harper, J. L. and Townsend, C. R., 1990,* Ecology: Individuals, Populations and Communities, *Blackwell Scientific Publications, Oxford; after Yorke, J. A. and London, W.P., 1973, Recurrent outbreaks of measles, chickenpox and mumps, II Systematic differences in contact rates and stochastic effects,* American Journal of Epidemiology, ***98***, pp. 469–482)*

When the proportion of immunes relative to susceptibles in the population is high (as shown earlier, in Figure 5.7c), the prevalence of the pathogen inevitably declines. It does not usually die out, however, because new susceptibles are being added to the host population.

□ There are two sources of new susceptibles: what are they?

■ New hosts are born who have not been exposed to the pathogen and so have not developed immunity. Immigration from other host populations brings in non-immune individuals from areas where the disease is not present.

The incidence of measles in New York shows a two-year cycle. This is much shorter than is typical for viral infections in natural populations, and is probably due to the high rates of immigration of people into this large population centre.

The impact of cultural evolution on resistance to infection

Another source of instability in host–pathogen relationships arises from the fact that a pathogen sometimes invades a new host species, which has no evolutionary history of interaction with it and, hence, has not evolved resistance. As mentioned above, and in Chapter 2, several human pathogens are thought to be derived from animal parasites. It has been suggested that HIV is derived from a virus of monkeys, for example. As described earlier, these *zoonotic* diseases are especially virulent in their newly-acquired human hosts, who have not had time to evolve effective resistance.

Various aspects of the inherent instability of the relationship between humans and their pathogens are well-illustrated by the history of infectious diseases introduced to North America from the Old World, a process that began with the arrival of Christopher Columbus in October 1492 (the article by Meltzer, 1992, listed under Further Reading tells the story). Following the arrival of Europeans, more native Americans died of a variety of infections than were born, a situation that has not been reversed until very recently. Estimates for the native American population in 1492 range from two to 18 million; by the end of the nineteenth century it had fallen to 530 000. (These figures refer to pure-bred native

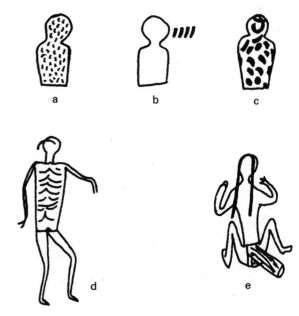

These Sioux Indian drawings were used to record the numbers who died primarily in epidemics of infectious diseases imported by European colonists and as a result of starvation through land loss. They represent (a) measles, (b) whooping cough, (c) smallpox, (d) starvation, and (e) cholera. (From American Indian Holocaust and Survival: A Population History Since 1492 *By Russell Thornton. Copyright © 1987 by the University of Oklahoma Press, Norman, Oklahoma and London, Figure 4.2, p. 81)*

Americans; there were, and still are, many people descended from matings between native Americans and Europeans.) The diseases that devastated the native American population included smallpox, measles, influenza, bubonic plague, diphtheria, typhus, cholera, scarlet fever, chicken pox, yellow fever and whooping cough.

This raises two questions. The more obvious one is: why did native Americans have so little resistance to the pathogens that caused these diseases? The less obvious question is: why did the invading Europeans not contract infectious diseases from the native Americans? The answers are thought to lie in the rather different cultural histories of the two human populations *before* they collided in 1492.

As described in Chapter 2, a critical stage in the social evolution of humans was the gradual abandoning of the hunter-gatherer form of subsistence, and the development of village life, with people forming dense populations in permanent settlements. Several species of wild animals were domesticated, including pigs, cattle and chickens, from which humans contracted certain infectious diseases. Smallpox is believed to be derived from cowpox, measles from rinderpest (a disease of cattle) or canine distemper, and influenza from viruses that originated in pigs. Over hundreds of years, these new diseases had sporadically devastating effects on settled agricultural and pastoral populations; large numbers of people died in epidemics, such as the Black Death (plague) in Europe in the fourteenth century. But the individuals who survived infection had a high level of resistance to the new diseases; as a result, settled populations of humans came to coexist in a broadly stable relationship with the pathogens derived originally from their domestic animals.

The transition from hunter-gatherer to agricultural and pastoral societies did not happen everywhere at once. It occurred much earlier in the regions we know today as Africa and Europe than it did in Asia. Evidence from the nature of their language, from anatomical features, and from analysis of their genes, suggests that native Americans originally came from Asia, crossing to America by a land bridge across what is now the Bering Strait about 11 500 years ago. They settled in a land that had a very diverse range of large mammals, such as mammoths, giant sloths, lions, sabre-tooth tigers, and bears. Some 10 800 years ago, 80 per cent of these large mammal species became extinct.

There is much debate as to whether these extinctions were caused by hunting by humans, or were due to climatic change, or a combination of the two. Whatever the cause, Meltzer suggests that one outcome of these extinctions was a shortage of species suitable for domestication by the 'immigrant' human population. Most of the surviving mammal species, such as the American bison, could not easily be domesticated and, in any case, were so abundant that they could easily be obtained by hunting. Native Americans, as a result, did not domesticate animals and so did not acquire infectious diseases from them or evolve any resistance to their pathogens.

The European explorers, then, brought to North America a wide range of infectious diseases, of relatively recent origin, to which the native Americans had never been exposed. Their lack of a history of domestication of animals meant that they had few unusual pathogens of their own with which they could return the compliment.

From this story emerge some interesting points about the *rate* at which host–pathogen relationships evolve. When a new pathogen enters a new host population, it tends to cause very high mortality, especially if the host population is very dense and the infection is transmitted directly. The resultant rapid decline in the size of the host population creates what is called a *genetic bottleneck*. The small population that survives a very serious epidemic contains a very high proportion of individuals that have high resistance to the pathogen, because they are descended from genetically-resistant parents. As a result, as the host population increases again, it has a much higher level of resistance than before the epidemic. This is exactly the same as the situation we described earlier for the evolution of drug-resistant strains of bacteria.

Total resistance, however, does not evolve. There is always variation in resistance among individuals in the host population, and genetic variation in virulence in the pathogen population, leading to the kind of unstable situation described above, in which minor outbreaks occur from time to time as mutations arise and more virulent varieties emerge among the pathogen population. The evolution of host–pathogen relationships tends therefore to be a slow process, with erratic shifts one way and then the other, punctuated by periods in which, through population crashes and genetic bottlenecks, evolutionary change may be very rapid in the short-term (Figure 5.10, *overleaf*).

During the coevolution of a pathogen and its host, adaptation by one and counter-adaptation by the other lead quite rapidly (in evolutionary terms) to their coming to coexist in unstable equilibrium. During the course of evolution, a single host species may undergo a series of events like that summarised in Figure 5.10, so that a host coexists with a large number of different pathogen species, with some of which it has an ancient association, with others a more recent one. We turn next to examine the long-term evolutionary results of this interaction between host species and a succession of diverse pathogenic parasites.[9] It may surprise you to learn that sexual reproduction may have evolved as a consequence of our relationship with pathogens.

---

[9]The material presented in this and the preceding section provides only a brief overview of a large and complex topic. A more extensive account of the evolution of human infectious disease is provided by Dobson (1992) and in greater detail by Anderson and May (1991).

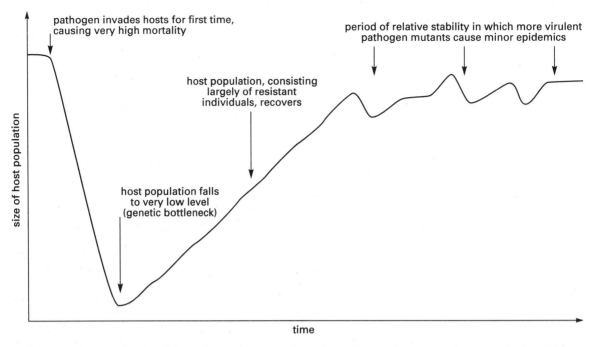

Figure 5.10 *Schematic diagram of the evolution of a parasite–host relationship over time.* (Remember to turn back to finish reading page 117.)

The evolution of sex

A current, unresolved problem in evolutionary biology is the evolution of sex. Relatively few pathogens reproduce sexually, that is, by the fusion of gametes from a male and a female (Chapter 4), but do so by some form of *asexual* reproduction, such as dividing into two. (There are many different methods of asexual reproduction, but they do not concern us here.) Many macroparasites, such as the tapeworm, reproduce sexually at some times in their life history, asexually at others. What evolutionary pressures determine which form of reproduction occurs?

□ Consider a female in a sexually-reproducing species.Whenever she reproduces, she passes on 50 per cent of her genes to each of her progeny, the other 50 per cent being provided by their father, or fathers. If she were to abandon sex and produce young asexually, what effect would this have on her offspring's genotype?

■ Each of them would contain 100 per cent of her genes. Thus, an asexual female in a normally sexual population has a two-fold advantage over other females: she passes her genes on to the next generation twice as effectively.

This leads to the general argument that, at the level of *individual* organisms, natural selection should favour asexual reproduction over sexual reproduction. This fundamental 'cost of sex' is often referred to as the cost of producing males. Much of the current debate amongst biologists about the evolution of sex is directed at identifying advantages that could offset this fundamental disadvantage of sexual reproduction.

Sexual reproduction differs from asexual reproduction in two important respects when viewed from an evolutionary perspective. First, as described in Chapter 4, the production of gametes (eggs and sperm) involves a form of nuclear division called *meiosis*, in which *half* the genes in the egg-producing or sperm-producing cell are passed on to each new gamete. Because the genes can be divided into a huge number of different 'halves', this generates great diversity in the genotype of each egg or sperm that a single individual can produce. Second, the fusion of two gametes, from genetically different parents, creates completely new combinations of genes. As a result of these two processes, sexual reproduction produces offspring that are much more genetically diverse than those produced by asexual reproduction. Asexually-produced progeny are genetically almost identical to their single parent and to one another ('almost' because small errors can occur when the genes are copied before cell division).

In the coevolution of pathogens and hosts, pathogens have a distinct advantage, as noted earlier. They typically have a very short generation time and a very high reproductive rate; a bacterium in the human gut can generate several dozen generations in a single day. Bacteria and viruses typically reproduce asexually and so show very little genetic variation between individuals of the same type. Their genotype is subject to mutation, however, so there is *some* genetic variation on which natural selection can act. Certain viruses, such as HIV and influenza virus, have very high mutation rates and so generate many, slightly different 'strains'. As a result, pathogens can evolve, that is become better adapted to the defences of their host, *within the lifetime of their host*. This is the key to the disadvantage of asexual reproduction among host species.

☐ Can you suggest what it is?

■ If the host reproduces asexually, it produces offspring genetically identical to itself and for which there is, therefore, a population of pathogens that are already adapted to infect it.

No such population of 'ideal' hosts (from the pathogen's viewpoint) is available if the host reproduces genetically-variable offspring by sexual reproduction. The hypothesis, then, is that sexual reproduction is an adaptation against pathogenic organisms. It ensures that at least some progeny are produced that are less susceptible to attack by those pathogens that have evolved during the lifetime of their parents.

Another important role for pathogenic parasites in the evolution of their hosts has been identified in the context of host sexual behaviour. W. D. Hamilton and Marlene Zuk published a highly influential paper in 1982 in which they suggested that exclusively male characteristics in certain species, such as bright coloration, elaborate visual displays, courtship songs, mating calls and odours, often act as 'revealing handicaps'. The argument is, first, that animals are subject to potentially debilitating parasites; second, that resistance to such parasites is heritable; and, third, that only those individual males that are resistant to parasites are able to express their sex-related characteristics fully. Consequently, females should evolve a mating preference for those males that have the best-developed sexual characteristics, because the offspring that result from such matings are likely to inherit greater resistance to parasites from their father. In recent years, numerous studies of a diverse array of animal species have demonstrated that females

do prefer those males with the most highly-developed sexual characteristics. Examples include long tail plumes in birds, complex calls in frogs and bright coloration in fishes. A number of studies have confirmed the predicted relationship between such characteristics and parasite infestations but, to date, only a small number of studies have confirmed that females preferring males with well-developed sexual characteristics produce progeny that are relatively free of parasites.

This line of argument has recently been taken further than accounting for the evolution of sex, by addressing the question 'What value are males?'. In many animal species, males make no contribution to reproduction other than the provision of sperm. In such species, there is typically intense competition among males for access to females, with a relatively small proportion of males actually mating, either as a result of being successful in fights with other males or by being very attractive to females. To achieve matings, males have to undertake energetically very demanding activities, like fighting and prolonged courtship, and only a few are successful. Males can thus be regarded as a 'dispensable caste' whose genotypes are 'screened' for disadvantageous genes during energetic sex-related behaviour.

At first sight, these arguments are of little, if any, obvious direct relevance to humans, though the general question 'What value are males?' is not without interest in a human context! Human males do not develop the kind of extravagant sex-related characteristics that are seen, for example, in peacocks and birds of paradise. Furthermore, at least during the early stages of human evolution, men probably contributed more to reproduction than the donation of sperm to women, though modern people vary greatly in the extent to which fathers contribute materially or culturally to raising their children.

Men and women do, however, look different; they show a number of secondary sexual characteristics that distinguish the two sexes. As described in Chapter 2, these differences are based largely on differences in the skeleton, the distribution of adipose tissue (fat), and patterns of hair growth. To some extent, these differences reflect the different roles of men and women in reproduction; the wider hips of women are an adaptation for giving birth to babies with large heads, for example. However, it is widely argued that certain sex differences in humans have become 'exaggerated' during evolution because of their role in sexual attraction. This process is called **sexual selection**, which is a form of natural selection that favours any characteristics that enhance an individual's ability, not to survive, but to obtain matings.

For example, adult women differ from all other mammals in having prominent mammary glands (breasts) at times when they are not feeding babies. In many cultures, breasts are attractive to men; evolutionary theory suggests that they have evolved as a 'permanent fixture' outside feeding periods because they increase the female's chance of obtaining a mate and passing on her genes. Yet more controversial is the suggestion that female sexual preferences may have favoured in men the accentuation of characteristics commonly identified by heterosexual women as being sexually-attractive. The fact that these characteristics vary somewhat from one population to another does not undermine the theory. Thus, while humans are clearly not as flamboyant in their secondary sexual characteristics as peacocks, they may, by a similar process, have evolved sex differences for which the sole basis is sexual attraction.

Biodiversity and the place of micro-organisms

The inevitable focus on human infectious disease in this chapter may have further reinforced the widespread misconception that micro-organisms are generally harmful to other life-forms. Bacteria in particular among the micro-organisms have had a bad 'image', which is at odds with their essential role in maintaining the rich diversity of life on Earth. Here we step back from the emphasis on disease and consider the diversity of organisms and their life styles and life histories. What is the relative importance of humans and micro-organisms in the wider scheme of things?

The word **biodiversity** has become part of the lexicon of environmentalism and 'green' politics in recent years. What does it mean? Crudely, it refers to the fact that a given type of habitat, such as a tract of tropical forest, a seashore, or a hedgerow, supports a large number of animal and plant species that vary greatly in terms of their way of life and their interactions with each other. As described at the beginning of this chapter, species interact with one another in many different ways. For example, plants are fed on by herbivores and herbivores fall prey to predators. Such interactions are often depicted as a 'food chain' with plants, described as *primary producers*, at the bottom and predators, called *consumers*, at the top (Figure 5.11). The chain analogy is a poor one, however; such is the number of species and the complexity of interactions among them that the phrase 'food web' is now more commonly used (Figure 5.12).

The organisms in a food web can be arranged in a vertical series of categories, according to how they obtain nutrients; these categories are called *trophic levels*. At the

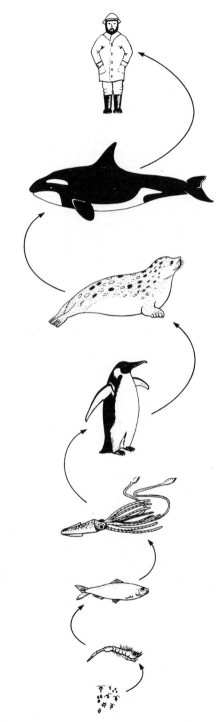

Figure 5.11 *An example of a food chain, in the oceans around Antarctica, involving plankton, krill, fish, squid, penguin, leopard seal, killer whale and human.*

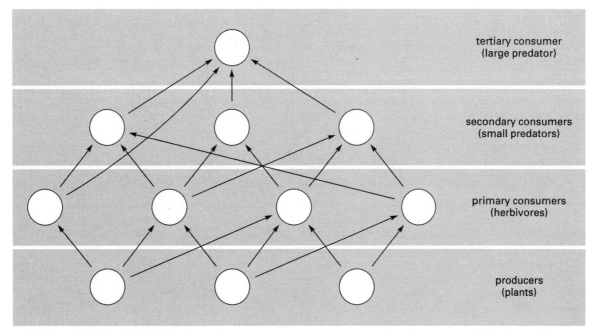

Figure 5.12 *A generalised food web.*

lowest trophic level are the producers: these are plants and *phytoplankton*, which use energy from the sun to convert simple chemicals into sugars, proteins and other complex substances and, in the process, produce vast amounts of oxygen. Phytoplankton ('fye-toe-plank-ton') are plant-like single-celled organisms that drift in the sea and are the basis of most marine food chains, like the one shown in Figure 5.11.[10] These primary producers are eaten by small, primary consumers, which are in turn eaten by larger secondary consumers, and so on.

When the number of species, and the total number of individuals at each trophic level is calculated, what is revealed is a broad-based *pyramid of numbers* (Figure 5.13a), in which there are many more species and individuals at lower levels than there are at the higher levels. More importantly, when account is taken of the body

mass (or **biomass**) of all the organisms at each level, what emerges is a *pyramid of biomass,* which shows that the total biomass of small organisms at the lower trophic levels greatly exceeds that of the larger organisms further up the food web (Figure 5.13b).

Humans occupy a position at the top of the global food web and we share this position with other large-

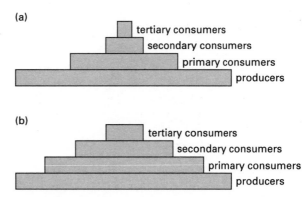

Figure 5.13 *(a) A typical pyramid of numbers. (b) A typical pyramid of biomass.*

[10]The general term 'plankton' covers both the drifting plant-like phytoplankton and the microscopic animal-like protistans that swim in the upper layers of the sea; multi-celled sea animals eat both, but only the phytoplankton are 'producers'.

bodied animals, but we and they are relatively insignificant in terms of total biomass. It is easy to lose sight of the enormous and vital importance of bacteria and other microscopic organisms simply because each individual is so small.

The shape of the pyramid of biomass arises largely because the transfer of energy from one trophic level to the next is very inefficient. As a rough estimate, only about 10 per cent of the energy potentially available at any one level actually finds its way up to the next, the rest being dissipated in various ways, including heat. This is shown graphically in Figure 5.14.

These simple ways of depicting biodiversity and the interaction between species make an important point. Communities of organisms are based ultimately on microscopic organisms, such as bacteria and plankton, which are so numerous that, despite their microscopic size, they make up much the largest proportion of the total mass of life on Earth. The main business of bacteria is feeding off dead plants and animals, not in causing disease in humans and our crops and livestock. Only a small minority of species and a tiny fraction of the bacterial biomass are symbiotic on or in larger animals and only a few of *them* are pathogenic.

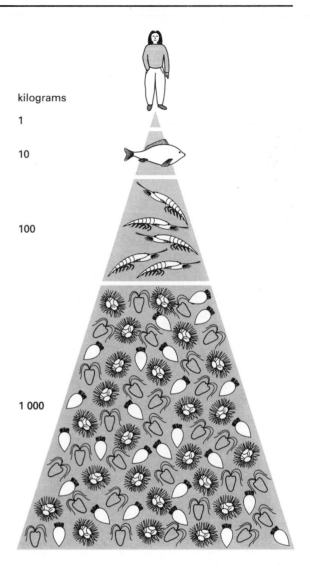

Figure 5.14 *A schematic view of a marine food web that supports humans. Such is the inefficiency of transfer of nutrients and energy from one trophic level to the next that, to produce one kilogram of a human, it requires 1 000 kilograms of plankton.*

OBJECTIVES FOR CHAPTER 5

When you have studied this chapter, you should be able to:

5.1 Give examples of the diversity of the pathogens that affect humans, and illustrate methods of classifying them in terms of their size, site of infection, mode of action and mode of transmission.

5.2 Explain what is meant by coevolution and give examples of different kinds of host–pathogen relationship that have evolved by coevolution.

5.3 Give a general account of the evolutionary consequences of the fact that pathogenic organisms have much faster generation times than their hosts.

5.4 Explain the role of factors that lead to instability in host–pathogen relationships.

QUESTIONS FOR CHAPTER 5

Question 1 (*Objective 5.1*)

Give brief definitions of the following terms: (a) microparasite, (b) vector, (c) virulence.

Question 2 (*Objective 5.2*)

Define the term coevolution and give an example of it in the context of host–pathogen relationships.

Question 3 (*Objective 5.3*)

List three adaptations of host species, such as humans, that are defences against pathogens, explaining in each case the significance of that defence.

Question 4 (*Objective 5.4*)

List four factors that may cause host–pathogen relationships to become unstable over time.

6 Surviving infectious disease

Before commencing this chapter, it would be helpful to look back at the discussion of cell membranes in Chapter 3 of this book and in particular at Figures 3.5 to 3.8. During your study of this chapter you will be asked to revise the Reader[1] article by Marc Strassburg, entitled 'The global eradication of smallpox', which was set reading for World Health and Disease, Chapter 3.

The threat of infectious disease

The fact that numerous species of pathogenic organisms co-exist with the human population in an unstable equilibrium in which neither becomes extinct is a matter of no interest to an individual suffering from an infectious disease. At the personal level, the important questions are 'Will I survive? And if I do, will I suffer permanent harm?' In Third World countries over 16 million people die from infection annually[2] and, as we pointed out in Chapter 5, over a billion people (or one-sixth of the world's population) are infected with protistans and parasitic animals ranging in size from single-celled organisms like the malarial parasite to tapeworms over a metre in length, causing chronic illness and disability. Infectious diseases are a relatively inconspicuous cause of death in the industrialised nations, killing around half a million people every year, but they cause significant episodes of illness for most people throughout their lives. Since the 1980s, awareness has grown that even in industrialised countries some infectious diseases regularly result in death.

[1]In Health and Disease: A Reader (1984 and revised edition 1994).

[2]Figure 3.1 in World Health and Disease presents mortality data from infectious diseases and other causes.

□ From attention to the news media, can you name some infectious diseases that cause deaths in the United Kingdom?

■ Among the most publicised are AIDS (Acquired Immune Deficiency Syndrome), some forms of meningitis, and legionnaires' disease. Many other infectious diseases are more likely to cause death in very young or very old people, than in other age groups (e.g. pneumonia and salmonella food poisoning).

In this chapter, we will look inside the human body at the highly-varied defence mechanisms which have evolved in response to the threat of infection and at the counter-measures evolved by different types of pathogen. You will get some idea of why certain pathogens are mildly inconvenient while others kill and why it is that certain individuals seem more susceptible to infectious disease than others. We will also briefly review some of the ways in which medical science is attempting to tilt the balance in favour of human survival.

This is the territory of the branch of biomedical science known as **immunology**, the study of the cells and molecules that interact in the bodies of multicellular animals to protect them from infection. This network of cells and molecules is collectively called the **immune system** and when it works successfully to eradicate pathogens in the body *before* they cause symptoms of disease, we say that the host has **immunity** to that type of pathogen. 'Host' is a general term meaning an organism that has pathogens living inside it, which will already be familiar to you from Chapters 2 and 5.

First, a word of caution about the language of threat and counter-attack which permeates every discussion of the biological responses to infectious disease. Elsewhere in this series, we discussed the usefulness and the pitfalls of biological *metaphors*.[3] A prime example is in the use of military terms as metaphors for the biological processes that occur when pathogenic organisms enter the body.

[3]See Studying Health and Disease, Chapter 9.

Pathogens are often described as 'invaders' or 'foreign cells' which sneak through the body's defences like undercover agents; ranged against them is an 'arsenal' of biological weapons, which search out and attack the invader with deadly accuracy, like a 'smart missile' homing in on its target. These are exciting images and close enough to some important features of the actual biological processes to justify their limited use. But overuse of military images has one serious drawback. It reinforces the wholly mistaken view that pathogens and the defensive mechanisms in the human body are literally engaged in warfare, with each side trying to outwit the other. In this make-believe world, as one side develops a new strategy, so the other counters it with an opposing move. Cells are portrayed as though they are knowledgable entities capable of intentional actions. For example, the human immunodeficiency virus (HIV) is frequently misrepresented as an adversary of frightening cleverness, which has 'disarmed' our biological defences and rendered them powerless to protect us.

□ What biological error can you identify in this use of military metaphors? You will need to think back to earlier chapters and the processes that underly evolutionary change.

■ HIV has not been cleverly designed to evade biological defences that it somehow 'knew' the details of in advance. It is the product of random mutations which occurred over time in the genetic material of 'ancestor' viruses. Mutation generated a range of slightly different viruses and HIV is simply the present-day survivor of a competition between earlier versions, which were 'selected against' because they were less successful than HIV at reproducing new virus particles and passing them on from one host to the next. In evolutionary terms, HIV is the version that is *best adapted* to survive and reproduce under *present* conditions.

Later in this chapter, we will look more closely at the specific interaction between HIV and human biology,[4] but we begin by taking a more general view of pathogenic organisms and the defences of their human hosts against infection. The first level of defence does not involve the immune system at all.

[4]There is also a multi-disciplinary case-study of AIDS, which includes more detailed discussion of the biology of this disease, together with sociological and political aspects and personal accounts, in *Experiencing and Explaining Disease* (Open University Press, revised edition, 1995).

Physical and chemical barriers to infection

The most effective way to survive an infection is not to let pathogens get into the body in the first place. Intact skin forms an impenetrable barrier to most pathogenic organisms and the acidity of sweat also inhibits the growth of many kinds of bacteria on the body surface. But we have to breathe, drink and eat, so it is inevitable that infection will enter in contaminated air, water and food, as well as through breaks in the skin. Humans reproduce sexually, which creates more opportunities for infection to be transmitted. Figure 6.1 illustrates the range of physical and chemical barriers to infection; most are in the respiratory and reproductive tracts and gut, as you might expect.

An example of a chemical barrier is an enzyme called *lysozyme,* which splits the chemical bonds that hold together the molecular components of bacterial cell walls. (Look back at Chapter 3, Figure 3.11b and imagine that the enzyme pictured is lysozyme.) Bacteria have a 'wall' of sugar-rich molecules outside their cell membrane, which gives some protection from chemical attack and dehydration in the often inhospitable conditions inside the body. These sugars are unique to bacteria, so

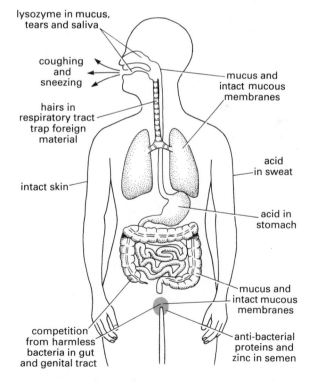

Figure 6.1 *Physical and chemical barriers to infection in the human body.*

the presence of lysozyme in blood, sweat and tears (and nasal secretions and breast milk) has no effect on human tissues, but it digests holes in the cell wall of many bacteria.

However, some types of bacteria have evolved yet another protective layer, a capsule of protein outside the sugar-rich cell wall, which lysozyme cannot penetrate. This example illustrates the point made earlier about the evolution of defensive mechanisms which in their turn are rendered ineffective by later evolutionary developments. Note, in passing, that viruses also have a tough outer envelope of proteins which is resistant to digestion.

Why is the immune system so complicated?

As you will see shortly, once bacteria breach the physical and chemical barriers and get into body tissues and fluids, they meet a range of cells and molecules that interact in a defensive network of bewildering complexity, collectively known as the immune system. In this short chapter we can do no more than sketch in some of the major features of the immune system and its response to infection, but before embarking on this task, it is worth reflecting for a moment on why such a complex system of defences has evolved.

The world is populated by millions of different organisms competing for habitats in which they can survive and reproduce. The bodies of multicellular animals contain numerous suitable niches for smaller organisms to colonise; the larger and more complex the body of the host becomes so the more varied are the habitats it contains, and the greater the number of species of smaller organisms it can support. Humans are composed of huge numbers of specialised cells of many different kinds with a stable temperature and constant food supply, so the opportunities for colonisation by bacteria, viruses, protistans, fungi and larger parasites are endless, as a glance back at Chapter 5, Figure 5.1, will confirm. Some of these organisms are harmless, some are even beneficial (for example, certain bacteria in our guts are essential partners in the process of digestion, as Chapter 7 describes), but many cause damage and disease.

Pathogens come in many shapes and sizes; their bodies are composed of a wide range of chemical substances, some of which are exactly the same as molecules found in the body of their host, but others (like the sugars in bacterial cell walls) are unique to that type of organism. Moreover, they have very different 'lifestyles'; for example, some reproduce *inside* the cells of their host (these *intracellular* pathogens are particularly difficult for the host to detect), whereas others live in the gut or the bloodstream; some reproduce very rapidly whereas

others are slow-growing or even lie dormant for many years before becoming active. And, most important of all, different pathogens have evolved quite different mechanisms to protect themselves from the host's defensive responses.

The biological inevitability of extensive infection by such a varied array of organisms has given a 'selective advantage' to animals which have evolved an equally extensive network of biological protection, which is capable of detecting and destroying or inactivating all these different pathogens. The success of the human species can be attributed partly to our immune system, which is a marvel of complexity. In this book we are concerned primarily with the health of the human species, so the account in this chapter focuses on the human immune system. But in describing the mechanisms by which we are protected from infection, you should bear in mind that the immune systems of other mammals, birds and adult amphibians are similar to those of humans. If humans have any advantage, it is in the size of the 'repertoire' of foreign cells and molecules to which our immune system can respond.

□ Compared to other mammals, humans are long-lived and produce few offspring, who mature very slowly (Chapters 2 and 5). How might these features of our biological evolution have contributed to the evolution of an exceptionally sensitive immune system?

■ In the course of our long lives we encounter a huge range of pathogens which, in the absence of a sensitive defence system, could damage our reproductive success. Juveniles must be protected during the long period before reproduction takes place.

□ In what ways has human *cultural* evolution been facilitated by a complex immune system capable of responding to a huge range of foreign cells and molecules? (Think back to Chapter 2.)

■ The ability to defend against infection by a huge range of pathogens has contributed to the successful colonisation by a single species, *Homo sapiens*, of nearly every terrestrial habitat, from snowfields to deserts and tropical rainforests. It has also enabled humans to eat an enormous variety of animals and plants, which carry micro-organisms and parasites into our bodies; the immune system (and the digestive system, the subject of Chapter 7) provide adequate defence. Most humans now live in settled communities, in close contact with other humans and with many species of domestic animals, eating, sleeping, expelling waste and depositing rubbish in close proximity; an effective immune system is essential in a situation that so encourages the transmission of pathogens between people and between ourselves and other species.

Other developments in human culture such as mass migration of labour during times of economic disaster or war, cheap air travel and package holidays to every part of the globe, have brought increasing numbers of people into contact with pathogens that were formerly restricted to a few locations. HIV is the prime example, but the spread of malaria carried by mosquitoes in the clothes and luggage of air travellers is another.

Moreover, the very fast generation time of most micro-organisms means that their genetic makeup (genotype) can change quite rapidly as mutations or 'mistakes' occur when DNA is copied during cell division. As the previous chapter described, high rates of reproduction and mutation give pathogenic organisms an advantage in that they can evolve a succession of new varieties, a few of which will be better adapted than their predecessors at surviving inside the human body. Thus, the human immune system not only has to cope with all the existing pathogens, but also with any that may evolve in the near future.

But there is another vitally-important reason why the human immune system has evolved such complexity. Like the pathogens that penetrate its outer barriers, the human body is composed of many different kinds of cells, and many of the molecules of which these cells are composed are common to humans and pathogenic species. Despite their structural similarities, the immune system has to distinguish accurately between the body's own cells and a harmful bacterium, virus or other parasite, and differentiate between an essential protein such as an enzyme or hormone and the harmful proteins (toxins) that certain bacteria secrete. More difficult still, it must detect a body cell that has become infected by viruses or other intracellular pathogens, while leaving untouched all neighbouring uninfected cells.

This problem is shared by all multicellular animals. In the jargon of immunology, the immune system of every species can tell the difference between 'self' and 'non-self', and maintain **self-tolerance** while mounting a vigorous destructive attack on pathogenic cells and molecules. Self-tolerance is the highly-selective *unresponsiveness* of the immune system to the cells and molecules that make up the natural body of the host. Unless the host's own cells have been invaded by pathogenic organisms, the *normal* immune system does not

respond to them; but if self-tolerance breaks down, then normal cells and molecules in the body can be attacked and destroyed just as if they were pathogens. The details of how the cells of the developing immune system in the embryo become tolerant to 'self' and responsive to 'legitimate targets' are beyond the scope of this book, but central to the process are precise recognition events between cells of the immune system, normal body cells and pathogens or other 'non-self' material. The general character of these events will be familiar to you from earlier in this book; they involve precise lock-and-key interactions between the exactly-matched surfaces of molecules secreted by or embedded in the surface membranes of living cells.

The evolution of immunity

The precise details of the cells and molecules involved in defensive reactions to infection in the human immune system have been worked out in large measure by extrapolating from research done on rats and mice.[5] It may seem rather implausible at first glance that these animals have much in common with us, but like us they are highly-successful *mammals* (warm-blooded, hairy animals that give birth to immature offspring, which are fed initially on their mother's milk); brown rats and house mice live in communal groups in close contact with humans in virtually every habitat on earth, and they eat an enormous variety of foods. Like humans, they have evolved a complex immune system to cope with the wide range of pathogens they encounter in their daily lives. They have the added practical advantage of breeding prolifically in laboratories as well as in their natural habitats.

The marked similarities in the immune systems of humans, rats and mice reflect strong similarities in their 'ways of life', but the need to combat infection is common to all parts of the animal kingdom (even bacteria are attacked by viruses, as noted in Chapter 5), and so you would expect to find similarities (albeit weaker ones) in the defensive mechanisms employed by organisms far removed from us in evolutionary terms. It is possible to trace the evolution of the complex immune system at work in present-day humans by looking at the biological defences of organisms that evolved before us.

You will recall that humans were late-comers on the evolutionary scene, arriving less than 2 million years ago, but the first worms had already been here for around 750 million years and reptiles preceded us by at least

[5]The use of animals as substitutes or 'models' for humans in biomedical research is discussed in *Studying Health and Disease*, Chapter 9.

500 million years. Echoes of some of the solutions they evolved to cope with infection can be found in the human body today. This is not to imply a direct lineage between ancient species and modern humans; it may simply be that similar solutions to the same problem have evolved independently in several different parts of the animal kingdom, in much the same way that birds, insects and bats independently evolved wings as a means of flight. But looking at other organisms gives an insight into the selection pressure exerted by the evolution of an increasingly varied array of pathogenic organisms. As time passed and yet more species of pathogen evolved, so the complexity of immune systems in their host species increased because only the 'fittest' survived to reproduce and pass on their genes.

Innate immunity

Even the most simple *invertebrates* (animals without backbones such as worms, jellyfish, sponges, insects and shellfish) can defend themselves from infection, using mechanisms that have striking similarities to those found in *vertebrates* (animals with backbones, such as fish, amphibians, reptiles, birds and mammals). These mechanisms have been given a collective name, **innate immunity**. 'Innate' means inborn or evident in all members of a particular species without the need for any prior learning experience. The term was chosen by the biologists who first began unravelling the mechanisms of the immune system because the similarities in the defences of animals as diverse as mice and earthworms were so striking that they seemed to have been 'programmed' into the earliest evolution of life on earth. Indeed, when the DNA of very diverse animals is closely examined, similarities are found in the nucleotide sequences of some of the genes involved in generating these innate immune responses. The suggestion is that these gene sequences appeared quite early in the evolution of life on Earth, and conferred such an advantage on their possessors that they were preserved as new species evolved from their common ancestors.

The basic mechanisms that contribute to innate immunity can be broadly divided into those based on defensive cells and those based on defensive proteins. First, we will look briefly at each of these mechanisms in turn. In humans, all the defensive cells are members of a group of cells collectively called the **white cells** (or *leucocytes*, 'loo-koh-sites'). (White cells are often misleadingly called white 'blood' cells because they are most easily detected in the bloodstream, but in reality they occur throughout the body.) Then we will 'sum up' by describing what happens if these mechanisms are all triggered at the same time in the same place, producing a chain-reaction known as an *inflammatory response*.

Defensive cells

Phagocytosis roughly means 'eating cells'.[6] In Chapter 3, you learned about the process called *endocytosis* in which cells take in large molecules or particles of food by enclosing a portion of the outside world in a bag of cell membrane (called a vesicle) and drawing the bag and its contents into the interior of the cell. (You may wish to look back at Figures 3.9a and 3.9b.) All multicellular animals, from sponges to the President of the United States, have *phagocytic cells* (or phagocytes for short), which use endocytosis to draw pathogenic organisms into their interior, where they are rapidly destroyed. The vesicle containing the pathogen fuses with a small membrane-bound packet (called a *lysosome;* Figure 3.5 shows several in a liver cell), which contains digestive enzymes and powerful chemicals akin to domestic bleach, which break up the molecules of which the pathogen is built. Some of the break-down products are simply used as nutrients by the phagocytic cell and the rest are dumped outside by the reverse process of exocytosis (Figures 3.9c and 3.9d). Figure 6.2 shows a phagocyte at work.

In humans, phagocytosis is a major contributor to our defence against infection. There are several different types of phagocytes, all members of the highly-varied white cell population (the best-known is called a *macrophage* ('mack-roh-fage'), which literally means 'big eater'. Some phagocytes are highly mobile and 'rove' around the body, squeezing between other cells to penetrate every tissue; others remain stationary in parts of the body where infection is highly likely to occur.

Cytotoxic cells are another general category of defensive cells; their method of attacking pathogens is not well represented by their name (which means 'cell poisoning' and is pronounced 'sigh-toh-toxic'). In fact they do not kill pathogenic cells with poisons, but by a simple mechanical device. They manufacture cylindrical tubes of protein which they can 'punch' through the outer membrane of the pathogen's cells, even if the membrane is protected by a wall of sugars or a protein envelope (as it is in some bacteria).

---

[6]You may need some help with pronunciation: *phagocytosis* ('fag-oh-sigh-tosis'); *phagocyte* ('fag-oh-sight'); but *phagocytic* ('fag-oh-si-tic').

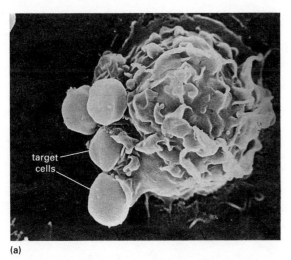
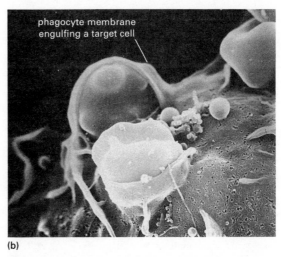

(a)　(b)

Figure 6.2　*This phagocyte is engulfing red blood cells from another species, which were 'fed' to it in the laboratory. (a) The red cells are ensnared by folds of cell membrane, which draw them towards the phagocyte (magnified about 5 000 times). (b) Red cells are being enclosed in a bag of membrane (magnified about 10 000 times). The 'packaged' red cell is then taken into the phagocyte's interior, where it is broken down by powerful enzymes and destructive chemicals. (Photos: courtesy of Drs S. Gordon and G. G. McPherson, Sir William Dunn School of Pathology, University of Oxford.)*

☐ The fluids inside a cell generally contain a more concentrated mixture of dissolved molecules than the fluid outside. This concentration gradient between the inside world and the outside world is maintained by the intact cell membrane which acts as a highly-selective barrier to the passage of molecules into and out of the cell (Chapter 3). What do you predict would happen to a cell that has been punctured by a cylindrical tube pushed through its cell membrane?

■ The cell would be unable to prevent the collapse of the concentration gradient as dilute fluids from outside the cell rush in through the puncture. (In Chapter 3, you learned that in the absence of an intact barrier, the concentration on both sides of a permeable membrane equalises as the molecules 'spread out' evenly through the available space.)

A cell that has been punctured in many places becomes so leaky that it swells and bursts under the pressure of in-rushing fluid. Cytotoxic cells can be found in all multicellular animals. Several different types exist in humans, including the memorably named *natural killer cells* (or NK cells for short); they are all members of the white cell population. They are particularly active against any of the body's own cells that have been invaded by intracellular pathogens (all viruses, many bacteria and certain protistans live and reproduce *inside* the host's cells). This ability to attack cells that appear to be 'altered self' is also demonstrated in the curious phenomenon of **graft rejection**.

If tissue is transplanted from the body of one person to that of another, as in a skin graft or kidney transplant, the graft is attacked and destroyed primarily by cytotoxic cells, even when the donor is closely related to the recipient. This ability is surprising since tissue transplantation is not a natural event, so why should a 'defence' against it have evolved? The likely explanation is that it is a side-effect of the ability to distinguish between self and non-self with such exquisite accuracy that even the cells of another member of one's own species are recognised as 'foreign'.

Graft rejection can be demonstrated in many kinds of invertebrates, including sponges, which may give a clue to an earlier evolutionary function. If two sponges are bound tightly together by a clamp, cytotoxic cells in each animal migrate into the area of close proximity and attack the cells of the other sponge until a zone of dead cells is produced between them. This mechanism forces sponges to 'keep their distance' and may serve to prevent overcrowding of habitats. It is a sobering thought (if true) that the problems faced by medical science in persuading a human body to accept a transplant from another person may partly be a consequence of mechanisms that first evolved in invertebrates like the sponge. Concern about the ethics of organ transplants are discussed in Chapter 9 of this book.

Defensive proteins

The third category of mechanisms that contribute to innate immunity are the many different proteins that directly or indirectly damage pathogens. All invertebrates have phagocytic and cytotoxic cells as part of their defences against infection, but proteins that damage pathogens are not found in the earliest animals to evolve (sponges, corals, jellyfish and flatworms). In more complex invertebrates like the octopus, sea-urchins, insects and shellfish, proteins can be detected that bind onto pathogens but do not bind to the animal's own cells. These *antisomes* do no direct harm to the pathogen, but they are believed to be the evolutionary precursors of the *antibodies* found in all vertebrate species.

Antibodies will be mentioned again later in the chapter, but their general function is to 'label' suitable targets for destruction by other mechanisms in the immune system. For example, phagocytic cells are able to engulf bacteria much more rapidly if the pathogens have antibodies bound to their surface. In invertebrates, the antisomes seem to have the same effect. Note that the binding protein does not *directly* damage the pathogen; it simply makes the pathogen more likely to be destroyed by other mechanisms.

You have already met one protein that does directly damage pathogens, lysozyme, the enzyme that digests bacterial cell walls. Another important example is a 'protein cascade' known as *complement*. Before we describe its action, it is worth dwelling for a moment on the general principle because **cascade reactions** are common in biological systems and you will meet another later in this chapter. In a cascade reaction, a series of molecules or cells exists in an *inactive* form; they remain inactive until a specific 'trigger' activates the first member of the series, which in turn activates the second member of the series, and so on, until the last member is activated. The final component of the series brings about a major change in the system. Generally, a 'scaling up' takes place as the sequence progresses, so that whereas only a few molecules or cells of the first member of the series were activated, they are able to activate many more molecules or cells of component two, and so on, as Figure 6.3 shows.

☐ What advantages can you see in cascade reactions?

■ First, the reaction can very rapidly generate a high concentration of the final component, because all the elements were pre-formed in the system just

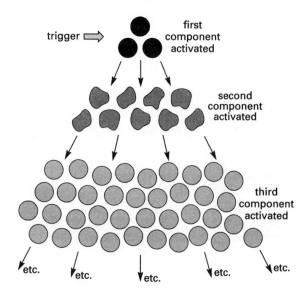

Figure 6.3 *Schematic representation of a cascade reaction in a biological system. The symbols might represent molecules or cells.*

waiting to be activated. Second, the large number of steps in the sequence gives several opportunities for 'negative feedback' (Chapter 3) to influence whether the cascade proceeds beyond that step. When the outcome of a completed cascade is a major change in the system, there is an advantage in having built-in failsafe mechanisms that could switch it off at an early stage.

The complement cascade reaction is a good example of why failsafes are advantageous. The term 'complement' refers to over 20 different inactive proteins found in certain body fluids including blood. Once activated, the proteins in the cascade build up on the surface of pathogens until the final component is activated. The final component is a cylindrical molecule rather like the protein tube produced by cytotoxic cells and with just the same function; it punctures the pathogen's cell membrane. It is vitally important that the cascade is *only* triggered by non-self cells, to avoid damaging the body's own cells, but if it *was* set off inappropriately at least there are several steps at which it might be stopped. There are two main mechanisms for triggering the complement cascade: it can be set off by unique configurations of sugar molecules found only in the walls of bacteria; also, when antibodies bind to the surface of non-self cells, they can trigger the cascade at that location.

The inflammatory response

The three general types of mechanisms that contribute to innate immunity (phagocytic cells, cytotoxic cells and defensive proteins, as described above) do not occur in isolation; if pathogens get into the body, all three mechanisms are triggered at once. The chemicals released by the various cells involved in innate immunity, and the unique sugars and proteins in the pathogen itself, trigger yet another type of white cell, called *mast cells*, to release a 'cocktail' of intensely irritant chemicals, including *histamine*. When these irritant chemicals are released, they cause the walls of nearby blood vessels to swell and become very leaky so that fluid and white cells flood out. The inflamed area feels puffy and hot and looks red because of the high blood flow.

□ Can you explain why this uncomfortable inflammation is adaptive, i.e. gives some survival advantage to organisms that possess it?

■ The inflammatory response causes the area of an infection to be flooded with phagocytic and cytotoxic white cells and a whole range of defensive proteins such as complement. Despite the temporary discomfort, this response can eradicate an infection before the pathogens have time to multiply sufficiently to cause damage and disease.

Unfortunately, the inflammatory response is easily triggered in some people by harmless plant and animal material such as pollens and cat fur, as any allergy sufferer can testify. In such cases, the person makes a special kind of antibody that binds to the *allergen* (a general term for whatever substance the person is allergic to) and this, in turn, binds to *mast cells*, which are abundant in the airways and around the eyes. You will learn more about antibodies shortly. In Chapter 10 we consider the possibility that chemical pollutants in modern industrial environments contribute to the incidence of allergies. But for the moment, focus on the effectiveness of the inflammatory response against pathogens.

Most of the mechanisms of innate immunity are more effective against bacteria and small parasites than against viruses and large parasites, which is one reason why viral infections are difficult to treat and parasitic infestations are generally long-lasting and may cause chronic illness and disability. The large parasites escape complete destruction primarily because they *are* large: it is a tall order for the immune system to destroy a worm or fluke composed of millions of cells. Viruses are simple protein boxes containing little more than a strand of genetic material (DNA or RNA), and are far less vulnerable to the puncturing techniques that damage true cells. Furthermore, if a phagocyte engulfs a virus it may simply be doing the virus a favour, by taking it inside a living cell which can then be 'taken over' by the viral genes and turned into a factory for new virus particles. One mechanism evolved by mammals to combat viruses is a protein called *interferon*, which 'interferes' with the process of making viral proteins in accordance with the code contained in viral genes.

Non-specific recognition of pathogens

Throughout the foregoing discussion of innate immunity, there has been a question lurking in the background which you may now be able to answer. How does a phagocyte, or a cytotoxic cell, or a protein that binds only to pathogens or damages them without harming the body's own cells, recognise legitimate targets?

□ Think back to the discussion of cell membranes in Chapter 3 and see if you can suggest an answer.

■ Interactions can be restricted to very specific 'partners' if a lock-and-key fit is required between the partners before a reaction results. Phagocytes and cytotoxic cells 'recognise' pathogens because pathogens have molecules in their structure that exactly fit the shape of receptors on the surface of a phagocyte or cytotoxic cell (as in Figure 3.10c). These molecules must be unique to pathogens (i.e. not found in the host's cells and body fluids). Similarly, a protein that binds selectively to or damages only pathogens, does so because it can only bind to molecular shapes unique to pathogens and is not present 'naturally' in the host.

Many of the molecules found only in the structure of bacteria and viruses, but not in the structure of multicellular animals, are complex sugars (or sugars with bits of protein or fat attached). There are relatively few different kinds of 'pathogen-sugars' and they are commonly found in the structures of a wide variety of different bacteria and viruses, so the ability to recognise a few unique sugars enables an animal's immune system to recognise a lot of different pathogens. Recognition is *non-specific* in the sense that the animal cannot distinguish between one kind of pathogen and another, since all it is able to 'see' are the sugars that are common to both.

Non-specific recognition of pathogens is a *defining characteristic* of innate immunity. Invertebrate animals are only able to recognise pathogens in this non-specific way, but it seems to give adequate protection from the relatively limited range of pathogenic organisms that infect invertebrates. Remember that 'adequate protection' simply means that, even though some individuals in the host species may die from the infection, many survive.

During the long evolution of animal species in close interaction with bacteria and viruses, animals that were able to 'recognise' pathogens and attack them were at a *selective advantage* (that is, they were more likely to survive and reproduce than animals that could *not* defend themselves from infection). Another way of saying the same thing, but at the *molecular* level, is 'animals whose cells carry receptor molecules, which exactly fit the shapes of complex sugars found only in the structures of bacteria and viruses, were at a selective advantage'.

☐ Can you rewrite the last sentence to describe how selection would operate at the *genetic* level?

■ Animals whose DNA includes genes that encode the instructions for making receptor molecules, which exactly fit the shapes of complex sugars found only in the structures of bacteria and viruses, were at a selective advantage.

The unique sugars and proteins commonly found in the structures of many bacteria and viruses have probably been extremely stable components of pathogen structure over millions of years of evolution. We can infer this from the fact that the relatively small number of different receptors required to fit (and hence recognise) all of these unique sugars and proteins can be found on the surface of defensive cells in animals throughout the animal kingdom. The widespread existence of these receptors and the genes that code for them are evidence for the co-evolution of pathogens and their hosts over a very long time-scale; so long that, even as new animal species evolved, they preserved the genes involved in recognising bacterial and viral structures.

But a feature of evolution that you should recall from Chapter 5 is increasing diversity. As time passes, so more species evolve and though some become extinct, new species are continuously forming. By 500 million years ago, all the major kinds of animals alive in the world today were already present. The evolution of large multicellular animals with backbones (fish, amphibians such as frogs and salamanders, reptiles, birds and mammals) created extremely varied habitats not only for new strains of bacteria and viruses, but also for single-celled creatures (protistans) and multicelled parasites such as worms and flukes. The strategies that had evolved

to protect invertebrates from infection were not adequate to defend vertebrates from this rapidly increasing and diversifying array of pathogenic organisms. Reinforcements were required.

Adaptive immunity

Innate immunity only recognises the *major* molecular differences between host and pathogen, such as unique sugars and proteins shared by many different types of bacteria and viruses, but never found as part of the host's cells. A more difficult problem for a multicellular animal's immune system is to recognise and attack a pathogen that is *itself* an animal (such as a tapeworm), rather than a bacterium or a virus, and which is therefore constructed from molecules that are mostly the *same* as those of the host's own body. Moreover, as more and more different kinds of microscopic pathogens evolved, many of them took to colonising the *inside* of the host's own cells, making them much more difficult to detect. Exquisite precision is necessary in these circumstances to distinguish between the cells and molecules of which the pathogen is constructed and those of the host.

The additional pathogen-recognition mechanisms evolved by vertebrates which enable them to achieve this 'fine focus' are known collectively as **adaptive immunity**, for reasons that will emerge later. These mechanisms are capable of detecting extremely small variations in the surface contours of molecules; they can recognise any molecular shapes that are even very slightly different from quite similar molecules normally found in the host. The principle of lock-and-key interactions between receptors on the host cells and unique molecular shapes on the pathogen's surface is the same as in innate immunity, but *millions* of different receptors are necessary to achieve the sensitivity of the adaptive immune system to the millions of tiny differences between the host's and the pathogen's molecules. This massive 'repertoire' of different receptors found on the cells involved in adaptive immunity is in sharp contrast to the relatively small range of receptors found on the cells involved in innate immunity.

Innate immunity only operates at the 'broad brush-stroke' level of distinguishing self from non-self, without being able to recognise more subtle distinctions between (for example) two strains of bacteria. But the adaptive immune system is capable of such highly *specific* recognition of tiny molecular differences between cells, that it can, in effect 'tell one pathogen from another'. We will explain how this remarkable ability is achieved.

Specific recognition of pathogens

The adaptive immune system in humans is the most sensitive in the animal kingdom. It has been estimated that each of us can detect at least *100 million different molecular shapes* that occur in the structures of cells other than our own. These tiny unique molecular shapes are collectively known as **epitopes** and any larger molecule or cell that contains an epitope in its structure is called an **antigen**. 'Foreign' proteins such as the toxins produced by certain bacteria typically contain several different epitopes, each constructed from tiny sections of the large protein molecule as it coils in space (see Figure 6.4a). Virus particles and whole cells, such as bacteria or protistans and the cells of larger parasites, may have hundreds of different epitopes in their structure (Figure 6.4b).

Each organism has a characteristic array of epitopes, which together make up a sort of 'call-sign' for that pathogen. Thus, the epitopes on the influenza virus are different from those on the measles virus; those on the bacteria that cause tuberculosis are different from those on the bacteria that cause pneumonia, and so on. And because each pathogen has a unique set of epitopes, it can be recognised quite *specifically* by the host's immune system. Unlike the non-specific recognition displayed by innate immune mechanisms, the adaptive immune mechanisms can distinguish not only between self and non-self but between one type of pathogen and another. What goes on in our bodies is analogous to what happens in a hospital pathology lab when a sample of infected blood or tissue is sent for analysis: the lab identifies exactly which strain of pathogen is causing the infection, and so can we.

So great is the capacity for non-self 'pattern recognition' that individuals can also distinguish between the molecules on the surface of their own cells and those of their closest family members. This capacity is demonstrated by the rejection of transplants, even between first-degree relatives, unless the graft-recipient's immune system is suppressed by drugs. The only exception is when the graft-donor and recipient are identical twins; since their genes are identical, all the molecules on the surface of their cells are also identical and the graft appears to be 'self' to the recipient.

The extraordinary capacity for recognising vast numbers of different non-self molecular shapes (epitopes) ensures that vertebrates have a high probability of detecting any pathogen they may encounter during their relatively long lives. Although humans can recognise the greatest range of different epitopes, other mammals and birds are not far behind. The range of recognition gets

(a)

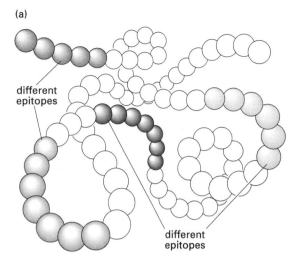

different epitopes

different epitopes

(b)

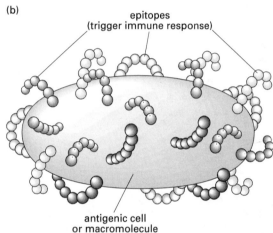

epitopes (trigger immune response)

antigenic cell or macromolecule

Figure 6.4 *An antigen is a large molecule or cell with one or more unique areas (epitopes) in its structure, which are recognised as 'non-self' by the host's immune system. (a) In this sketch, a large molecule contains four different epitopes, each of which is recognised as non-self because cells in the host's immune system have receptors that exactly fit these epitopes. The rest of the molecule does not trigger an immune response because the host's own body contains these same molecular configurations; they appear to be 'self'. (b) A single-celled pathogen has many copies of several different epitopes in its structure.*

steadily more restricted in the earliest vertebrates to evolve, such as reptiles and sharks, and, as described earlier, in invertebrates recognition is restricted to a few large and unusual molecules commonly found in many bacteria and viruses.

However, the need to recognise at least 100 million different epitopes poses the human genotype with a packaging problem. Each unique epitope fits into the binding site of just one unique receptor shape, which means in practice that there must be at least 100 million different receptors on the surface of cells in the human immune system, each of which exactly fits an epitope that might occur somewhere in nature—past, present or future. 100 million different receptors ought to mean 100 million different genes, each one encoding the structure of one receptor, but human DNA only contains about 100 *thousand* genes altogether, with much else to do besides detecting pathogens. How can so few genes contain the codes for so many different receptors? The solution to this problem takes us back for another look at DNA.

Shuffling genes to create diversity

In Chapters 3 and 4 we described the way in which the instructions for making a unique protein are contained in the sequence of nucleotides of a single unique gene. At this point we have to confess that the notion that 'one gene makes one protein' is an oversimplification. The study of the adaptive immune system brought about a minor revolution when it was recognised that certain large and complex proteins involved in the immune response to pathogens were actually assembled from several smaller proteins, each coded for by different genes. This discovery proved to be the key to the puzzle of how the human immune system could make 100 million different receptor proteins with apparently far too few genes for the task.

Imagine that you had just a few hundred different genes to play with, but you needed 100 million different proteins. If each of those proteins was assembled from sections encoded by about six different genes, then how many *different combinations* of six genes could you get from a pool of several hundred? Hundreds of thousands of different proteins could be generated by shuffling the combinations of a few hundred genes. Then imagine that when the sections of protein were assembled, they could be spliced together in a variety of ways. This process introduces yet more diversity, more than enough to produce over 100 million different receptor proteins, each one capable of binding to just one epitope shape.

The genes that code for the receptors involved in pathogen-recognition are 'shuffled' early in embryonic development in members of the white cell population called **lymphocytes** ('lim-foh-sights'). The lymphocytes are the principal cells on which *adaptive* immunity rests.

The embryo contains versatile **multipotent stem cells**, so-called because they give rise by cell division to all the lymphocytes and to the many other kinds of white cell that take part in immune responses (such as phagocytes and cytotoxic cells), and also to red blood cells, and platelets, which are part of the blood-clotting mechanism.

In their DNA, the stem cells have several hundred genes that contain the coded instructions to make several hundred different sections of possible receptors that could bind to different epitopes. As the stem cells divide and mature to give rise to new lymphocytes, all but five or six of these several hundred receptor-genes are lost from the DNA that is passed on to each of the 'daughter' cells. The losses are *random* and as a result each daughter lymphocyte inherits a *unique* set of five or six genes, just enough to code for a single uniquely-shaped receptor. The surviving genes are 'spliced' together by special enzymes that join the broken pieces of DNA (see Figure 6.5). The joins are somewhat haphazard, which introduces yet more variation into the gene sequence that each lymphocyte inherits.

By shuffling a few hundred genes and 'dealing them out' to the lymphocytes in random combinations, at least 100 million different receptors can be generated, enough to fit every epitope likely to be encountered in a lifetime. But the random nature of the shuffle creates another problem: it is inevitable that it will also generate receptor shapes that 'fit' parts of the molecules from which the host's own body is made. Unless these 'self-receptors' are eliminated, the immune system turns on the host.

Self-tolerance

Early in embryonic life, when millions of different receptor shapes are being randomly generated as new lymphocytes form, these receptors inevitably collide with complementary shapes on cells and macromolecules in the embryo. All the molecular shapes that these receptors encounter are part of 'self'. Each time a receptor binds to part of a self-molecule in the embryo, the lymphocyte that carries that receptor undergoes profound changes in its ability to respond to that epitope. The mechanisms underlying this 'self-learning' process are complex and beyond the scope of this chapter, but the overall effect is that by the time of birth, all the lymphocytes in the body have become *unresponsive* to the body's own cells and molecules. The immune system is **self-tolerant**, usually but not always for life.

The breakdown of self-tolerance is a serious business. Several important human diseases, including rheumatoid arthritis and juvenile-onset diabetes, involve self-destruction of body tissues by the immune system, because the mechanisms that maintain self-tolerance have failed.

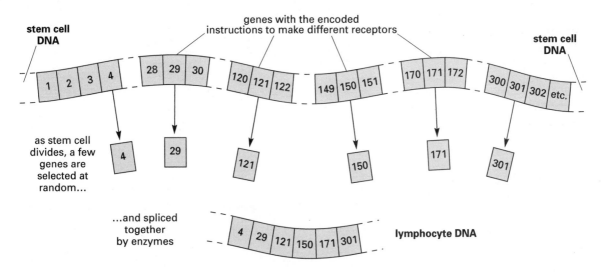

Figure 6.5 *Each lymphocyte inherits a unique combination of a few receptor-genes from the pool of several hundred receptor-genes in the stem cell's DNA. It then has the coded instructions to make one receptor shape and hence to bind to one specific epitope. (The dashed lines indicate where long sections of DNA have been omitted from the drawing to save space.)*

Fortunately, these *autoimmune diseases* are relatively rare occurrences. In the normal course of events, lymphocytes are responsive only to cells or molecules that have, in their structure, the 'non-self' epitope that fits into the lymphocyte's receptors. Once the lymphocyte has bound to that epitope, a series of reactions is set off in the immune system which culminate in the destruction of the pathogen or the toxic molecule of which that epitope was a part.

Scaling up the adaptive immune response

It may have been puzzling you why the additional protective mechanisms evolved by vertebrates are called 'adaptive'. The term is a little unfortunate because it has one meaning in evolutionary biology, which is already familiar to you, but another in immunology which has yet to be explained. Adaptive in its evolutionary sense describes a characteristic that increases the likelihood that an organism will survive long enough to reproduce, and this is clearly true of all aspects of the immune response to infection. Having an immune system is certainly adaptive in that sense of the term.

But immunologists use it to describe an adaptation which takes place in response to infection *during the lifetime* of an organism. In other words, the term is being used to describe a *developmental* rather than an evolutionary feature. So how does the adaptive immune system adapt?

Think back to the previous discussion about shuffling genes and remember that each lymphocyte carries on its surface a number of receptors that bind to just one shape of epitope and, between them, the entire population of lymphocytes has receptors for 100 million different epitopes. A single lymphocyte would not be enough to mount an effective immune response against a pathogen that was actively reproducing; many millions of lymphocytes capable of recognising that pathogen are required. But the human body is not large enough to accommodate 100 million sets of lymphocytes, each consisting of millions of cells. Moreover such a mechanism would be a very wasteful solution to the problem, because only those sets that recognise the pathogens that were *actually* encountered during a lifetime would ever be called upon for protection. All the rest would be a waste of space. A much more economical solution has evolved, which is known as **clonal selection**. Figure 6.6 (*overleaf*) shows the sequence of events.

First, the few lymphocytes that had the correct receptors to bind to unique epitopes on the pathogen multiply by numerous cell divisions. Replication is not simply triggered by contact with the pathogen, but also requires several chemical signals from other types of white cell. Every daughter cell derived from this replication process is identical to the parent, so all the new lymphocytes have the same surface receptors and bind to the same unique epitope (and hence to the pathogen) that triggered the original cell.

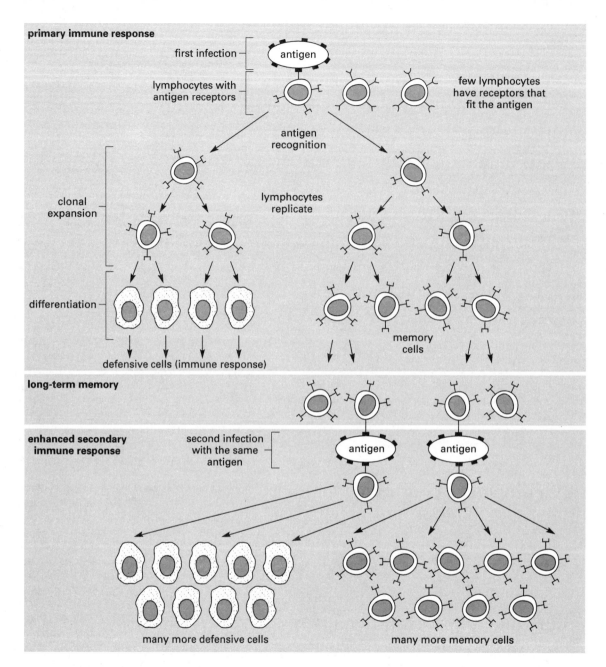

primary immune response

first infection — antigen

lymphocytes with antigen receptors

few lymphocytes have receptors that fit the antigen

antigen recognition

clonal expansion

lymphocytes replicate

differentiation

defensive cells (immune response)

memory cells

long-term memory

enhanced secondary immune response

second infection with the same antigen

many more defensive cells

many more memory cells

Figure 6.6 *Clonal selection is a defining characteristic of adaptive immunity. It enables the immune response to a pathogen to be 'scaled up' as the original lymphocyte replicates to give a clone of active cells. The formation of memory cells enables any subsequent encounters with the same pathogen to be even faster.*

Together, these identical lymphocytes are called a *clone*. It takes a few days before a large enough clone of defensive lymphocytes has been generated to mount an effective attack; this is called the **primary immune response.** During the delay, the pathogen could multiply sufficiently to cause illness.

All the defensive lymphocytes engaged in the original attack die within a few days of eliminating the pathogen, so they are unable to contribute to an immune response if the same pathogen re-enters the body. However, as the original clone enlarges, thousands of these lymphocytes differentiate (change) into *memory cells,* which survive for months or even years after the pathogen has been eliminated. If that pathogen gets into the body again, the memory cells can multiply far more quickly than was possible the first time around. This **secondary immune response** may be fast enough to prevent symptoms from occurring, and it generates even more memory cells so that a third infection has even less chance of taking hold. This ability to adapt and improve the response as a consequence of an encounter with a pathogen underlies the term *adaptive* immunity.

□ When children are immunised against common infectious diseases such as whooping cough and diphtheria, they are usually given three injections of the vaccine at intervals of several months. What do you think the vaccine might contain? Why do three, spaced injections give better protection than one?

■ The vaccine contains samples of the unique epitopes found in the structure of the pathogens you wish to protect the child against. The first injection triggers off a primary immune response, in which the few lymphocytes capable of recognising those epitopes multiply into a large clone and long-lived memory cells are formed. The second and third injections trigger the production of even more memory cells, so that if the live pathogen ever gets into the body it will be eliminated before it can cause illness.

Adaptive immunity is a very specific form of defence. Pathogens that get into the body once are likely to get in again, so it is advantageous to be 'primed and ready' for them. But the adaptation that follows an infection or a vaccination with a specific pathogen (such as measles) does not change the number of lymphocytes capable of recognising most *other* pathogens. So, for example, immunity to measles does not improve the immune response to the polio virus, or the bacteria that cause TB, or the malarial parasite, or anything else you might think of. However, there are a few closely-related pathogens that have some epitopes in common, so immunising against one of these pathogens gives some protection against the other. The most famous example is illustrated by the work of the English country doctor Edward Jenner who, at the end of the eighteenth century, protected people from smallpox by scratching their skin and introducing matter from cowpox pustules; the viruses that cause the two diseases are closely related.

The mechanisms of adaptive immunity

The principal way in which lymphocytes protect us from infection is by directing the mechanisms already described for innate immunity to much greater effect. Lymphocytes manufacture and secrete dozens of different signalling proteins, some of which act on the phagocytes and cytotoxic cells of the innate immune system, greatly increasing their activity and effectiveness, while other proteins (including the antibodies, which we mentioned earlier) stick onto the pathogens and label them for destruction, or set off the complement cascade.

Lymphocytes come in two main 'families': the *T cells* and the *B cells* ('T' and 'B' refers to 'thymus' and 'bone-marrow' respectively, the sites in the body where these cells mature). Each of these families of lymphocyte has a very diverse range of functions, which are the subject of weighty textbooks; we have space here for only the most basic details. Each T cell or B cell has receptors on its surface for a single epitope shape and they all undergo clonal selection, clonal expansion and memory cell formation after the original contact with their matching epitope (as in Figure 6.6).

B cells synthesise and secrete **antibodies**: complex proteins which contain binding sites for the epitopes found on pathogens. Each B cell produces only one kind of antibody, with binding sites for only one shape of epitope, so the interaction between an antibody molecule and an epitope is highly specific. For this reason, the presence of antibodies in a person's body which can bind to a certain pathogen can be taken as an indication that the person is, or has recently been, infected with that pathogen. This is the basis of the HIV test, which detects antibodies in the person's bloodstream which bind selectively to samples of HIV particles in a laboratory test. The virus particles themselves are not detected directly, but their presence is inferred from the presence of specific 'anti-HIV' antibodies in the blood.

Antibodies have become an important research tool because of their ability to 'pick out' their matching epitope and bind to it in laboratory tests, even when the epitope is in a complex mixture of other molecules. This is precisely what happens in life, where antibodies bind only to their matching epitope even though faced with a massive array of other molecular shapes on all the cells and molecules of the body. This specificity is a consequence of the precise lock-and-key fit between binding sites on the antibody and the matching shape of the epitope. At the end of this chapter, we will look briefly at ways in which this specificity may be harnessed by medical science.

The other family of lymphocytes on which adaptive immunity depends are the **T cells**. They come in three basic types.

Cytotoxic T cells function in much the same way as the cytotoxic cells described earlier under innate immunity, but with much more precision in their selection of targets. They have evolved in response to pressure from pathogens that replicate inside the host's own cells, where only the most subtle recognition systems can detect them.

Helper T cells secrete over twenty different signalling molecules with the general property of enhancing the effectiveness of all the other contributors to an immune response.

Suppressor T cells have the opposite effect, damping down the immune response when the need for it has passed. The roles of all these cells are shown in Figure 6.7.

It would be misleading to suggest that the helper and suppressor T cells are the only regulatory influence on the immune system (for example, the helper T cells themselves require a whole range of chemical signals from certain phagocytes, which are in evolutionary terms a much 'older' type of cell), but they are pivotal in tilting the balance of survival in the host's favour. In industrialised nations, before the arrival of AIDS, we might have assumed that infectious diseases had declined to the point where lethal infections no longer exist in the environment. This complacency has been shattered by AIDS, which kills mainly young and otherwise healthy people, who succumb to a wide range of infectious diseases normally not seen in the developed world.

People with AIDS are vulnerable to so-called *opportunistic infections*, involving pathogens that are quite commonly found in the environment but which are unable to reproduce sufficiently to cause symptoms in people whose immune system is functioning normally. When the immune system collapses, as in AIDS, these pathogens have a rare opportunity to cause disease. The principal effect of the virus that underlies AIDS is the destruction of helper T cells.

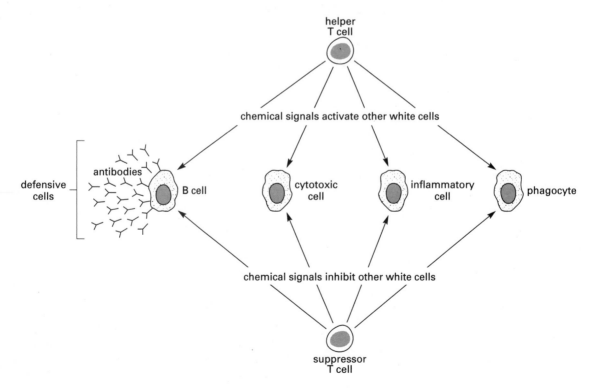

Figure 6.7 *Both the innate and adaptive mechanisms in the immune system are regulated by the activity of helper and suppressor T cells. (Other regulatory mechanisms exist, but they do not concern us here.)*

◻ How can the destruction of just one cell type bring about the collapse of such a complex and multi-faceted immune system?

■ Figure 6.7 gives the answer: without the activating signals produced by the helper T cells, all the other mechanisms in the immune response become less effective or cease altogether.

Policing the body

So now you have a general picture of innate and adaptive immunity and can view the adaptive mechanisms as a later evolutionary development that can 'piggy-back' on the older innate responses to infection, giving them more direction and impact. But there is a vitally-important aspect of the immune response in which the adaptive mechanisms are reliant on the innate mechanisms; this has to do with maximising the chances of a pathogen that gets into the body 'meeting' the few lymphocytes that can recognise it. Before the primary immune response to a certain pathogen is triggered by the first encounter, there are only about 100 lymphocytes in the body with the correctly-shaped receptors capable of recognising it. The chance of a random encounter between the pathogen and one of these few cells is not high, especially because lymphocytes (both T cells and B cells) spend less than 10 per cent of their lives circulating around the body in either the bloodstream, or the equally extensive but rarely mentioned lymphatic system (Figure 6.8).

The rest of the time the lymphocytes stay in the various *lymph nodes* (solid masses of white cells, bounded by a membraneous wall) which can be found throughout the body but are particularly noticeable in the neck, armpits and groin (they can be felt as 'swollen glands' during certain infections), or in major organs such as the spleen, thymus and bone marrow, or in the sheets of membrane that join together loops of gut in the abdomen.

All these sites of static lymphocytes have a blood supply and a lymphatic supply, so any pathogens that get into either of these circulatory systems will be swept along and eventually reach a lymph gland or organ. There the pathogen may 'bump into' a lymphocyte that has the correct receptors on its surface to fit its unique epitopes, which all sounds rather 'hit and miss'. The human body is a vast assembly of suitable habitats for a huge variety of different organisms, some of which are lethal if allowed to reproduce. It would not be an adequate strategy simply to wait for a chance encounter with the immune system. A better method of policing the body evolved quite early in evolutionary history, based on the highly mobile *phagocytes*.

Phagocytic cells can move freely around the body, either in the bloodstream or by squeezing between

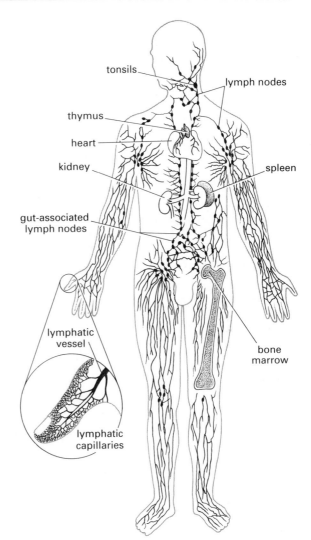

Figure 6.8 *The human lymphatic system consists of solid masses of white cells in numerous lymph nodes and in the bone marrow, spleen and thymus, connected by an extensive network of capillaries containing a fluid (lymph) in which white cells and nutrients are transported.*

the cells of which all our tissues are made. Apart from the cornea (lens of the eye) there is nowhere they cannot reach; they can even get into the brain. Phagocytes come in different kinds, each of which has a particular 'territory', but all take the same action whenever they encounter a pathogen. First they engulf it, then they break down its structure into small sections and transport those sections back to the cell surface, where they expose bits of pathogen on their own cell membrane. Finally, they head for the nearest lymph gland or organ, to 'present' the foreign epitopes they have acquired to the helper T cells.

This is an essential step in the immune response, known as *antigen presentation*. Without it, the precise mechanisms of the adaptive immune response fail to operate. For example, B cells cannot produce antibodies without signals from helper T cells, but the T cells will not 'turn on' until they have been presented with the correct foreign epitopes by the phagocytes. Moreover, in the act of presenting epitopes to the T cells, the phagocytes also give information about *where* the original infection can be found. We mentioned earlier that each type of phagocyte has a particular territory, so the T cell has only to identify which type of phagocyte has arrived to know something about its 'usual address'. This mechanism assists in directing the adaptive immune response to the correct location.

Pathogens fight back

The versality of the human immune system, combining both innate and adaptive mechanisms, has exerted selection pressure on the array of human pathogens; those that have evolved strategies to counteract the host's immune response are at a selective advantage and increase in the population, generation by generation. As we described in Chapter 5, humans and their pathogens have *coevolved*. A vast number of different mechanisms have been evolved by successful species of animal parasites, protistans, and bacterial or viral strains, which increase their chance of survival. We have space here to review only a few of these so-called *escape mechanisms*, but their variety testifies to the random nature of the mutations that generated such diverse solutions to the same problem: how to survive in the hostile environment of the host's body.

For example, some pathogens conceal their unique epitopes from the immune system under a coating of other molecules that resemble those of their host. *Ascaris lumbricoides,* the most common roundworm infesting the gut, has a coating of molecules that closely resemble human collagen, a component of human cartilage and the deeper layers of the skin. More effective still are those pathogens that 'borrow' molecules from their host to coat themselves with. The surface layer of the bacterium *Staphylococcus aureus,* which causes abscesses, secretes an enzyme that coagulates clotting components in human blood, which then adhere to the bacteria. Various species of *Schistosoma* flukes, which cause the tropical disease schistosomiasis, coat themselves with a whole range of their host's proteins and sugars.

An entirely different strategy is to change the shapes of the unique epitopes on the pathogen's surface very frequently, a process known as *antigenic drift*. This is one of the escape mechanisms displayed both by HIV and the influenza virus.

☐ How would it help a pathogen to evade destruction by the immune system if it changed the shapes of its epitopes?

■ The first time the host's lymphocytes encountered that pathogen, they would mount a relatively slow and ineffective *primary* immune response, which usually gives the pathogen enough time to replicate successfully and move on to a new host. If the same pathogen is encountered again, the *secondary* immune response may be strong enough to eradicate the pathogen. But if it has changed the shape of its epitopes between the first and second encounter, the immune system responds to it slowly, as though meeting it for the first time.

In HIV, the genes that encode the surface epitopes are highly unstable and prone to mutate. HIV changes its epitopes so fast that, even within the same person, an increasing number of new strains of the virus are generated the longer the infection persists. The waves of influenza that sweep across a country from time to time are the result of a new variant of the influenza virus that no one has encountered before. Antigenic drift is an illustration of the fact, emphasised in Chapter 5, that pathogens can evolve faster than their hosts because of their much shorter generation time.

☐ How does the 'escape' mechanism of antigenic drift create difficulties for vaccination programmes to prevent outbreaks of influenza?

■ The vaccine can only contain samples of epitopes from influenza strains that already exist. It cannot protect people from new variants that arise by mutation. (If a vaccine against HIV is ever developed, it will have to overcome the same problem.)

The most common escape mechanisms might be summed up as 'resisting arrest'. Many kinds of pathogens synthesise and secrete chemicals that deter phagocytes or cytotoxic cells from approaching or getting a grip on them. Others secrete enzymes and 'blocking' proteins that break down or inhibit the important molecular defences in the immune response, such as complement, lysozyme and antibodies. The bacteria that variously cause tuberculosis, leprosy, legionnaires' disease and certain tropical fevers reproduce inside the host's cells, where they are very difficult for the immune system to detect or attack. These bacteria are engulfed by phagocytes and enclosed in a vesicle, but are able to prevent fusion of the vesicle with the lysosomes, which (as Chapter 3 described) are packets of enzymes and other destructive chemicals.

Balancing the survival of host and pathogen: bacterial endotoxin

These varied escape mechanisms illustrate the delicate balance that has been struck between 'host kills pathogen' and 'pathogen kills host'. A good example of what happens when this equilibrium is disturbed is provided by the many types of bacterial infection associated with high fevers and shock (a medical term meaning malfunction of major organs as a result of severe disturbances in the circulation of blood). All the bacteria associated with these potentially fatal symptoms have a layer of *endotoxin* molecules covering their outer surface. Endotoxin is formed from a sugar and a fat, both of which are unique to bacteria. The structure varies somewhat from one bacterial strain to another, but the basic plan is the same. (Rietschel and Brade, 1992, and Moltz, 1993, review the state of knowledge about endotoxin and fever at the time of writing.)

As long as endotoxin stays on the surface of the bacteria it causes no harm to the host, but it is a potent target for immune attack because it contains unusual epitopes not found in animal cells. So in this location it tilts the balance of survival against the bacteria. When the bacteria reproduce by cell division, they release a few molecules of endotoxin, but a *low* concentration of 'free' endotoxin molecules sets off cascade reactions in the host, which stimulate the immune response locally and tilt the balance even further against the bacteria. However, the pendulum is about to swing back the other way.

As the immune response builds up, increasing numbers of bacteria are killed by it and their cell walls disintegrate, releasing a *high* concentration of endotoxin molecules. The more successful the immune response against the bacteria becomes, so the higher the concentration of endotoxin rises and the further it is swept around the body in the bloodstream. Widespread endotoxin causes widespread inflammatory activity in the host's immune system, which may fail to respond effectively as a consequence. This interference with the immune response tilts the balance of survival back towards the bacteria, which may recover lost ground. The inflammatory activity dispersed over large areas of the body leads to fever and, if severe and prolonged, shock and death. Even if the host dies, the infection may still be passed on. But there is inconclusive evidence to suggest that a *moderate* fever may enhance the ability of the immune system to eradicate the bacteria, demonstrating yet another counter-measure in the struggle for survival. Medical science may have the last word, however, because the ability of low concentrations of endotoxin to *enhance* the immune response may be harnessed in the design of a new class of anti-bacterial drugs.

Variations in immune responsiveness

Before leaving the inner world of infection and response, you might look back to Chapters 4 and 5 and think about the information contained there about variation in the susceptibility of populations and individuals to disease. Each of us has a unique genotype and just as this affects our ability to withstand or sustain lung damage from tobacco smoke, or to produce the enzymes necessary for adequate digestion and nutritional health, so too it affects our resistance to infection. The frequency with which a population encounters a certain pathogen over many generations results in the selection of genotypes that confer some resistance to that pathogen. Similarly, where a pathogen is rare, there is only a very weak selection pressure to favour the increase in the population of genes that confer some protection against this pathogen. Thus, as mentioned in Chapter 5, the arrival of colonists in the Americas resulted in devastating infection among the indigenous populations from pathogens to which the colonists were relatively immune.

Even within a single population, there is enormous variation between individuals, as you might expect. At one end of the spectrum can be found rare individuals with genetic defects in their immune system that are so severe they can only survive in highly-protected environments. At the other end of the spectrum, the differences between one person's susceptibility to infection and another's are so subtle that they can only be inferred by extrapolation from studies of laboratory rats and mice. In rodents, it is clear that the immune responsiveness of each animal has a 'personal profile' in which certain pathogens are attacked more effectively than others. Thus, each individual may be a 'good responder' to certain pathogens, but have less effective responses to certain others, and may not be able to respond at all to a very few. The pathogens that provoke high or low responses vary from one individual animal to the next. It seems likely that the same is true for humans.

Immune responsiveness varies not only between individuals, but within the same person at different times in their lives.

□ When would you expect a person to be most vulnerable to infection in their lifetime and why?

■ In early life, when every pathogen is being encountered for the first time, so that all responses are of the slower *primary* type.

Babies and infants are also more vulnerable to infection because certain features of the immune system take up to two years to mature. But they are born with pre-formed antibodies already circulating in their bloodstream, which came across the placenta from their mother's circulation. Her immune system makes antibodies to any pathogen she has encountered in the previous few months, which she 'donates' to the baby while still in the uterus and, after birth, in her breast milk (which, by the way, is pathogen-free). The antibodies in breast milk survive digestion in the baby's gut and give some protection against those pathogens most likely still to be in the local environment.[7]

At the other end of the lifespan, the effectiveness of the immune system to respond to encounters with new pathogens gradually declines in old age. Elderly people usually retain their immunity to any infection they have previously encountered and successfully eliminated, but may succumb to new infections, particularly those affecting the respiratory system. This vulnerability may partly be due to a lifetime of breathing pollutants (particularly tobacco smoke) and partly due to 'shallow' breathing which leaves parts of the lungs inadequately inflated and creates suitable habitats for bacteria to multiply. Other aspects of changed biology in old age are discussed in Chapter 8 of this book.

A possible cause of variation in susceptibility to infection that has created much speculation is *stress* (Cohen and Williamson, 1991, gives a review). This 'catch-all' term has so many different meanings that it is extremely difficult to be certain whether or not the normal stresses encountered in everyday life have any *significant* effect on immune responsiveness. It is commonly believed that at times of emotional stress, people are more likely to get minor coughs and colds, but this effect has been very hard to demonstrate conclusively in well-designed experiments on human subjects living 'normally' stressful lives. Too many other variables get in the way; for example, a few studies of students show that they have higher concentrations of bacteria in throat swabs during exam periods than at other times of the year.

□ One interpretation of this result is that exam stress made the immune system less efficient and allowed more bacteria than usual to grow in the students' throats. Can you think of an alternative interpretation?

■ They may have been *behaving* differently than at other times of the year, with the effect that they were more exposed to infection (for example, they may have smoked more cigarettes than usual, creating a sore throat where bacteria can get in).

Even though the experimental data linking stress to suppression of the immune system are not conclusive, the mechanisms by which stress could *in theory* increase vulnerability to infection are at least understood. A defining characteristic of the response to stress is the secretion of hormones from the adrenal gland which increase the mobilisation of stored fats and sugars and their conversion into usable energy. This is an adaptive response to stress (adaptive is used here in its evolutionary sense), and is part of what is generally known as the 'fight or flight' reaction. However, it seems to have an unwanted side-effect in that these same adrenal hormones reduce the effectiveness of the immune response. There is a trade-off between preparing for evasive action against an immediate threat and being ready to repel an infection that might not in fact materialise. But despite consistent experimental evidence showing that stress inhibits the immune response somewhat, there is no consensus about whether this actually results in greater susceptibility to infection.

The evidence concerning the effects of intense *exercise* on the immune system is also contradictory (Caren, 1991 is a useful review). Some studies have shown no difference in the rates of infection among elite athletes in training for major competitions, nor in relatively unfit individuals who begin strenuous training for an unfamiliar sport. Others have shown that the incidence of respiratory-tract infections is greater during training and competition than at other times, especially for endurance events like the marathon.

---

[7]In Chapter 7 of this book you will learn more about the role of breast milk in childhood nutrition and intolerance to milk in adults.

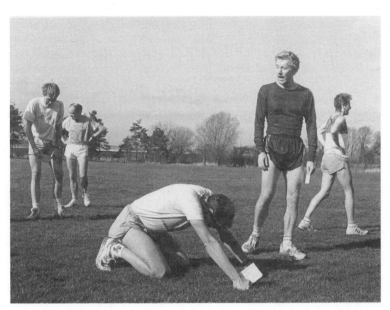

The evidence about whether intense exercise affects the immune system is contradictory. (Photo: Mike Levers)

☐ Can you suggest an explanation for the positive correlation between strenuous training and respiratory infections that does *not* involve an exercise-induced deficiency in the immune system?

■ Athletes in training may come into contact with more infection than at other times, or their respiratory tract may be damaged by gasping for air during strenuous training, especially when the athlete trains on roads polluted by traffic exhaust fumes. This may create more points of entry for pathogens.

This example illustrates how difficult it is to prove 'cause and effect' in such a complex system.

Harnessing the immune response

Finally, we offer a glimpse into the many ways in which medical science is attempting to harness the immune response in the prevention and treatment of disease, not all of which are infectious. You already know about vaccination, a technique which has achieved some remarkable successes, most notably in 'The global eradication of smallpox', the title of an article in the Reader by Marc Strassburg.[8] The smallpox story illustrates the extent to which the biology of the pathogen can profoundly affect the ability of medical science to act against it.

[8]This was set reading for *World Health and Disease*, Chapter 3, but you could usefully re-read it now.

☐ What features of the smallpox virus made it particularly vulnerable to eradication by a vaccination programme?

■ It can only reproduce in humans; there are no reservoirs of infection in other species. It has a short incubation time and it does not produce 'carrier' states in which people who seem well are actually infectious (like Typhoid Mary, mentioned in Chapter 5), and it spreads from person to person fairly slowly.

Other pathogens have proved harder to counter by vaccination because they have none of the above features. An additional problem arises where it is difficult to obtain adequate or stable samples of the pathogen's epitopes to use as the basis of the vaccine. This is the case with leprosy, where the bacteria have proved extremely difficult to grow in bulk. A vaccine against malaria has been delayed because it is so hard to stimulate an immune response with killed *Plasmodium* (the protistan that causes malaria). These difficulties may be overcome by the technique of genetic engineering, which is being applied to produce large amounts of epitopes from several pathogens (including *Plasmodium*). The gene coding for an epitope that is unique to the pathogen is removed from the pathogen's DNA and inserted into the DNA of harmless, fast-growing bacteria, which then manufacture the epitope in bulk as though it was one of their own proteins. Genetic engineering is discussed in more detail in Chapter 9.

Perhaps the most exciting potential applications of knowledge about the immune system relate to the major degenerative diseases, such as cancer and arthritis. It used to be thought that the immune system was on general 'surveillance' for abnormal cells, generated by mutation during an individual's life, which might become malignant. This theory has been disproved and the immune system has little natural role in cancer control, except for those few cancers which are themselves triggered by pathogens that the immune system can detect. The reason is simple: cancer cells are not 'foreign' material, but self-cells that behave in an abnormal manner. The immune system is tolerant of self-cells and thus cannot 'see' cancerous ones, but it might be made to do so.

In theory, it might be possible to generate anticancer antibodies from B cells which have been given additional genes in the laboratory. If antibodies can be made that bind only to cancer cells, they might also be used as carriers of toxic molecules or radioactive isotopes, which could then be targeted onto the cancer very precisely. It might also be possible to harness the many chemicals involved in inflammation reactions and direct those more effectively against cancers. The natural killer (NK) cells we mentioned earlier can be induced to kill cancer cells under certain circumstances, but there are very few of them in the body. One strategy might be to remove some NK cells from a patient, stimulate them to undergo repeated cell divisions in a laboratory vessel, and then return this greatly expanded population to the patient.

Instead of enhancing the immune response, the reverse process would be beneficial in arthritis, where inappropriate inflammation is the source of the disablement. Here the goal is to direct the various *suppressor* mechanisms (such as suppressor T cells) to the inflamed joints and even to use antibodies to 'knock out' the immune cells that are causing the inflammation.

In Chapter 9, we explore further the manipulation of human biology for therapeutic ends and ask what ethical dilemmas are raised by 'tinkering with nature'? But this book has other aims before we turn towards the future. The story of human evolution and its impact on human health and illness is more than the interaction between humans and their pathogens. In the next chapter, we move on to a completely different but equally vital aspect of human biology: how people deal with food and the products of digestion and absorption.

OBJECTIVES FOR CHAPTER 6

When you have studied this chapter, you should be able to:

6.1 Describe the basic mechanisms involved in the innate and adaptive responses of the human immune system to an infection and comment on the evolutionary pressures that may have shaped this system.

6.2 Illustrate some general consequences of the primary and secondary immune response to pathogens and give examples of states of deficiency or inappropriate activity of the immune system.

6.3 Give examples of ways in which variation in the biology of either the human host or the pathogen can affect the outcome of an infection, illustrating the unstable equilibrium between survival and destruction.

QUESTIONS FOR CHAPTER 6

Question 1 (*Objective 6.1*)

The human immune system is capable of recognising at least 100 million different epitopes, which may occur in the structures of pathogens or the molecules they secrete. What other features of human biology and culture have contributed to the evolution of this enormous repertoire, or have been facilitated by it?

Question 2 (*Objectives 6.1 and 6.2*)

The common cold is caused by *rhinoviruses,* of which there are several hundred different kinds. Children suffer repeated colds, often several in one year, but adults get fewer and fewer colds and they have become a rarity by old age. Explain this phenomenon.

Question 3 (*Objectives 6.2 and 6.3*)

In what ways does the human immunodeficiency virus (HIV) 'escape' destruction by the immune system? What light does HIV infection shed on the effectiveness of the *intact* immune system?

7 *Digestion and dietary change*

This chapter is about the biological mechanisms that convert food into biochemically usable nutrients. We relate these processes to the changes in the human diet that have taken place during the last 10 000 years. You may find it useful to refer back to Chapter 2 of this book and remind yourself of the impact of cooking, agriculture and pastoralism on diet. The account given here of the regulation of blood glucose concentration builds on the discussion of measuring blood glucose in Chapter 9 of Studying Health and Disease. *The content of the present chapter also relates to Chapter 11 of* World Health and Disease, *which is about nutrition and the contribution of diet to growth and maturation and to the role of diet in certain diseases. During your study of this chapter you will be asked to read the article 'The history of pernicious anaemia from 1822 to the present day' by Irvine Loudon, which is in the Reader.[1]*

Introduction

All living organisms need food; most plants can synthesise nutrients from water and other minerals when they are exposed to light, but animals eat only other organisms, either while they are still alive (e.g. the animal tissues eaten by certain parasites, and plants eaten by grazing and browsing animals) or when they are dead. Eating and digesting other organisms presents three major kinds of biological problems.

First, all organisms consist of large, chemically complex molecules, which are at least as complex, and often chemically very similar, to those of the eater. So digestion requires breaking down food without harming oneself. Second, if food is to be broken down, and the breakdown

---

[1] *Health and Disease: A Reader* (1984 and revised edition 1994).

products absorbed, intimate contact between the eater's tissues and those of other organisms is almost unavoidable. Such contact is hazardous; as pointed out in Chapter 6, tissues such as the skin, that are exposed to other organisms, some of which are pathogens, are adapted to excluding, or at least inactivating, them.

Third, food is often available only infrequently and in large chunks, more so, of course, for lions or polar bears, which eat for perhaps 20 minutes twice a week, than for sheep or deer that graze for about 18 hours of every day. However, *metabolic activity* (all the biochemical activities necessary for breathing, moving, thinking, etc.) goes on continuously: we use a bit less biochemical energy while asleep in a warm bed, and more during strenuous exercise, but most of the processes that keep us alive go on all the time. So the body faces a dilemma: its food supplies arrive intermittently, but usage of the nutrients is more or less continuous. This chapter explains how human digestion and metabolism deal with these problems.

As we said earlier, most food consists mainly of large, chemically complex molecules that, for reasons outlined below, must be digested (broken down) into much smaller molecules before they can be absorbed into the body and utilised; **digestion** and **absorption** are separate processes and it is important to consider them individually. From the point of view of digestion, the constituents of food can be classified as *fats* (including oils), *carbohydrates* (starches, sugars) and *proteins* (e.g. lean meat, fish, egg white). Most natural foods are mixtures of these major constituents, plus smaller quantities of *vitamins*, *minerals* (sodium, iron, calcium, etc.) and various non-nutritive components that are discussed later.

The principal agents of digestion in all organisms (micro-organisms, fungi and some green plants as well as all animals) are *enzymes*, protein molecules that facilitate the making or breaking of chemical bonds between other molecules. Most enzymes are effective only for one particular, or a few very similar, kinds of chemical reactions, and often particular molecules can be joined or severed only by one unique enzyme. Once in use, a typical enzyme remains active for a few hours, often only for a few minutes. The first step in enzyme activity is specific binding of the enzyme to certain parts of the molecule (or molecules) involved in the reaction that the enzyme catalyses (speeds up), by mechanisms of the 'lock-and-key' type described in Chapter 3 (see Figure 3.10).

Most of the hundreds of different kinds of molecules that animals take in as food are so large and chemically robust that several different digestive enzymes operating in succession are necessary to break them down into fragments small enough to be absorbed. The names of most enzymes end in -ase. For example, the many enzymes that attack different parts of protein molecules are collectively known as *proteases*. The enzyme *lactase* binds to and splits one particular bond in the sugar lactose, breaking it into two almost equal-sized, but chemically slightly different sugars called glucose and galactose. Later in this chapter, you will learn the significance of this reaction for human nutrition.

All enzymes are synthesised inside cells in the same way as other protein molecules. As soon as they are formed, the enzymes (often in a non-active form) pass to a structure called the *Golgi body*, where they are enclosed in an envelope of membrane. Thus parcelled up, they move to the edge of the cell and are *secreted* (expelled into the surrounding medium) when required. Any cell or organ whose main function is secretion is called a **gland**.

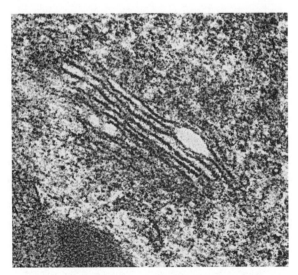

A section of part of a nerve cell showing a Golgi body, magnified 65 000 times by an electron microscope. Golgi bodies are 'stacks' of internal membranes in which secretions such as digestive enzymes are modified, stored or wrapped in membrane before being expelled from the cell. (Photo: Heather Davies)

☐ Why do you think digestive enzymes are thus parcelled up?

■ The material to be digested is chemically very similar to the cells that produce the digestive enzymes. If the enzymes were not contained in this way, they would digest the cell itself.

As pointed out in earlier chapters of this book, intimate contact with other organisms, whether living or freshly dead, is very risky; micro-organisms can cause disease and foreign proteins can stimulate the immune system to make an inappropriate response. When a cat eats a freshly-killed mouse, its meal consists of much more than just mouse tissues; the mouse's skin and gut may harbour many symbiotic bacteria (as ours do), and it may be infested with several kinds of macroparasites (see Chapters 2 and 5). Cooking kills most living organisms (and freezing kills some of them), but all fresh or cold food is 'contaminated' with micro-organisms that fall on it from the air. Some foods, such as cheese, yoghurt and beer, are made by culturing micro-organisms, which give them a distinctive taste and texture.

☐ What food (other than very hot food) is normally completely free of micro-organisms? (Think back to Chapter 6.)

■ Breast milk, as long as it passes directly from the mother to the infant.

However, milk is an excellent culture medium for micro-organisms and most animal milk is contaminated by the time it reaches the human consumer (see Chapter 2). Eating normal food inevitably involves intimate contact between the eater's tissues and those of a variety of other organisms, and an essential part of the process of digestion is inactivation of potentially harmful foreign organisms.

The digestive system

The gut is a series of chambers and tubes lined by cells with contrasting properties. As it passes along the gut the food comes into contact with many different enzymes and different chemical environments. Our next task is to describe the structures and functions of the gut from end to end. Figure 7.1 (*overleaf*) shows the main features of the gut and the organs associated with it.

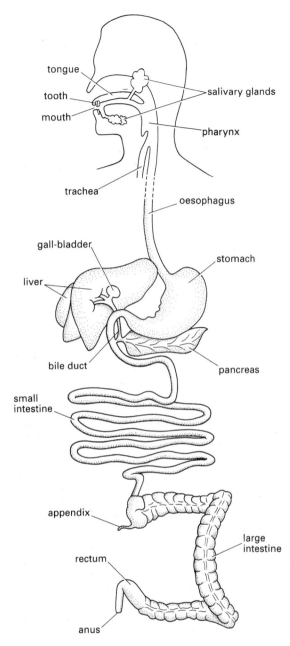

Figure 7.1 *The anatomy of the human digestive tract and associated organs.*

In humans, digestion starts in the *mouth*; chewing breaks up the food and an enzyme secreted from the salivary glands attacks certain bonds in starches. A complex muscular action called swallowing compresses the food into small balls and propels it through muscular,

non-secretory portions of the gut called the *pharynx* and *oesophagus*, and down to the stomach. Swallowing is greatly facilitated by the secretion of mucus, a watery lubricant, from the salivary glands. Figure 7.1 shows that the pharynx is also the route through which air moves from the nose and mouth to the trachea (windpipe) on its way to the lungs.

☐ Look at Figure 7.1; what happens when we choke on food?

■ A piece of food goes 'the wrong way', entering the top of the trachea where it immediately provokes powerful, unsuppressable contractions of the breathing muscles (coughing) which propel the food back into the gut.

A gulp of water stimulates swallowing, which helps to convey the misdirected piece of food down to the stomach. Choking is most likely to happen when we try to eat in strange postures, such as while lying down, and in infants, in whom coordination of swallowing and breathing is imperfectly developed.

The *stomach* is a highly distensible bag, expanding in adults from an empty volume of only about 0.05 litres to as much as 1.5 litres after a large meal. Special cells in the lining secrete water, hydrochloric acid and enzymes, particularly proteases that are adapted to work efficiently in an acid environment. On a normal diet, the stomach lining of an adult secretes about 2 litres of fluid per day into the stomach. The digestive action of these secretions is assisted by rhythmic, sometimes powerful, contractions of the muscles of the stomach wall, which break up the food and mix it with the acid and enzymes. The hydrochloric acid makes the mammalian stomach one of the most acidic environments known in any biological system. Some components of food are broken down directly by the acid. Stomach acid dissolves pieces of bone, tooth or eggshell, in the same way as vinegar or bleach dissolves chalk. And, of course, all but a very few kinds of micro-organisms die instantly in a strongly acid environment.

☐ What happens to the remains of the micro-organisms killed by the stomach acids?

■ Micro-organisms are chemically very similar to plant and animal tissues, so the dead cells are digested in exactly the same way as 'proper' food.

The cells lining the stomach wall are protected from the acid and their own digestive enzymes by secretions of thick *mucus*. Most nutrients cannot cross this protective layer but a few, notably alcohol and certain fats, diffuse through it and the cellular lining of the stomach, whence they pass into the blood.

☐ What are the implications of this property for the action of alcoholic drinks?

■ Alcohol enters the blood, and hence reaches the brain, within a few minutes of being swallowed, much faster than most other components of meals.

Under some abnormal circumstances, the mucus layer is breached and the enzymes and hydrochloric acid erode the stomach wall, causing a painful disorder called a peptic ulcer.

Passage through the stomach takes 2 to 6 hours depending upon the quantity of food and its chemical composition. Food consisting mainly of carbohydrate passes through more rapidly than that rich in protein, while fatty meals remain in the stomach for the longest time. The contents of the stomach leave in 'pulses', via the pyloric valve, as a homogeneous mixture of food and enzymes with the consistency of a fairly thick soup.

The next structure in the digestive tract is the *small intestine*, which is a coiled, muscular tube approximately 6.4 metres long and 2.5 centimetres in diameter, lined with many different kinds of cells. It is divided into three anatomically distinct segments: the duodenum (about 20 centimetres long), jejunum (2.5 metres) and ileum (3.7 metres).[2]

Secretions from the liver and the pancreas enter the duodenum through a shared duct a few centimetres from the pyloric valve. The liver secretes a yellow fluid called *bile* (about half a litre a day in adults) which is stored and concentrated in the gall bladder, a small sac under the liver, until eating stimulates its discharge. The active ingredients of bile are not enzymes but complex salts that emulsify fats (break them up and make them miscible with water) in much the same way as soap does, and thereby make them accessible to enzymes that operate best in a watery, rather than a fatty, environment.

The *pancreas* (the pancreas of cattle and pigs is sold by butchers as 'sweetbreads') is a much smaller gland than the liver. It secretes about 1.5 litres of pancreatic fluid per day, containing a mixture of several different enzymes that digest fats, proteins and carbohydrates. Bile and pancreatic fluid also contain salts that neutralise the acid from the stomach, so the contents of the duodenum

are only slightly more acid than the blood. The secretory cells in the lining of the small intestine itself also secrete over 1.5 litres of fluid daily, containing various enzymes that digest carbohydrates and proteins.

All these enzymes can only function in a non-acidic environment. Together they break up digestible carbohydrates into small sugars, mostly glucose and galactose, fats into fatty acids, and proteins into the 20 different amino acids of which they are composed, or into short chains of up to six amino acids. The scale of the operation is enormous: many common proteins in meat and grains contain thousands of amino acids, and the bonds that join them together are severed during digestion.

Mammalian digestion is very efficient; the combination of stomach acidity, enzyme activity and muscular churning at 37 °C breaks down food very fast and thoroughly. Consider how long meat, cabbage, etc. take to rot on a compost heap, compared to how long it takes a similar meal to go through you, or, even more impressive, through a cow or a sheep. Even at 100 °C, an Irish stew takes many hours to be reduced to a smooth soup!

☐ What do you think would happen to the stomach enzymes that were produced by the cells lining the stomach when they reach the small intestine along with the food they have been digesting?

■ Being adapted to work in a strongly acid environment, they would be ineffective in the much less acid small intestine. They are broken down by proteases of the small intestine in exactly the same way as the proteins in food, and thus their molecular constituents are 'recycled'.

As in the stomach, the secretions of mucus lubricate the food and protect the lining of the small intestine from being digested by its own enzymes. Rhythmic muscular contractions of the intestine wall, called *peristalsis* (pronounced 'perry-stall-sis'), aid digestion and absorption by stirring the gut contents and propelling them along. The time spent by gut contents in the small intestine is very variable and difficult to measure because this region is the main site of absorption of nutrients from the gut contents and sometimes little of the original food remains.

☐ Why are endoparasites such as tapeworms and roundworms (see Chapters 2 and 5) more likely to settle in the small intestine than in the stomach?

■ The stomach is too acid for parasites to live in. The small intestine is much less acidic and so it is a more congenial environment for parasites.

---

[2]There is no need to memorise these names (or the lengths of these sections of gut), but you might want to know how to pronounce them: *duodenum* ('dew-oh-deen-um'); *jejunum* ('jeh-joon-um'); *ileum* ('ill-ee-um').

By this stage, the gut contents are more thoroughly digested, making the nutrients in it more easily absorbed by the parasite as well as by the person. Parasites such as tapeworms (*Taenia*) and *Toxocara* (nematode parasites of dogs and cats, which can also affect people, Chapters 2 and 5) enter the body through the mouth, as eggs or dormant cysts, encased in a tough, impermeable shell that can resist hours of exposure to stomach acid and enzymes. After hatching in the small intestine, tapeworms attach themselves firmly to the gut lining, thereby resisting expulsion by peristaltic movements, and grow into soft, flattened 'tape'-shaped animals, which gain maximum contact with the nutritious gut contents. A few bacteria, among them *Vibrio cholerae* (which causes cholera), have also evolved the ability to form cysts that protect them from digestion by their host.

Absorption of nutrients

As well as completing the digestion of food, the small intestine is also the main site for absorption of the digested nutrients into the blood. On a regime of small, regular meals, most absorption takes place in the duodenum and jejunum, but the ileum is also absorptive, and acts as 'spare capacity' for absorption, becoming functional following very large meals. The whole of the small intestine is pleated and lined with tiny finger-like projections called *villi* (pronounced 'vill-eye', singular: villus, shown in Figure 7.2), whose surface is further frilled out to form microvilli, which maximise the surface area in contact with the intestinal contents.

The inner layer of cells forming a villus contains a mosaic of secretory and absorptive cells. The secretory cells are of two types. One kind secretes mucus that acts as a protective barrier against the digestive enzymes in the intestine and the other secretes the digestive enzymes. At the base of the villi there is a layer of muscles whose contractions churn the intestinal contents and move them down its length. A further outer layer contains secretory cells which lubricate its external surface and lets the gut glide easily against other organs.

The cells lining the small intestine are packed tightly together, which prevents leakage of the intestinal contents into the central region of the villus, where there are vessels of the blood system (Figure 3.21) and the lymphatic system (Figure 6.8). In the gut, the lymph transports fats from the gut lining to the bloodstream, as well as removing fluids and bacteria, and the cell debris that

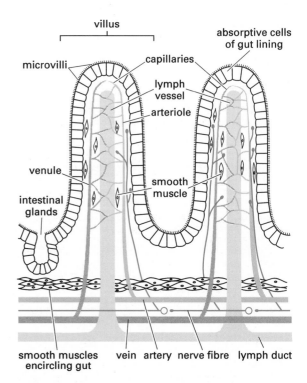

Figure 7.2 *The general structure of the lining of the small intestine. Each villus projects about 1 mm into the gut cavity.*

results from the body's immune responses to infection. The small intestine is also richly perfused with blood which then flows through the liver (where some of the newly absorbed nutrients undergo important chemical modifications), before passing through the heart and on to the lungs, limbs and peripheral tissues. After a heavy meal, a large proportion of the total blood volume in the body may be around the intestine and in the liver.

Cell membranes are made of fatty, rather than watery, materials (see Chapter 3), so fatty acids enter the gut lining quite well by passive diffusion, although they are mostly larger molecules than glucose and amino acids. Most other fat-soluble nutrients, such as vitamins A, D, K, and E, are also absorbed passively through the cells lining the small intestine, as are the major ingredients of bile, which are taken up by the liver and 'recycled' to produce more bile. Some larger particles are engulfed by endocytosis (see Figure 3.9a and b); membranes of cells lining the small intestine form a vesicle around the particle into which digestive enzymes are secreted and the nutrients thus released are absorbed by the cell.

including glucose and all the common amino acids, transport is not only restricted to particular sites on the cell membrane but is also 'active'; metabolic energy is necessary to convey each molecule from the gut contents into the tissues. Absorption of the minerals calcium and iron also involves specific transporter mechanisms. However, the gut of newborn infants is very much more permeable than that of adults and admits quite large molecules fairly indiscriminately. The sites of active transport into the cells lining the gut are identified by specific protein molecules called receptors, which are embedded in the cell membrane and 'match' the chemical structure of their target molecules, as described in Chapter 3. The mechanism of transport is complicated and need not concern us here. You should picture the lining of the small intestine as a mosaic of many different channels, each specific to a particular kind of molecule, that act as a sort of molecular 'escort service'. Nutrients are picked up from the gut contents and conveyed, molecule by molecule, into the blood.

□ What would happen if the uptake mechanism for a particular nutrient were defective?

■ The person would be unable to absorb that particular nutrient properly but would be otherwise physiologically normal and so, on an appropriately modified diet, could lead a more or less normal life.

The inherited disease, cystic fibrosis, is an example of a disease that arises from a deficiency in a transport protein. The incidence of the disease in families and careful analysis of the DNA of affected people indicate that cystic fibrosis is due to the inheritance of two defective alleles of a single gene (see Chapter 4). This gene codes for a protein that regulates the channel through which chloride (a constituent of common salt) passes across cell membranes. The most troublesome symptoms of the disease involve the accumulation of thick mucus in the respiratory system, but people with cystic fibrosis also experience digestive disorders that can be attributed to defects in chloride absorption.

As you have seen, digestion and absorption are both very complicated processes involving many different kinds of molecules. Some, such as enzymes and receptor molecules, are unique proteins, each coded for by a different gene. If the gene is absent or (more commonly) significantly modified, either no protein is produced, or it is present but malformed, so it cannot do its job properly. You will not be surprised to learn that defects of digestion, arising from the inability to synthesise certain digestive enzymes, or of absorption, due to the absence or abnormality of a receptor protein, are among the commonest kinds of genetic diseases in humans.

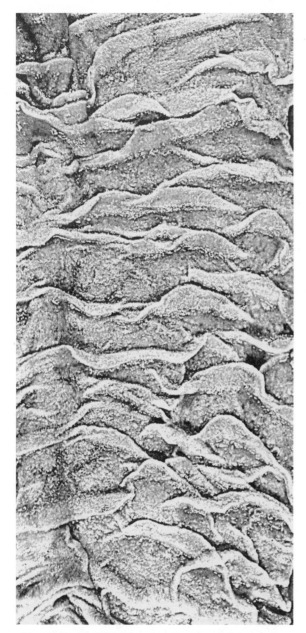

The inner lining of the human small intestine, showing the rough pleated surface (approximately actual size). The villi are too small to be visible. (Photo: Dr H. M. Gilmour, Department of Pathology, University of Edinburgh Medical School)

Many other kinds of molecules do not enter cells by passive diffusion and can pass only through specific channels in the cell membrane. For some nutrients,

As explained in an earlier book in this series,[3] *vitamins* and *minerals* are essential to nutrition. The mechanisms by which these chemically varied molecules are absorbed are complicated and in many cases incompletely understood. It is clear, however, that factors produced higher up in the gut can be essential to the uptake of iron, and possibly other minerals, in the small intestine. If such factors are lacking, absorption may be so inefficient that, even if the diet contains more than enough of the essential mineral, almost none of it is taken up by the gut lining and into the blood. The root cause of *pernicious anaemia* is now believed to be the lack of such factors for the absorption of vitamins. The story of how physicians and scientists reached this conclusion, after many confusing observations and erroneous theories, is told by the medical historian Irvine Loudon in the Reader article entitled 'The history of pernicious anaemia from 1822 to the present day'.[4] You should read it now.

☐ Give examples from Loudon's article of contradictory observations or experiments which indicate that (a) defects of the stomach were the *root cause* of pernicious anaemia, and (b) defects in the stomach were a *secondary* consequence, not a primary cause, of the disease?

■ (a) The stomachs of people who had died of pernicious anemia were found to be atrophied and they lacked hydrochloric acid. (b) Large reductions in the numbers of the red blood cells were found in people in the early stages of pernicious anaemia, long before they complained of digestive problems. Feeding patients with hydrochloric acid improved their digestion but did not cure the disease.

The example of pernicious anaemia illustrates the complexity of the mechanisms governing absorption from the gut. Even if the diet contains adequate amounts of iron, it cannot be absorbed unless several other mechanisms are working properly.

As pointed out above, the gut lining, liver and pancreas secrete large quantities of *water* into the gut, where it facilitates the digestion and movement of the food. Water is much too precious to be expelled with the undigested remains of meals, so most of it is reabsorbed. There is no active transport system, or indeed any specific channels, for water uptake; salts, particularly sodium,

[3]*World Health and Disease,* Chapter 11.

[4]In *Health and Disease: A Reader* (1984 and revised edition 1994).

potassium and chloride, are absorbed actively and the water follows passively to equalise the concentration of salt solutions between the lining of the intestine and the gut contents.

Even with the help of specific receptors and transport systems for most nutrients, absorption inevitably involves intimate contact between the intestinal lining and the gut contents, which includes digestive enzymes. Such contact between the intestinal cells and the gut contents does not normally stimulate the immune system (see Chapter 6) because by this stage, the food has been digested into molecular fragments too small to elicit an immune response.

A certain amount of undigested material in the gut contents is normal, and indeed may be essential to maintaining strong peristaltic activity, which keeps the contents moving along the gut. However, if key digestive enzymes are deficient or absent, or if the food contains much indigestible material, large proteins and carbohydrates may reach the ileum, and elicit an immune response, particularly if the lining of the gut is abnormally 'leaky', enabling foreign materials to penetrate deep into the villi. Such mechanisms may underlie certain 'food allergies', but their existence, together with the perception that they are becoming increasingly common in the Western world, remains controversial.

The delicate lining of the small intestine erodes rapidly, and so is continuously renewed. In adults, the entire lining is replaced with newly formed cells about every five days, with the loss into the gut of about 250 grams (half a pound) of dead cells from the old lining. Because renewal of the lining of the small intestine is so dependent upon newly formed cells, any agents that impede cell division, such as starvation, high fever and certain anti-cancer drugs, quickly impair both the digestive and the absorptive functions of the small intestine.

The large intestine

The last section of the gut is the *large intestine,* so called because it is broad (about 6.5 centimetres wide) but relatively short (about 1.5 metres long). It includes the colon or bowel, which extends from the junction with the small intestine near a functionless protrusion called the appendix, followed by the rectum and the anus, through which the faeces are expelled (look back at Figure 7.1). Digestion and absorption are almost complete by the time the intestinal contents reach the large intestine, but there is still a variable quantity of undigested food remaining and unreabsorbed material released from the gut, including secretions and debris of dead cells from the lining of the small intestine. The brown colour of faeces is due mainly to a pigment in bile (formed from the breakdown of red blood cells) that is not reabsorbed or broken down and so is eliminated as waste.

Symbiotic bacteria

The distinctive feature of the colon is the presence of numerous symbiotic bacteria (see Chapter 5). Micro-organisms can often synthesise a wider range of enzymes than can larger, anatomically more complex organisms, and these symbionts digest some components of the host's food, mostly carbohydrates, that human enzymes cannot break down.

The bacteria take up the carbohydrates thus digested, metabolising them to gases (flatus) that distend the bowel and eventually emerge as farts. Adults on a mixed diet expel 1–3 litres per day of such gases. The colonic bacteria are also an important component of faeces. Before being thus expelled, they help in the synthesis of several vitamins, including B vitamins and vitamin K, which are absorbed passively through the lining of the colon. Cells in the lining of the large intestine may also take up and, with the help of phagocytic cells (see Chapter 6), digest whole bacteria.

☐ How would this process promote good nutrition?

■ The bacteria are themselves nourished by the residues of the food that the human gut has not digested. Taking up such bacteria into the lining of the colon and digesting them is an excellent way of increasing the extraction of nutrients from otherwise indigestible food. Such mechanisms may be particularly important for people on diets that are low in proteins and essential fats.

You know already that almost all active micro-organisms are killed by the stomach acids and the digestive enzymes as they pass through the upper portions of the gut, so you may be wondering how the symbiotic bacteria survive to reach the large intestine. They form protected spores or cysts and only 'hatch' to proliferate when they reach the more benign environment of the large intestine.

At birth, babies have very few symbiotic or pathogenic bacteria, but they quickly acquire some from the mother. The process is quite efficient in newborns because their stomach is much less acid than that of adults, and they secrete only enzymes that are adapted to digest milk and are not very effective on bacteria. But in weaned children and adults, large or frequent doses of powerful antibiotics can destroy the symbiotic bacteria in the bowel, causing abnormal faeces and, if doses

are prolonged, vitamin deficiencies. The bowel is only slowly recolonised by 'new' bacteria taken in with food or water, because all but the best protected micro-organisms are killed and digested in the stomach and small intestine.

☐ What features of the infant gut make infants more susceptible to pathogenic bacteria such as *Vibrio cholerae* that enter the body with water and food?

■ The less acid stomach and the lack of 'generalist' enzymes that digest non-milk proteins make infants much more susceptible to such infections.

The formation of faeces

The active absorption of salts from the gut contents into the tissues continues in the large intestine in much the same way as in the small intestine.

☐ How would the composition of the gut contents be affected if they have a lower concentration of salts than exists in nearby tissues?

■ Water in the gut contents would diffuse across the gut lining into the tissues, thereby concentrating and drying out the gut contents, which are condensed to form faeces. (If you are unsure about why this process happens, look back at Figure 3.8; water 'follows' the salts into the tissues, thereby equalising the salt concentration in the contents and lining of the gut.)

The gut contents normally remain in the colon for about 18 to 24 hours, but the longer they remain, the drier the faeces become. Normal faeces contain about two parts water to one part dry solids. They move into the rectum, from where they are expelled by a complex series of movements called defaecation, that involve abdominal and thoracic (chest) muscles as well as those of the gut itself and, except in young children, are normally under voluntary control.

☐ The gut responds to the presence of toxic materials and organisms by accelerating and strengthening peristalsis. How would the composition of the faeces be affected?

■ Stronger and more frequent peristalsis hastens the passage of the gut contents through the small and large intestines, shortening the time available for reabsorption of salts and water, and so producing the watery, unformed faeces that we know as diarrhoea.

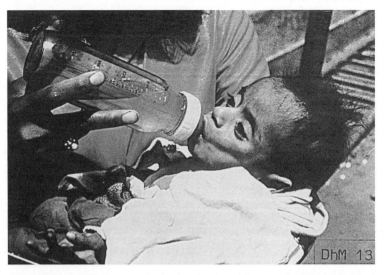

Severe diarrhoea causes the loss of so much water and salts that the tissues become flaccid, producing the characteristic wizened appearance of this baby. Replacement of water and salts may achieve a complete recovery. (Photo: courtesy of Teaching Aids at Low Cost (TALC), P.O. Box 49, St Albans. Details of TALC materials sent free on request.)

Peristaltic movements sometimes become vigorous enough to override the voluntary control of defaecation. We are all familiar with the noticeable, sometimes painful, contractions of the gut muscles that precede diarrhoea, which sometimes happens uncontrollably.

☐ Why are brief bouts of diarrhoea an effective response to the presence of harmful materials or parasites in the gut?

■ The powerful contractions expel the potentially dangerous gut contents quickly, before their toxic components have time to be absorbed through the small intestine.

The presence of potentially toxic material in the gut often causes severe depression and distress, but as soon as it is expelled, the person feels better remarkably quickly, often within a few minutes, and recovers completely within hours. Mild diarrhoea is thus a natural, adaptive mechanism for preventing the absorption of toxic substances. In more severe forms of diarrhoea, notably that caused by the pathogenic bacterium *Vibrio cholerae*, the channels through which salts are reabsorbed in the lower intestine are also impaired.

☐ Why is diarrhoea potentially lethal, especially in small children?

■ Salts and water are expelled as faeces instead of being reabsorbed. Secretion from the stomach, liver, pancreas and duodenum continues, so unless the salts and water are replaced, the body rapidly becomes severely dehydrated.

Over the last decade or so much attention has been paid to the role of dietary fibre in maintaining good gut function, with recommendations that fibre additives, such as bran, are included in the diet. Bran is a by-product of the process of milling grains like wheat. The bran residue, and many other plant fibres, consist of a carbohydrate called cellulose, which the human gut cannot digest. It retains water and adds bulk to the contents of the intestine, increasing the volume by 40–100 per cent and supports the growth of symbiotic bacteria in the bowel, many of which can digest cellulose. By increasing the volume of the gut contents, its presence gently stimulates peristalsis and so *decreases* the transit time of the intestinal contents, thereby slightly reducing the efficiency of digestion.

Absorbing fewer nutrients may not matter in well-nourished people, but consuming larger quantities of fibre can result in dietary deficiencies because fibre can absorb minerals such as calcium, iron, magnesium and phosphorus, making them unavailable for absorption into the blood supply. The advantage of faster transit is that food residues, some possibly carcinogenic (cancer-causing or promoting), spend less time in the gut.[5]

[5]The controversy about the value of dietary fibre is briefly reviewed in *World Health and Disease*, Chapter 11.

Digestion of other components of food

As pointed out in Chapter 2, obtaining food is a physio-logically complex process, to which different kinds of organisms have found a wide variety of solutions. Evol-ution normally proceeds towards preventing organisms from eating other organisms and their component parts, in other words, to frustrate the transfer of energy up the food chain (see Chapter 5). Mice (and other prey species) avoid cats (and other predators) by running away or hiding. Plants, micro-organisms and some animals (e.g. mussels and oysters) cannot move, but they deter other organisms from eating them by being hard, tough, spiky or poisonous. You may have seen a squirrel's attempts to penetrate a hard nutshell, and noticed that sheep and cattle readily eat grass and dandelions while avoiding the thistles, stinging nettles, alder and other nasty-tasting or toxic plants.

Toxins are any substances that delay or disrupt any biological process in the cells or tissues of an organism. However, many toxic substances only produce notice-able effects if present at high concentrations. The human diet, especially that of adults, includes a great many such potentially toxic compounds: indeed, we have come to like, at least in small quantities, the pungent flavours that they impart to our basic foods. Pure flour, rice or potato and unseasoned meat tastes bland and unappetising; most of the strong flavours we use in cookery come from plants, particularly seeds (e.g coffee, pepper), leaves (e.g. tea, mint, sage) and roots (e.g. ginger). Simple flavours such as salt, sweet and sour (i.e. acidic) are due to small, simple molecules, but many others arise from chemically complex molecules that are either not digested at all or are only partially digested by the normal digestive enzymes, so they yield no nutrients. Some such large substances dissolve quite well in fats and hence pass through cell membranes and into the blood. Others, notably certain ingredients of tea and coffee, reach the small intestine almost unchanged, and inactivate enzymes by binding onto them.

□ How would drinking a lot of tea or coffee affect a person's digestion and nutrition?

■ Inactivation of enzymes would impair the efficiency of digestion and (since enzymes are pro-teins) would squander the body's protein reserves.

However, this effect is only a significant cause of malnu-trition if people drink very large quantities of tea or coffee, and eat very little.

Many non-nutritious molecules enter the blood, so reaching the brain (e.g. caffeine in tea and coffee) where,

in small quantities, they may alter mood or the sensation of pain and, in large doses, may produce serious mental and physical symptoms such as hallucinations and impaired control of movement. From a physiological point of view, such substances are toxins; the liver takes them up and converts them into harmless components (or wraps them up in protein molecules), which are then excreted through the kidneys. Alcohol is unusual in that it both acts directly on the brain to impair movement and affect mood and it is converted into glucose as a source of energy. Inactivating and eliminating potential toxins uses both energy and proteins and the liver cannot cope with unlimited quantities or variety of such materials. Delicious though they are in small quantities mixed with bland-tasting foods such as meat or flour, one cannot live on a diet that consists only of sage, coffee, garlic, pepper, cinnamon, ginger, turmeric or similar ingredients.

In general, the livers of grazing and browsing mam-mals, which eat leaves, seeds or roots, can cope with a wider range of potentially toxic substances more efficiently than those of fruit-eaters or carnivores, particu-larly specialised predators such as lions, cats, wolves and polar bears.

□ Can you suggest an evolutionary reason for these facts?

■ The diet of predators that eat other mammals, birds, fish, etc. contains few non-nutritious, poten-tially toxic molecules, but grazing and browsing mammals ingest a wide variety of toxins from the plants in their diet and so have very efficient livers.

□ Would people's capacity to deal with toxins from plants and micro-organisms be similar to that of the predators, or that of the grazing and browsing mammals?

■ As pointed out in Chapter 2, most primates eat fruit and flowers rather than tougher, more indigest-ible plant parts, and very little animal food. However, humans are exceptional among primates in that we went through a long period (probably at least a million years) in which other large mammals formed a major part of the diet, so you would expect the human digestive system and liver to resemble that of both fruit-eaters and carnivores, and to be *less* efficient at dealing with toxins than those of plant-eaters.

As mentioned in Chapter 2, cooking renders many poten-tially toxic foods more palatable and digestible. Indeed, the habit probably first developed as a means of dealing with plant foods rather than for cooking meat. Cooking enabled people to eat a wider range of plants, so their diet became more diverse, and hence more adaptable to changes in climate and season. The human diet changed even more rapidly during the last 10 000 years, with the rise of agriculture and animal husbandry.

It is very difficult to determine exactly when and why new foods were added to the human diet; plant fragments and even animal bones rot so quickly that few remains survive for us to study. Recently, anthropologists have tried to determine what ancient people ate by examining fine scratches and patterns of wear on teeth. Experts differ in their interpretation of these observations but everyone agrees that the human diet has changed in the recent past, and is still changing as new foods, and new ways of processing food, are discovered.

In view of the rapid, relatively recent changes in diet, we should not be surprised that certain natural and artificial flavours, preservatives and other non-nutritive ingredients of foods are indigestible for some people or, more seriously, that they pass unnoticed into the blood where they remain for some time because the person's liver cannot deal with them and so they are only slowly excreted. Examples include certain artificial flavourings, preservatives and colouring agents that are apparently harmless to most people, but have been implicated in the causation of behavioural problems such as hyperactivity or depression in others.

It is important to emphasise that natural substances in foods that have only recently entered our diet are often as indigestible and harmful as some synthetic food additives are believed to be. For example, some people (and many animals) dislike the taste of beetroot, which arises partly from the chemical that gives the plant its red colour. This substance is not digested and so passes unaltered into the blood, where it is usually harmless at low concentrations. Some people's liver can break it down and so they can eliminate it as colourless products, but that of others cannot, and so the red colour appears in their urine a few hours after eating beetroot. Such physiological differences do not matter for people's ordinary lives, but they illustrate the genetic diversity within the human population and help us to understand different people's food preferences and dietary needs.

The brain and the gut

The gut is a major secretor of body fluids, a major user of proteins in the synthesis and secretion of enzymes and is an important interface between our bodies and the outside world. Not surprisingly, the activity of such an important structure is constantly monitored and controlled by the nervous system (Figure 3.22) and by numerous hormones, mostly in ways of which we are normally unaware. These elaborate and largely unconscious interactions between the brain and the gut mean that its secretions and muscular activity, and related behaviour such as appetite and food preferences, are sensitive indicators of the well-being of the body as a whole. At least since the time of the ancient Greeks and probably much earlier, physicians have diagnosed illnesses by listening to and feeling the gut and studying its effusions.

The presence of food in the stomach triggers the release of various hormones that stimulate secretion of enzymes and bile, and activate peristalsis in muscles further down the gut. Thus many people find that eating breakfast stimulates defaecation about an hour later.

☐ Why would it be efficient for secretion of enzymes to be turned on and off by hormones?

■ Energy and materials are used for the synthesis and secretion of enzymes, and once free in the gut, any one molecule does not remain active for very long. It is therefore more economical to secrete enzymes only as and when required.

As mentioned above, small quantities of digestive enzymes are stored in the Golgi bodies of cells lining the gut for some time before being secreted. Digestion of a large meal always requires enzyme synthesis, which takes some time (around 10 to 20 minutes). So 'early warning' signals to the gut, some generated just by seeing or smelling food, speed up digestion while also avoiding unnecessary wastage of the relatively large quantity of the body's energy and materials that are deployed in the synthesis of gut secretions.

☐ Why is precise coordination between secretions in different regions of the gut essential to efficient digestion?

■ Most enzymes work efficiently only in certain chemical environments and in the correct order.

For example, if the quantity of neutralising bile salts secreted does not match the acid produced in the stomach, the duodenal contents may be too acid (or not acid enough), thereby impairing the action of the many important enzymes secreted by the pancreas and small intestine. The pancreatic enzymes cannot digest fats properly until they are emulsified by the bile.

Control of gut activity by the nervous system and certain hormones is essential, particularly if, as is often the case with modern humans (and probably also our hunter-gatherer ancestors), each meal is different in composition from the last. Imperfect coordination between parts of the digestive system, if serious or prolonged, could lead to valuable reserves of protein, energy and water being squandered on synthesising secretions that are unable to digest food efficiently, as well as to pain and the various other unpleasant symptoms that we call indigestion.

Communications and interactions between the brain and the mouth and stomach (and to a lesser extent other parts of the gut) are numerous and complex, and frequently intrude into everyday life. The brain receives much information about the chemical composition, texture and quantity of food in the stomach as well as from the mouth and throat, although the exact mechanisms involved are far from clear. We have all experienced eating things that 'make you feel sick' almost at once (though rarely causing actual vomiting), and being aware that a snack is nutritious (or unsatisfying) within a few minutes of eating it.

☐ Why are such observations evidence for the existence of sensors that detect the presence of food in the stomach itself?

■ The sensations could not arise from absorption into the blood of significant quantities of nutrients from the food. Very little passes through the stomach wall and it takes hours rather than minutes for the food to pass into the absorptive regions of the small intestine.

Such sensory feedback is very important in food selection and the regulation of appetite. Experience makes our responses quicker and more accurate; newly weaned children often have 'food fads' and have to be trained to eat 'what is good for them', establishing habits and preferences that last a lifetime. However, the mechanisms are not infallible: as the confectionery and 'junk' food industries know well, we are easily tempted to eat more of very appetising foods whether or not they are nutritious. Distortion of sensory perception of food leading to excessive (i.e. physiologically unreasonable) appetite is believed to be a major cause of overeating, and hence of obesity. Some poisons, notably those in certain fungi, have no taste or smell and hence are undetectable. People, especially children, can often be persuaded to eat large quantities of foods that 'do not agree with them', sometimes with disastrous consequences.

Vomiting is a reversal of the muscular movements of the stomach and upper part of the duodenum, aided by powerful contractions of the breathing muscles of the chest. The primary function of vomiting is the expulsion of food that is sensed to be harmful before it reaches the absorptive region of the small intestine.

☐ What happens to potentially harmful gut contents that fail to stimulate vomiting?

■ They may be detected in the small intestine, where they may cause more vigorous peristalsis, perhaps leading to diarrhoea.

Many such substances elicit both mechanisms for expelling harmful materials from the gut. However, as described below, other toxins and pathogens evade detection, enabling them to enter the blood or establish themselves in the small intestine.

Many other factors, including excitement, pain, fear, motion sickness, noxious smells, some kinds of brain and spinal injuries and infections, and a variety of drugs, including many general anaesthetics and painkillers, often produce nausea (feeling sick) and vomiting, whether or not any food has been eaten. The physiological mechanisms are intricate and, in spite of intensive study, scientists know little about how they work, and why the connection between, for example, motion and nausea has evolved. Consequently, there are few really effective remedies for these unpleasant and inconvenient symptoms.

Anorexia (loss of appetite, not to be confused with anorexia nervosa, a mental disorder characterised by self-starvation) is a common symptom of a wide range of maladies from mild depression and anxiety to lethal fevers and chronic cancers.

☐ In view of this account of digestion and its control by the nervous system, can you suggest why anorexia is such a common feature of feeling unwell?

■ Eating is an energetically expensive, often hazardous physiological process; digestion, absorption and the regulation of the concentrations of nutrients in the blood require large quantities of materials and energy, and there is always a risk of absorbing pathogenic organisms or toxic substances. Under almost all forms of stress, it is physiologically easier to live on reserves of energy and protein, at least for a few hours or days, than to embark upon the energetically expensive and risky activities of eating and digesting food and of absorbing the nutrients.

Babies and young children, and almost everyone else when feeling unwell, prefer bland-tasting food and small, nutritionally balanced meals. Alcoholic drinks, highly spiced dishes and large quantities of meat or sugary food may be appetising to healthy teenagers and adults but are much less attractive to, and suitable for, infants, invalids and elderly people. These dietary preferences arise from the intricate relationship between the brain and the gut.

The control of fuels absorbed into the blood

As mentioned in the introduction to this chapter, regulation of the levels of nutrients absorbed into the blood is essential to efficient metabolism, the more so in animals, such as humans, which eat large, infrequent meals. Although digestion and absorption are relatively slow compared to the time taken actually to eat meals, nutrients still enter the blood as abrupt 'pulses' rather than as a continuous trickle.

The major source of energy for movement and most biochemical activities is the precisely-controlled breakdown of glucose and fats, in combination with oxygen obtained from the atmosphere as we breathe, to yield carbon dioxide, water and energy. (This reaction is termed *oxidation*, so in biological terms you would say that energy is obtained from the oxidation of glucose and fats.) On a normal diet of frequent meals rich in sugars and starch, much of the glucose that is oxidised to generate energy is absorbed directly from the gut, but the liver can also *synthesise* glucose from amino acids absorbed from the diet, or derived from the body's own tissues, which it does extensively in periods of starvation.

The muscles, brain and other 'consumers' of the products of digestion work best with a steady supply of glucose and other nutrients. Both too much and too little glucose in the blood make one feel unwell and are harmful if prolonged. As well as their roles in digestion, the liver and the pancreas make essential contributions to the **regulation of glucose** concentration in the blood.[6]

As explained in the previous section, digestion is coordinated and speeded up by hormones released by the early stages of eating that stimulate the lower regions of the gut. Similarly, food intake triggers the release of other hormones, notably **insulin**, that stimulate adjustments in the metabolism of many tissues, including the liver, muscles and *adipose tissue* (the white or yellowish,

greasy component of meat, popularly called 'fat'; it is a tissue specialised for storing energy as fatty molecules.). These responses accommodate the sudden flood of nutrients entering the blood through the small intestine, thereby preventing damage to vulnerable organs such as the brain and kidneys.

The passage of blood with a slightly elevated concentration of glucose through the pancreas stimulates it to release more insulin into the blood (several other factors, including certain amino acids and some of the hormones produced by the gut also stimulate insulin secretion, but they do not concern us here). Insulin has many different effects on many different tissues. The best known is the promotion of glucose disposal by stimulating the muscles and the liver to take up the 'extra' glucose that cannot be used immediately for energy production and to convert it into harmless large molecules such as *glycogen* ('glye-koh-jen'). Glycogen is a large, insoluble molecule formed from hundreds of glucose molecules linked together (see photograph on page 160).

Insulin also inhibits the release by the liver of glucose made from the breakdown of glycogen and greatly reduces the rate of breakdown of fats stored in adipose tissue to produce fatty acids as fuels. Figure 7.3 summarises the major role of insulin in regulating the body's energy supply.

☐ Why is curtailing the release of glucose from the liver, and of fat from adipose tissue, important in regulating the concentration of glucose in the blood?

■ In the absence of fuels from these internal stores, all the other tissues (e.g. the muscles) have to use *dietary* glucose absorbed into the bloodstream from the gut, thereby helping to prevent its concentration in the blood from getting too high.

Insulin also stimulates the synthesis (in humans, mostly in the liver) of storage fats from glucose and from the fatty acids that were released by the breakdown of dietary fats and absorbed through the gut, and promotes their transfer to adipose tissue.

☐ Why do people become obese from persistently eating too much sugar and starch, or by eating a very fatty diet (or both)?

■ Once absorbed into the blood, all these energy-providing molecules are either oxidised (i.e. broken down as fuels for muscular movement, etc.), or they are converted into storage fats that accumulate in the adipose tissue. They cannot normally be eliminated from the body in any other way.

[6]Other simple sugars such as galactose are also absorbed, but the liver converts them at once to glucose, so from the point of view of the regulation of fuel levels in the blood, we need only consider glucose.

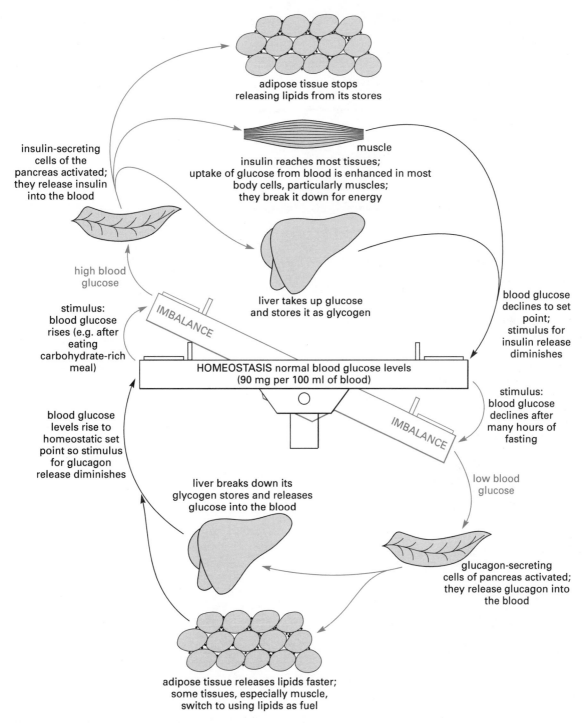

Figure 7.3 *Diagram summarising the principal mechanisms in humans for maintaining homeostasis of the concentration of glucose in the blood.*

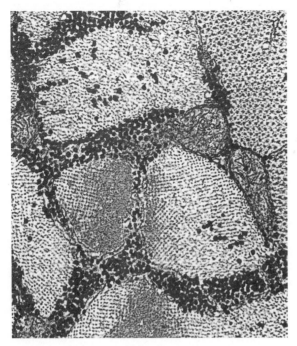

Electron micrograph of a fragment of calf muscle from a person who has recently eaten a meal rich in sugars and starch. The carbohydrates were broken down in the gut into simple sugars such as glucose, which were absorbed into the bloodstream and circulated around the body. The glucose was transported into the muscles, where it was converted into insoluble glycogen which forms tiny granules, here stained dense black. The energy for muscle contraction is generated in the mitochondria that can be seen packed around the contractile elements of the muscle; the contractile elements are seen 'end-on' in this photograph, which is magnified 45 000 times life-size. (Courtesy of Dr M. J. Cullen, Muscular Dystrophy Research Group Laboratories, Newcastle General Hospital, Newcastle upon Tyne)

Insulin is a relatively small, highly soluble molecule that freely permeates most tissues. Its action on cells depends upon it binding with receptor molecules that are specific for insulin (bind to it alone), and which are produced by the cells with which it interacts. There are several different kinds of insulin receptor molecules, that, when bound to insulin, have different effects on different biochemical processes. Insulin can thus have different effects on different kinds of target cells; most of the many kinds of cells that respond to insulin produce only some of the kinds of insulin receptor molecules and thus have only certain responses to the hormone. Furthermore, the target cells' responses to insulin can depend as much upon the abundance of receptors that they themselves have produced and sequestered in their surface membranes, as upon the concentration of insulin secreted by the pancreas.

☐ A big meal increases the influx of glucose into the blood. What normal activities would deplete the blood of glucose?

■ Prolonged vigorous exercise or other muscular activity such as shivering.

The muscles use large quantities of glucose (and fats) during exercise and shivering, so in order to maintain supplies to important tissues such as the brain and the kidneys during such activities, the mechanisms that remove dietary glucose from the blood must be reversed.

☐ How could such reversal be achieved?

■ By reducing the secretion of insulin.

Insulin secretion is curtailed (it is almost impossible to stop any biochemical pathway completely and instantly), and the pancreas releases another hormone called *glucagon* ('glue-ka-gon'; look for it in the flow diagram in Figure 7.3).[7] Glucagon appears in the blood after about 24 hours of fasting; it stimulates release of glucose from the liver by breakdown of the glycogen stored there, and it also promotes the breakdown and release of fat from adipose tissue, and several other biochemical adjustments that ensure that all essential tissues have adequate fuel supplies. Information about the levels of glycogen in the liver and muscles, and other nutrient stores reaches the brain and contributes to appetite and hence to replenishing the body's glucose supply by eating (Figure 7.3). Glucagon stimulates the opposite responses to insulin in the liver, muscles and adipose tissue.

This account of the control of fuel levels in the blood is greatly simplified but it illustrates some principles of physiological *homeostasis* (which we discussed earlier, in Chapter 3). A system in which changes in the input cause modifications in the output that *oppose* the change in input is called a *negative feedback* control system. The classic example is the thermostat used to control domestic central heating. When the room temperature falls below the temperature setting on the thermostat, the boiler is switched on and when the set temperature is reached the boiler is switched off.

The living situation is much more complicated than a simple thermostat. As illustrated in Figure 7.3, there are two opposing negative feedback systems (secretion of insulin and secretion of glucagon) that combine to maintain the level of glucose in the blood within a range that supplies the body's immediate energy requirements.

[7]Three different kinds of cells in the pancreas secrete insulin, glucagon and pancreatic fluid, respectively.

Major deficiencies in the secretion of insulin, or in the tissues' ability to respond normally to the hormone, produce a disease called *diabetes mellitus* (commonly abbreviated to **diabetes**).

☐ How could the effects of diabetes be relieved by changing the diet?

■ Insulin specifically regulates blood glucose concentration, which is altered by the uptake of glucose produced by the digestion of carbohydrates. So the symptoms of diabetes can be ameliorated by reducing intake of all dietary carbohydrates, and particularly by avoiding eating large quantities of glucose-containing foods in a short period of time.

The form of diabetes that is due to defective insulin production can be rectified, though not cured, by administering insulin regularly and taking small, frequent meals that contain a more or less constant amount of carbohydrate. However, insulin doses must be carefully controlled; too much insulin lowers the blood glucose too far, starving the brain of vital fuel and leading to fainting and coma. An excessive blood sugar level, sustained for long periods, caused by too little insulin (or a weak response to normal concentrations) is also harmful to the brain and to many other tissues.

In spite of the well-known defects in the storage and regulation of energy-releasing substances (glucose and fats), it is important to stress that they are stored in larger quantities, and their concentration in the blood is more efficiently regulated, than is the case for most other essential nutrients. An adult of average weight and body build has enough energy reserves to support at least six weeks of sedentary living on a total fast, as long as water is available. Protein is stored in the liver (and probably also in the muscles), but reserves are small, so symptoms of protein deficiency, such as shabby skin and hair, appear after only a few weeks on a very low protein diet.

Just as too much glucose harms many tissues, too much of certain amino acids can also disrupt the functioning of the brain, kidneys and immune system. For example, a sudden excess of particular fatty acids or amino acids is probably the main cause of the headaches and general malaise that some people experience 4 to 12 hours after eating a lot of certain foods such as cheese, shellfish or chocolate. Symptoms disappear in a few hours as the liver takes up or detoxifies the culprit nutrients.

Many essential nutrients (e.g. iron, used in the synthesis of the red blood pigment haemoglobin, and many vitamins) are too toxic to be stored in large quantities.

They must be supplied regularly in the diet in a readily absorbable way.

Our brief account of the digestive system and the mechanisms of absorption, detoxification and energy balancing ends here. In the rest of this chapter, we take a wider view of the human diet and its effects on health via a case study which also illustrates the central theme of this book: the interaction of biological and cultural evolution.

Evolutionary adaptation to a novel diet

As pointed out in Chapter 2, human habits and diet have changed greatly during the last 10 000 years with decline in large prey animals and the rise of agriculture and animal husbandry, from which we now obtain most of our food. Not merely the flavours but the dietary staples of our food have changed.

☐ Did these changes in diet and habits require corresponding changes in eating, digestion and metabolism?

■ We know that the teeth of *Homo sapiens* became smaller during its evolution and that dental caries, which was rare in hunter-gatherers, became much more common following the rise of agriculture (Chapter 2).

There may well have been changes to other parts of the digestive system as well, but such soft tissues are very rarely preserved in fossils, so we know nothing about them. In the absence of such information, we can deduce something about the adaptations that enabled people to live on the new diet from comparison of inherited adaptations of the gut and liver in different groups of modern people.

New crops and domestic animals were gradually introduced to different parts of the world, and they became established only where the climate proved suitable for them, so different groups of people did not all switch from hunting to farming at the same time. As mentioned earlier (in connection with the red colour of beetroot), some people have the biochemical capacity to deal with certain foods that others lack. The modern human population is thus a rich mixture of diverse peoples who live in different climates, and have different cultures, diets, habits and genetically determined abilities to deal with foods. One of the most thoroughly studied examples of this diversity in diet, habits and physiological capacity is the ability of weaned children and adults to digest fresh milk.

Lactose malabsorption and lactose intolerance

Milk is usually considered to be the most natural food; all female mammals suckle their young, sometimes for considerable periods, during which time the young grow rapidly. Milk consists of small globules of butterfat suspended in a solution containing lactose, proteins and various minerals including calcium, chloride and sodium. In common with other newborn mammals, human infants (with rare exceptions) are born with the ability to secrete, in the small intestine, the enzyme *lactase*. This enzyme digests lactose, the main sugar in milk, splitting it into two smaller molecules, galactose and glucose. You might wonder about the advantages of splitting lactose into these smaller molecules. Like other sugar molecules, lactose does not dissolve in fatty cell membranes and so cannot pass through the gut lining 'unescorted', but the lining of the small intestine contains active transport sites that convey both galactose and glucose from the gut into the blood.

The proportions of the different components of milk differ greatly between species (and may change as the suckling young matures). For example, cows' and ewes' milk contain much more fat and less water and lactose than that of women or mares. All mammals are born with the ability to secrete lactase in the small intestine, and thus to digest lactose, but the capacity declines sharply at weaning and is usually absent in adult mammals.

□ Would you expect human babies to secrete more or less lactase (in proportion to their size) than calves or lambs?

■ More. Human milk contains much more lactose (and less fat) than the milk of all domestic animals from which milk is harvested, except the mare.

The Milk Marketing Board continually extols the virtues of 'getting enough bottle' for all age groups, but milk is not an adequate food for adults: for example, it is deficient in dietary iron and is an inadequate source of vitamin C. The picture of milk as a 'natural', universal food suffered a further blow in 1965 when Cuatrecasas, Lockwood and Caldwell published the paradoxical findings from their study of teenagers and adults in Baltimore, Maryland, USA, in which they compared blacks and whites. Cuatrecasas *et al.* reported that the major sugar in milk, lactose, was not efficiently digested by 73 per cent of the black subjects nor by 16 per cent of the whites studied. Further studies on different ethnic groups living in various parts of the world have revealed the existence of white-skinned and black-skinned populations with widely different proportions of people who can, or cannot, digest

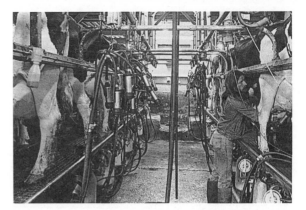

Cows' milk has become a standard component of human diet, especially for infants and children, in most parts of the industrialised world. (Photo: Mike Levers)

lactose after weaning. People who cannot digest lactose are called *lactose malabsorbers* and the condition is known as **lactose malabsorption**. People who can digest lactose throughout their lives are called *lactose absorbers*.

□ Is lactose malabsorption likely to be due to a defect in the gene that codes for the lactase protein itself, or to a change in the mechanism that regulates the activity of this gene? (Think back to Chapter 4.)

■ People in whom the gene that codes for lactase is defective would be unable to digest their mother's milk (or formula milk) and so would not survive infancy. The normal gene must exist in lactose malabsorbers and must have functioned effectively when they were babies. But after weaning, the gene is 'switched off' and lactase is no longer produced, or only in very reduced amounts.

Infants who are unable to produce lactase at all are known to medical science, but they are very rare. Rearing them has only become possible in the last 30 years, with the development of synthetic substitutes for milk (e.g. manufactured from soya beans).

□ What do you think are the consequences of lactose malabsorption for the digestion of milk?

■ The fats and proteins in milk are digested and absorbed normally, but the lactose remains in the gut contents.

Gut contents containing large quantities of lactose retain more water than is normal, thus diluting the digestive enzymes and disturbing normal digestion.

☐ What would happen to the lactose when it reaches the large intestine?

■ Like other residual carbohydrates, it would be digested by the symbiotic bacteria (most species of which can produce lactase).

☐ Could the resulting glucose (and galactose) pass through the gut lining and into the blood?

■ No. There are no glucose (or galactose) transporters in the lining of the large intestine.

The gut contents are not normally moved 'upstream' back to the small intestine, so, instead of being absorbed into the person's blood, the products of lactose digestion mostly support the proliferation of the lactose-digesting bacteria. The abnormally large numbers of bacteria thus maintained produce much more carbon dioxide and other gases than is normal, leading to a condition called *lactose intolerance*; the symptoms include flatulence (wind), intestinal cramps and, in severe cases, diarrhoea, nausea and vomiting. Lactose intolerance is usually mild in adults because many lactose malabsorbing people have enough residual lactase activity to enable them to eat small quantities of whole milk (i.e. in a cup of tea, or as an ingredient of cake) without causing symptoms, but lactose malabsorbers who eat a lot of lactose-containing food over a short period may become ill.

☐ Would you expect lactose malabsorbing people to choose foods containing fresh milk?

■ No; there is efficient communication between the gut and the brain that makes people aware of and so avoid foods that, for one reason or another 'do not agree with them'.

Under normal circumstances, it is possible to avoid such foods without fuss, and indeed many people do so without being aware of their physiological condition. Most populations with a high proportion of lactose malabsorbers either do not collect milk from their domestic animals, or they routinely ferment it into cheese or yoghurt. Whole milk is regarded as 'baby food' and is not drunk by adults or older children.

Fermentation of milk into cheese is an ancient skill that probably began shortly after people domesticated large mammals. When milk is allowed to stand in a warm place, micro-organisms in the air colonise it, and their enzymes turn the lactose to lactic acid, which precipitates most of the protein and fats to form a thick, nutritious curd that is easily separated from the thin, watery whey. Three processes may reduce the lactose content of cheese, making it edible to lactose malabsorbers: the

micro-organisms convert the lactose into lactic acid; they secrete the enzyme lactase which splits lactose into glucose and galactose; lactose, like other sugars, is very soluble in water, so any remaining is removed in the whey.

This ancient method of separating milk is still used to make pot cheese and cottage cheese. Different conditions, especially temperature, favour the proliferation of different kinds of micro-organisms that confer different flavours and textures on the cheese. Thus, cheese production is a cultural practice that allows lactose malabsorbers in dairying populations to obtain most of the nutrients of milk without any of the symptoms of lactose intolerance. Important nutrients thus obtained from milk include calcium, which promotes the development of healthy bones and teeth, and fats, some of which have recently been shown to be essential for normal brain development and functioning.

☐ Would lactose malabsorbers be healthy on a varied diet that excludes whole milk?

■ Yes. The lack of one particular enzyme, lactase, impairs only the ability to digest lactose. All other digestive processes may be normal, so lactose malabsorbers suffer no ill-effects if they avoid taking in large quantities of whole milk.

The problem of lactose intolerance usually does not come to light until famine or mass migration force people to eat milk-containing food in abnormally large quantities.

Distribution of lactose intolerance

Since the original study by Cuatrecasas *et al.,* there have been many attempts to measure the proportions of lactose absorbers and lactose malabsorbers in a wide variety of human populations. Populations can vary between 0 per cent lactose absorbers, where no weaned children or adults produce sufficient lactase, and 100 per cent where everyone can digest lactose. Conventionally, a population with 30 per cent or fewer lactose absorbers is described as lactose malabsorbing. In a review of the distribution of lactose absorbers and malabsorbers from 197 populations, F. J. Simoons of the University of California at Davies concluded that:

…high prevalences of lactose malabsorbers, from about 60–100 per cent of the persons studied, are typical of the overwhelming number of ethnic groups around the world…including all American Indians and Eskimos studied so far, some New World Mestizos, most sub-Saharan

African peoples and their relatively unmixed overseas descendants, most Mediterranean and Near Eastern groups, most subjects whose origins are India, all peoples of Southeast and East Asia, as well as the two Pacific groups, New Guineans and Fijians, who have been studied. (Simoons, 1978, p. 964)

A minority of the world's peoples, primarily northern and western Europeans and their descendants in the Americas and Australia, but also certain peoples of the Mediterranean and Near East, three pastoral groups of Africa (Tussi, Hima, and Fuiani), and several groups living in the western parts of the Indian subcontinent, have low proportions of lactose malabsorbers (from 0 to 30 per cent).

Only a few present-day groups have intermediate prevalences of lactose malabsorbers (30 to 60 per cent), probably arising from a mixed absorber/malabsorber ancestry. Most relatively unmixed ethnic groups of the world fall into two categories: lactose absorbers (0 to 30 per cent frequency of lactose malabsorbers) and malabsorbers (60 to 100 per cent frequency of lactose malabsorbers).

We can learn about the genetic aspects of lactose malabsorption by observing the frequency with which the children of normal absorbers and malabsorbers inherit their parents' characteristics. In Chapter 4, we described the typical pattern of inheritance of characteristics due to a single gene, which can occur in two alternative forms (alleles), one dominant and one recessive.

☐ What would be the *phenotype* of a person who inherited both the dominant and the recessive allele

of this gene, one from each parent? (Remember, phenotype can be roughly translated into 'the way the person turned out'.)

■ The person's phenotype would be that produced by the dominant allele, which masks the effect of the recessive allele.

In Table 7.1, the *observed* frequency with which children inherit lactose malabsorption from their parents is compared with the *expected* frequency (right-hand column) of the inheritance of a characteristic due to the presence of two recessive alleles of a single gene. As you can see, lactose malabsorption tends to run in families, which suggests that its underlying cause may be genetic. The observed proportions of lactose malabsorbing children of LA × LA, LA × LM and LM × LM parents are very close to the expected values, showing that the LA phenotype is due to the presence of at least one dominant allele, and that the LM phenotype is due to two recessive alleles.

☐ About a quarter of the children born to parents who are *both* lactose absorbers (LA × LA) turn out to be malabsorbers; what can you conclude about the genotypes of the parents?

■ The parents must be heterozygous (see Chapter 4) for the gene that controls lactase production after weaning; they each have one copy of the dominant allele and one copy of the recessive allele. A quarter of the offspring born to these heterozygous parents are homozygous for the recessive allele (they have two copies of the recessive allele, having inherited one copy from each parent) and hence are lactose malabsorbers.

Table 7.1 Evidence for the inheritance of lactose malabsorption in humans: observed frequency compared with frequency expected if the condition is a recessive characteristic

Parental phenotypes	Number of families studied	Number of children born	Offspring with LM phenotype	Observed proportion of LM offspring	Expected proportion of LM offspring
				%	%
LA × LA	10	31	8	25.8	25
LA × LM	60	196	101	51.5	50
LM × LM	76	220	208	94.5	100

Parental phenotypes are listed as LA, lactose absorption phenotype, and LM, lactose malabsorption phenotype; the 'x' denotes the 'cross-breeding' between two parents of the phenotypes listed. (Data adapted from Durham, W. H., 1991, *Coevolution, Genes, Culture and Human Diversity*, Stanford University Press, Stanford, California, Table 5.2, p. 239)

The union of heterozygous parents with homozygous lactose-malabsorbing parents (LA × LM) produces half the children as lactose malabsorbers (homozygous recessives) and half as lactose absorbers (heterozygotes). (If you are unsure about how such parental genotypes produce these offspring, draw out a grid like the ones in Figures 4.8 and 4.13 to check the prediction.) The surprise in Table 7.1 is that the union of two lactose malabsorbing parents (LM × LM) should not result in *all* their children also being malabsorbers: the twelve children in this group who can apparently absorb lactose may be cases of misdiagnosis, or perhaps of misreported parentage.

☐ Referring back to Chapter 2, do you think that the hunter-gatherer peoples who lived before the rise of agriculture and pastoralism were lactose absorbers or lactose malabsorbers?

■ It is, of course, impossible to know for sure, but since all other weaned mammals are lactose malabsorbers, and there is no evidence that pre-agricultural people ever used animal milk, most were almost certainly lactose malabsorbers.

Thus, lactose absorbers are the result of a relatively recent evolutionary change that almost certainly evolved as an adaptation to the modern diet based upon agriculture and animal husbandry. An explanation for the evolution of the adult capacity for lactose absorption proposed by Simoon suggests that the decline in the production of lactase at weaning is controlled genetically, but in some people the decline can be delayed, so they retain the ability to digest lactose into adulthood. This ability is part of the normal, and largely inconsequential, genetic variation within a population. If the population was placed under some stress which gave people with the ability to absorb lactose an advantage that led to greater reproductive success, then the genes involved would be favoured by natural selection and would thus gradually increase in frequency in the population (see Chapters 3, 4 and 5).

It is not known exactly when dairying cultures first emerged; a conservative estimate of the time since milk first became important as food for adults is 5 000 years or around 250 generations. If lactose absorbers managed, on average, to raise 1 per cent more children than lactose malabsorbers (which is not unreasonable), this time is sufficiently long for gene frequencies to have been altered substantially by natural selection.

What were the stresses that led to the genes involved in lactose absorption becoming advantageous within particular populations? William Durham tried to answer this question in 1991 by choosing for detailed study 60 of the populations reviewed in Simoon's article (introduced above), which between them represented the full range of ability to absorb lactose. Table 7.2 shows Durham's sample together with information about the normal diets those 60 populations had consumed for generations before recent contact with other cultures caused a switch to modern, mass-produced foods. The 60 populations in Table 7.2 are categorised by their dairying culture (they rear animals for their milk) or lack of it. The third column in Table 7.2 shows the percentages of lactose absorbing people in the populations and the fourth column shows the number of populations sampled.

Table 7.2 The 60 populations chosen by Durham, categorised by their normal diet, showing the percentages of lactose absorbers in the populations in each category

Category	Nature of subsistence	% lactose absorbers	Number of populations sampled
A	hunter-gatherers traditionally lacking dairy animals	12.6	4
B	non-dairying agriculturalists	15.5	5
C	recently dairying agriculturalists	11.9	5
D	milk-dependent pastoralists	91.3	5
E	dairying peoples of North Africa and the Mediterranean	31.8	16
F	dairying peoples of northern Europe (above 40 °N)	91.5	12
G	populations of mixed dairying and non-dairying ancestry	56.2	13

Data derived from Durham, W. H., 1991, *Coevolution, Genes, Culture and Human Diversity*, Stanford University Press, Stanford, California, Table 5.1, p. 234.

□ Look at the distributions of lactose absorbers among the seven populations A–G in Table 7.2. Is there a relationship between the normal diet and the percentage of lactose absorbers?

■ At first sight there seems to be a relationship: the populations in the A and B categories who do not rear or use dairy animals have low percentages of lactose absorbers, whereas the D and F populations who have dairying cultures and consume dairy products have high proportions of lactose absorbers. The 'mixed' populations in category G have intermediate proportions of absorbers and malabsorbers.

□ From Table 7.2, can you propose an explanation, in terms of natural selection, for the high proportions of individuals with the lactose absorption phenotype in categories D and F?

■ A plausible hypothesis is that when populations that had established a dairying culture were placed under some dietary stress (e.g. a shortage of other food sources), people who were able to digest milk when adult were more successful in evolutionary terms (i.e. they raised more offspring) than those with the lactose malabsorption phenotype. This characteristic therefore became more common in the population in each successive generation.

□ Do the data from the category C populations support or contradict this hypothesis?

■ The finding that agriculturalists who have only recently turned to dairying have a low percentage of lactose absorbers supports the general hypothesis.

The evolution of the ability to digest lactose, like all evolutionary changes, takes a relatively long time and it may not yet have happened in those populations that have recently adopted dairying.

□ Milk has been a major food for the dairying peoples of North Africa and the Mediterranean (category E) for at least 5 000 years. How can the finding that they have relatively low proportions of lactose absorbers be accommodated into the basic hypothesis developed above?

■ This finding appears to cast doubt upon the hypothesis: it shows that the ability to digest lactose does not depend upon that population using milk as a dietary constituent, even if the habit has been established for a very long time.

Dairying populations with a low proportion of lactose absorbers use whole milk only for babies. For adult consumption, it is converted into cheese or yoghurt, thereby avoiding putting the large proportion of lactose malabsorbers at a nutritional disadvantage compared with absorbers. Some dairying populations adopted this strategy (and so remained mainly lactose malabsorbers), while the ability to digest lactose when adult gradually became common in others.

Latitude and vitamin D production

As you have seen, many populations that have long practised dairy farming contain different proportions of lactose malabsorbers and lactose absorbers. The question of interest is: if a cultural solution (cheese-making) was available to lactose malabsorbers that allowed them to obtain adequate nutrition from dairy farming, what were the additional selective pressures that favoured lactose absorbers? In the absence of such additional pressures, you would not expect the proportion of lactose absorbers to increase, since they derived no advantage from their ability; yet clearly the proportion *has* risen in most dairying cultures.

To answer this question, William Durham extended his earlier study to investigate the locations of the homelands of the 60 lactose absorbing and malabsorbing populations, which formed the basis for Table 7.2 earlier. He found an association between the proportion of lactose absorbers in a population and the *latitude* of their homelands; the majority of the populations with high proportions of lactose absorbers live in latitudes greater than 30 degrees north or south of the Equator. Exceptions to this relationship are milk-dependent peoples of East Africa and Saudi Arabia and the Eskimo populations of Greenland. We will return to these anomalies later, after we consider Durham's evidence of a significant relationship between latitude and diet. But first we must describe the biology of vitamin D. The relevance of this vitamin to lactose absorption and latitude will soon become apparent.

Vitamin D

Vitamin D is very important to health and normal growth: it facilitates the transport of calcium through the lining of the small intestine into the blood, it controls the deposition of calcium in the bones during growth, and it maintains adult bone structure. The consequences of **vitamin D deficiency** are well known. With less calcium available, the skeleton fails to develop normally. The most obvious symptom is the bowing of the long load-bearing bones in the lower limbs, producing the condition called rickets. Children with vitamin D deficiency grow more slowly and may become smaller adults which, in women, has serious consequence because the pelvis may end up so small or misshapen that normal birth is severely impeded.

Vitamin D can be absorbed through the gut; dietary sources of vitamin D include fish and fish livers, mammal livers (e.g. pig, calf), shellfish and egg yolks. In the 1920s, Sir Edward Mellanby showed that vitamin D added to the diet could prevent the development of rickets, thereby providing a scientific basis for the folklore that cod liver oil (a rich source of vitamin D) is effective in preventing rickets. Under the right conditions, the human body can also synthesise the vitamin for itself. A band of ultraviolet light called UV(B) radiation promotes the synthesis of essential precursors of vitamin D in the human skin. The precursor molecules are transported in the blood from the skin to the liver and kidneys, where they are converted to the biologically active form of vitamin D. Under the control of hormones, vitamin D is released from the liver and kidneys into the circulation.

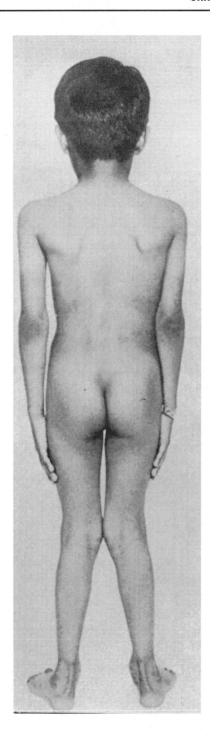

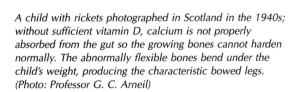

A child with rickets photographed in Scotland in the 1940s; without sufficient vitamin D, calcium is not properly absorbed from the gut so the growing bones cannot harden normally. The abnormally flexible bones bend under the child's weight, producing the characteristic bowed legs. (Photo: Professor G. C. Arneil)

Lactose absorption, vitamin D deficiency and skin depigmentation

Until the invention of special kinds of electric lights earlier this century, the only source of UV(B) was sunlight. As shown in Figure 7.4, the amount of UV(B) (and other components of sunlight) to reach populations living at latitudes above 30 degrees north or below 30 degrees south of the Equator is a lot less than the amount of UV(B) experienced by people living in equatorial regions. People living above or below 30 degrees from the Equator receive between 40 and 88 per cent less UV(B) radiation than equatorial peoples, depending on how far north or south they live. As a consequence, people living at high latitudes have a lower capacity to synthesise vitamin D in the skin than those living nearer the Equator. (Remember, the equator has a latitude of 0 degrees, so latitude gets 'higher' the further you move away from the Equator to the north and to the south.)

□ Is vitamin D deficiency therefore inevitable for people living permanently at very high latitudes?

■ No. If their diet provided sufficient vitamin D, they would not develop symptoms of vitamin D deficiency.

□ What factors other than high latitude would inhibit vitamin D synthesis in the skin?

■ Dark pigments in the skin and wearing clothes both shade the skin from the UV(B) light essential for forming the precursors of vitamin D.

If the skin is frequently exposed to plenty of sunlight, more than enough vitamin D is synthesised, even if the skin is partially shaded by dark pigments. Indeed, the pigment is essential to protect the skin cells from being damaged by too much radiation.

□ Did ancestral people have pigmented skin?

■ Almost certainly yes. As explained in Chapter 2, humans evolved on the sunny grasslands of eastern and southern Africa, where protection from excess light and heat is essential and more than enough UV(B) radiation reached the skin for vitamin D synthesis. Early people were probably as dark as their modern descendants now living in these regions.

However, if dark-skinned people migrate to a cloudy climate, and/or adopt the habit of wearing clothes that cover a large part of the body, they may risk vitamin D deficiencies not experienced by their tropical ancestors.

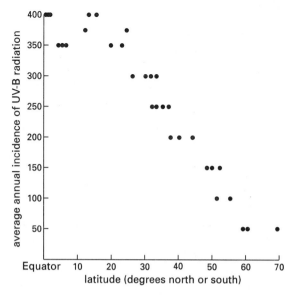

Figure 7.4 *The amount of UV(B) radiation at the earth's surface decreases as latitude increases, either north or south. (From Durham, W. H., 1991,* Coevolution, Genes, Culture and Human Diversity, *Stanford University Press, Stanford, California, Figure 5.8, p. 259.)*

□ When did people begin to change their habits in these ways?

■ About 0.1 million years ago, when they spread out of the sunny parts of Africa to dense tropical rainforest, and north to Europe and Asia, where the climate is cooler and cloudier (see Chapter 2).

We can now tie together all the strands of the lactose malabsorption story. Durham (1991) suggested a causal link between the evolution of paler skin, the ability to absorb lactose after weaning and vitamin D deficiency. His theory, which is one of several possible interpretations of these observations, proposes that vitamin D deficiency in populations living in high latitudes was a factor in giving a selective advantage to people who had somehow acquired the ability to absorb lactose from milk throughout their lives, compared with people who could not.

Figure 7.5 shows the relationship between latitude of origin and skin colour of the populations described in Table 7.2. The skin of indigenous populations, as judged by a skin-colour index devised by other anthropologists, is lighter in people native to higher latitudes. A comparison of Figures 7.4 and 7.5 shows that people's skin becomes paler with increasing latitude, which corresponds to the reduction in UV(B).

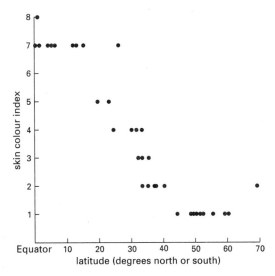

Figure 7.5 *The relationship between skin pigmentation and latitude of origin for the populations featured in Table 7.2. (From Durham, W.H., 1991,* Coevolution, Genes, Culture and Human Diversity, *Stanford University Press, Figure 5.10, p. 262)*

This comparison strongly suggests that natural selection has favoured lighter skins among peoples living in places that received low amounts of UV(B). Evolutionary theory predicts that lighter-skinned people at these high latitudes were at an advantage due to their greater efficiency at synthesising vitamin D in the skin; compared with darker-skinned people, they were more successful at raising children, who inherited the genes that made their skin lighter, and so the genes spread through the population over many generations. The advantage of light skins at high latitudes was perhaps compounded by people switching to diets that were low in vitamin D.

We can sum up Durham's explanation for the highly variable prevalence of lactose malabsorption in populations around the world. Durham argues that lactose malabsorption, which was the normal condition of our ancestors 10 000 years ago, became a 'problem' after people adopted farming and animal husbandry as their major source of food. He believes that there was, from time to time, stress on populations caused by dietary deficiencies and by crowding and insanitary living conditions that fostered bacterial infection and parasitism. A cultural solution to this dietary stress in dairying communities was to make cheese and yoghurt, which lactose malabsorbers could digest. In this way, additional sources of calcium, fat and other nutrients in the milk became

available. An alternative (or additional) biological solution involved natural selection, which favoured the spread of the lactose absorption phenotype, and, so Durham argues, may have arisen because of the additional stress on populations living in very cloudy climates or at high latitudes. In these latitudes, there was additional stress produced by the lower availability of UV(B) radiation.

☐ Why would natural selection favouring pale skin be stronger in northern Europe and Central Asia than in dense, dark tropical rainforests?

■ Because the climate in northern Europe and Asia is not only darker than in tropical regions but also much colder, which necessitates wearing dense, all-covering clothes.

As mentioned in Chapter 2, people began using animal skins as clothes when they colonised these northern

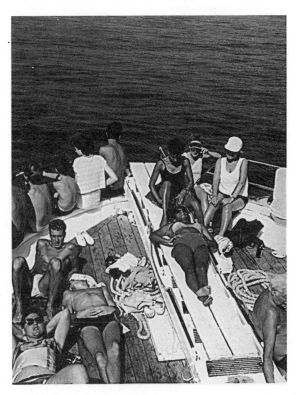

Prolonged exposure to sunshine stimulates the formation of vitamin D and protective dark pigments in the skin. The fashion for suntans is believed to be a major cause of the recent increase in skin cancer among light-skinned people. (Photo: P. W. Keer-Keer)

regions at the end of the last Ice Age, when the climate was even colder (and probably also cloudier) than it is now. When thus dressed, only a small fraction of the whole skin, perhaps only the hands and face, is exposed to sunlight, so vitamin D synthesis there must be as efficient as possible. It is important to point out that sunbathing is a modern habit. Most people who wear heavy clothes never undress outside. Pale-skinned people can produce several months' supply of vitamin D in an hour or two of sunbathing in bright sun.

Durham's explanation for the natural selection of the lactose absorption phenotype is intuitively plausible and fits the facts of the geographical distributions of indigenous lactose absorbing and lactose malabsorbing populations. The inheritance of lactose absorption and lactose malabsorption (Table 7.1) conforms to accepted genetic theories, suggesting that the capacity to absorb lactose depends upon a single gene for which there has been favourable natural selection. The period since dairying became established in northern climates (approximately 5 000 years) is thought to be sufficient for this evolutionary change to have occurred. Further, the evidence for

parallel selection for pale skin in populations native to high latitudes provides additional circumstantial support for Durham's hypothesis.

Earlier in this story, two populations were identified as not conforming to the explanation for the selection for lactose absorption at high latitudes: the Eskimo populations of Greenland and the milk-dependent peoples of East Africa and Saudi Arabia. The Eskimos do not keep dairy animals and so have no sources of lactose after weaning. They are predominantly lactose malabsorbers who nevertheless live successfully at 69 degrees north with moderately dark skins, heavy clothing, and low and periodic levels of sunlight.

□ Think back to the discussion of Eskimos in Chapter 2. Can you suggest an explanation of how traditional Eskimo societies avoided vitamin D deficiency?

■ The Eskimos remained healthy because their native diet consisted almost exclusively of fish and meat, which are rich in vitamin D.

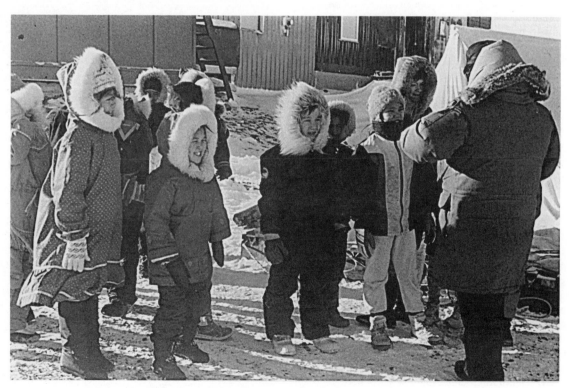

Humans are basically tropical, so clothes are essential in cold climates, but they shade as well as insulate the body and thereby restrict light-facilitated vitamin D synthesis in the skin. The natural diet of Eskimos is rich in vitamin D, compensating for the fact that very little of their skin is ever exposed to sunlight. (Photo: C. M. Pond)

Thus, this example does not provide a challenge to Durham's hypothesis that reduced levels of UV(B) can produce a stress on a population's health and fitness; the natural diet of Eskimos compensated for the lack of UV(B), so there was no pressure for cultural changes such as cheese-making or for the evolution of lactose absorption throughout life.

☐ In the last 40 years, most Canadian Eskimos have abandoned their traditional diet and habits and live almost entirely on food imported from southern Canada; how will this change of diet test Durham's hypothesis?

■ If Eskimos eat a diet containing less raw fish and meat, and hence less vitamin D, Durham's hypothesis predicts that over many generations the proportion of lactose absorbers in the population would rise.

The existence of pastoral communities in East Africa and Saudi Arabia who live at latitudes below 30 degrees (i.e. approaching the Equator), and have a long history of milk use, but who have high proportions of lactose absorbers in their populations, remains to be explained. These populations are inconsistent with Durham's hypothesis that lactose absorption spread in *higher* latitudes as a result of natural selection. It might be argued that other conditions unique to the culture or environment of these Equatorial populations contributed to the selection of the lactose absorption phenotype. Alternatively, there may have been selection for some other (as yet unknown) consequence of inheriting the gene involved in lactose absorption. If so, there would be no selection pressure *against* the spread of this gene in these populations, because the ability to digest lactose is beneficial rather than harmful to milk-drinking adults.

The lactose paradox and a solution

At the heart of the lactose absorption story is a biological paradox: why does the female mammal go to the 'trouble' and 'expense' of synthesising the lactose in breast milk from galactose and glucose, when it then has to be broken down into these constituents by lactase before it can be absorbed by the infant? The solution to the paradox comes from the observation that suckling babies are protected against vitamin D deficiency. Recent research indicates that young children do not depend upon vitamin D for calcium absorption for as long as they are breast fed (or given animal milk). Babies can maintain normal levels of calcium in their blood even if their mothers are deficient in vitamin D.

The explanation for this protection against vitamin D deficiency is that lactose acts directly on the cells in the lining of the gut to facilitate the absorption of calcium; in effect lactose in milk-fed infants is behaving like vitamin D. Studies on adults have shown that lactose promotes calcium absorption only in lactose absorbers and only in those regions of the gut that produce the enzyme lactase. The finding that lactose acts like a vitamin D supplement in promoting the uptake of calcium from the gut provides a partial explanation for why mammalian milk contains lactose rather than glucose or galactose.

☐ How does the evidence about the reduced availability of UV(B) at high latitudes and the fact that lactose acts like a vitamin D supplement support the view that lactose absorption spreads within certain populations as a result of natural selection?

■ The fact that some dairying populations adopted a cultural solution (cheese-making) to the 'problem' of lactose malabsorption suggests that lactose intolerance was not a sufficient stress on those populations to result in positive selection of the lactose absorption phenotype. But in dairying populations who did not obtain sufficient UV(B) radiation, the adults were under stress from vitamin D deficiencies, and the beneficial effects of lactose in facilitating absorption of calcium could favour the spread of the gene involved in lactose absorption.

Conclusion

Eating is one of the most expensive physiological processes in terms of the materials and energy required for digestion, the risk incurred of absorbing harmful organisms or substances and the necessity of counteracting abrupt changes in concentrations of nutrients in the blood. Food is not easy to deal with: the brain and its senses and the gut and associated organs such as the liver and pancreas work together to choose it and digest it. The first half of this chapter provided a brief sketch of the many different organs and processes involved in digestion and absorption; this knowledge may help you to appreciate why appetite, food preferences and eating habits can reveal so much about a person's mental and physical health.

The account of the association between lactose intolerance and vitamin D synthesis is still not universally accepted as the only possible interpretation of the facts (and doubtless new facts will come to light in the future that might discredit Durham's hypothesis), but it does illustrate some interactions between the physiology, geography and evolutionary history of our species. Collaborative research between anthropologists, biochemists and geneticists is helping to explain more of our habits and physiological capacities and limitations.

The lactose story also shows that there is often more than one way of obtaining essential nutrients, so what is a healthy diet in one place could prove inadequate under other circumstances. Humans are one of the most widespread large animals that have ever existed and our diet is correspondingly varied. We have recently adopted diets to which we may not be physiologically well-adapted.

People are still undergoing evolutionary change, and habits and diet are continuously changing as new foods, and new ways of preparing existing foods are added to our diet. Groups of people differ not only in dietary habits but in their genetic capacity to digest, absorb and metabolise certain foods. These biological facts cannot be ignored in recommending changes in diet and food preparation. Dietary deficiencies and factors such as the incidence of UV(B) radiation affect nutrition and health, thereby providing selection pressures for both cultural change and genetic evolution.

OBJECTIVES FOR CHAPTER 7

When you have studied this chapter, you should be able to:

7.1 Outline the gross structure and normal operation of the major components of the human digestive system.

7.2 Outline the main processes involved in the digestion and absorption of proteins, fats, carbohydrates and non-nutritive components of food.

7.3 Briefly describe some mechanisms involving the nervous system and certain hormones that control eating and digestion under normal circumstances and when food contains harmful components.

7.4 Describe the roles of the major organs and hormones involved in regulating the concentration in the blood of glucose absorbed from the gut.

7.5 Describe the biology of lactose absorption and lactose malabsorption and their possible relationship to the evolution of skin colour.

QUESTIONS FOR CHAPTER 7

Question 1 (*Objective 7.1*)

Describe in a few sentences the roles of (a) the stomach, (b) the pancreas, (c) the liver, and (d) the small intestine in the digestion and absorption of food and the regulation of blood composition.

Question 2 (*Objective 7.2*)

Describe briefly the roles in normal human digestion of (a) muscles, (b) enzymes, (c) secretions other than enzymes, and (d) symbiotic micro-organisms.

Question 3 (*Objective 7.3*)

Describe some factors that contribute to appetite and food selection. Why are short-term anorexia, vomiting and diarrhoea considered to be *adaptive* mechanisms that protect the body?

Question 4 (*Objective 7.4*)

List the factors that (a) increase, and (b) reduce blood glucose.

Question 5 (*Objective 7.5*)

Outline briefly the cultural and evolutionary changes involved in the origin and spread of (a) lactose absorption in adults, and (b) paler skin.

8 *On living longer*

This chapter briefly reviews the biological changes associated with ageing. It contains essential background material for the chapters on the health experience of older people in the present-day United Kingdom, which occurs in another book in this series, Birth to Old Age: Health in Transition.[1] *You will find it helpful to consult* World Health and Disease *while reading this chapter, which refers to several diagrams in the earlier book.[2]*

Introduction

The wiser mind
Mourns less for what age takes away
Than what it leaves behind.
(William Wordsworth, 1770–1850,
from *The Fountain*, published 1800)

In Chapter 2 of this book you read that humans live longer than any other mammal. You also read that there are age-related changes in some physiological abilities, such as a decline in running speed and maximum grip strength. Scientists can measure the decline in function and describe the cellular changes that commonly occur as the body ages, but they have not yet identified a *core mechanism* of ageing. Biologists and doctors are still at the stage of cataloguing the physical and psychological changes without knowing if they are causes or consequences of age. Nevertheless, humankind still seeks the secret of eternal youth through an understanding of the mechanisms of biological ageing, in the hope that, once understood, it might be possible to prevent or at least delay these changes taking place. This chapter gives a brief review of ageing from a biological perspective, drawing on theoretical debates about the evolutionary significance of 'living longer' as well as laboratory research on the possible mechanisms that may underlie the ageing process.

A person's physical appearance changes during the course of their life. From maturity onwards these changes are often described as *ageing*, a word that has a negative connotation in some cultures and a positive one in others, where age is venerated.

□ Can you give an example of an age-related change in physical appearance that is not necessarily socially disadvantageous, even in British society? (The discussion in Chapter 2 on the evolution of soft tissues may help you.)

■ Changes in the distribution of body hair, hair colour and facial wrinkles can bring higher status (though more commonly to men than to women in present-day Britain); a man with grey hair is more likely to be described as 'distinguished looking' and a face with some wrinkles may be said to have 'character' or 'laughter lines'. A person may need a 'mature' appearance in order to achieve promotion or a position of authority.

People often refer to someone as 'not looking their age', the implication being that ageing is a sequence of milestones, each of which should be reached by a specific chronological age. The reality is different. Ageing does not start at any one time, nor does it proceed at a constant rate; rather, the gradual accumulation of cellular and tissue changes over time has external signs and effects that become increasingly evident with age. These changes can result from a number of biological phenomena, which we describe later in this chapter: there are changes in cells themselves and in proteins in the fluids between cells; 'degenerative' changes occur in whole organs; and the effects of diseases can contribute to the ageing process. But each of these manifestations of the ageing process does not affect everyone, nor do they occur in a specified order, even in people who do experience them at some stage in later life; there is considerable individual variation.

[1] *Birth to Old Age: Health in Transition* (Open University Press, 1985 and revised edition 1995).

[2] *World Health and Disease* (Open University Press, 1993).

The correlation between the occurrence of these biological changes and chronological age also varies between species. Similar changes occur in all mammals, but they occur at very different points in the lifespan when different species are compared, and do not correlate well with the closeness of death. If we are to look at ageing as a biological phenomenon, we need to formulate a **biological definition of ageing** that does not depend on specific aspects of the process as it occurs in humans, as these may not occur in other species. Thomas Kirkwood of the Medical Research Council in Manchester gives such a definition:

> …ageing is a progressive, generalized impairment of function resulting from a loss of adaptive response to stress and in a growing risk of age-related disease. (Kirkwood, 1992, p. 35)

Ageing is not a uniquely human phenomenon, but the physiological and behavioural manifestations of old age are very much less apparent in natural populations of other animals than they are among humans.

☐ Explain why this should be so (think back to the discussion of human growth and life history in Chapter 2).

■ Most animals die in the wild before they reach old age. Among those that do not, any slight decline in the ability to survive caused by ageing increases their risk of death through predation, starvation or disease. Humans are better protected from such natural hazards, especially in prosperous societies where the majority live to old age.

Death is a separate issue from ageing. It is a matter of common observation that death can occur at any age, but in the United Kingdom and other industrialised nations it gradually becomes more likely after about forty years of life and the chance of dying accelerates quite rapidly after the age of seventy. However, this relationship between age and death is not true for all countries and historical periods. Consider the United Kingdom in the sixteenth century and many Third World countries today.[3]

☐ Which age group is most at risk of death in these examples?

■ Children under the age of five years.

Childhood mortality has been dramatically reduced in developed countries, and has fallen in most Third World countries in recent years, and as a consequence *average* life expectancy has increased. Until recently, scientists accepted that each species has an 'in-built' or genetically-programmed *maximum* lifespan, which can be estimated by recording the age at which the oldest members of that species die. For humans, this is around 115 years in well-documented cases. However, the idea that there are typical species-specific maximum lifespans has been challenged by two very different lines of evidence: experiments on fruit-flies and the analysis of Scandinavian church records from the eighteenth century (both of which are discussed later in this chapter). The risk of death in these examples does not show an indefinite exponential rise with age, but tends to 'level off' at advanced ages. This finding is important when we consider (below) the *evolutionary* mechanisms underlying ageing and (at the end of the chapter) the relationship between ageing and death, because it suggests that death in old age is not necessarily a genetically-programmed event.

There are a number of different theories about the evolution of ageing, which can be divided into those suggesting that ageing is *advantageous* in evolutionary terms, and those that view ageing as *deleterious* or, at best, neutral; we discuss these theories next. The middle of the chapter deals with biological processes and ageing. We describe the way in which cells change with age and examine the extent to which these cellular changes explain some age-related changes in the appearance and functional abilities of individual people; we consider the various biological mechanisms that have been proposed as the underlying 'driving forces' of ageing. Finally, we look at the relationship between ageing and death.

The evolution of ageing and death

> Since everything was made for a purpose, everything is necessarily for the best purpose. (Voltaire, 1759)

This optimistic view, expressed by Dr Pangloss in the novel *Candide*, is often accepted by romantics surveying 'wondrous Nature'. It parodies the mistaken belief, in the context of evolution by natural selection, that *every* characteristic of the organisms we see surviving today

---

[3]See Figure 5.5 in this book, and also *World Health and Disease,* where age-specific mortality rates can be found in Figure 2.3 (Brazil in 1987) and Figure 6.3 (Zimbabwe in 1986 compared with a sixteenth-century London parish); for comparison see Figure 9.10 (England and Wales in 1990).

must be *adaptive*; that is, every characteristic has in some way increased the chance of the organism surviving to leave offspring that in their turn also reproduce. According to this view, surely it must be possible to understand the adaptive value of ageing and death? You should, by now, be able to detect the fallacy in this assumption: some characteristics *are* adaptive in the present environment, but others are deleterious and some are neutral.

As you would expect, there *are* hypotheses that ageing is adaptive and that it evolved through natural selection, but they do not withstand critical examination. Natural selection operates on the *individual* and no hypothesis has been advanced that seriously suggests that it is an advantage to individuals to be dead.

There are, however, several hypotheses that ageing evolved through natural selection, but which argue that ageing is deleterious and thus *non-adaptive*. At first sight, this appears to be a contradiction: how could natural selection lead to the evolution of a non-adaptive characteristic? You have already met one such hypothesis in Chapter 5 of this book: it states that *late-acting* deleterious genes cannot be eliminated by natural selection.

□ How 'late' must the activity of these deleterious genes be in an individual's lifespan, according to this hypothesis?

■ The genes must have a deleterious effect only after some reproductive activity has taken place, thus ensuring that these deleterious genes have had a chance to be passed on to progeny.

Another hypothesis that ageing is non-adaptive but evolved through natural selection is based on the fact that many genes have multiple effects (for example, the gene responsible for the disease *phenylketonuria*, PKU, described in Chapter 4, affects mental function, hair colour and skin tone). If a gene with multiple effects is involved in ageing, it might have favourable effects early in an organism's life but deleterious effects later. Natural selection will favour the spread of such genes because of their beneficial early effects, leading inevitably to the accumulation of genes with deleterious late effects. This hypothesis does not specify which particular genes are likely to be responsible for the process of ageing, but another hypothesis is more specific about the nature of the ageing processes.

The **disposable soma theory** is named after a Western economic phenomenon and the Greek word *soma* meaning 'body'. Motor cars and other machines are typically designed and built to last for a certain length of time. It is possible to make cars that last a very long time, but they are expensive to make and, such are the realities of consumer taste and wealth, have only limited market appeal. Generally, rather little investment is made by machine manufacturers in durability. By analogy, it is suggested that organisms derive little benefit from investing resources in increasing their lifespan beyond a certain point.

Two arguments are involved here. First, the fundamental trade-off between *somatic effort* and *reproductive effort* (discussed in Chapter 5), means that somatic effort will never be maximised because, to do so might be to pass up the chance to reproduce at all. Thus, some durability must be sacrificed to achieve reproduction. Second, all organisms are subject to accidental death, through a variety of hazards, and so have only a finite expectation of life, even if they do not age. To invest in survival in the expectation of eternal life is inefficient, because the inevitability of eventual death through some kind of accident means that resources that could have been put into reproduction will have been wasted. Thus, the disposable soma theory argues that the *optimal* level of investment in the soma (body) is *less* than would be required for the indefinite survival of the individual. Consequently, organisms show the various manifestations of ageing because they do not invest resources in preventing them from occurring.

These *non-adaptive* explanations of the evolution of ageing are not mutually exclusive. The disposable soma theory is consistent with the basic tenets of *life-history theory* (see Chapter 5), and does not present any counter-arguments to the other non-adaptive hypotheses mentioned above. It seems likely that ageing occurs through a combination of harmful genetic effects, the pattern of investment in the soma throughout life, and also to by-products of normal cellular activity. The relative importance of these three factors probably varies greatly from species to species, and between individuals, but there are some aspects of the ageing process that are common to all organisms. The common cellular signs of ageing are described next.

The cell and age

All cells undergo some changes with age, though age does not necessarily mean the same thing for the many different types of cell in the bodies of large multicellular animals such as ourselves. Some cells are short-lived and are rapidly replaced by others: for example, in humans this is true of skin cells, cells that line the gut (Chapter 7) and red blood cells. For these cells, ageing occurs over a few weeks; they change in form and function and are then shed or destroyed. Other cells, such as the nerve cells (neurons) in the brain, cannot be replaced after birth, so they tend to be long-lived and brain-ageing occurs over the lifespan of the individual.

One method of studying ageing in normal cells is known as *tissue culture*.[4] Cells are isolated and grown outside the body in containers of nutrient medium. The 'growth potential' of these cells is measured by the number of times the population of cells doubles in number, in other words, by the number of cell divisions. In general, the growth potential of cells in laboratory cultures decreases slightly with increasing age of the donor from whom the original cells came, but all cultured cells have a period of normal growth followed by a period of ageing when they divide less frequently. Another method of studying cellular age-related changes is to compare the appearance, biochemistry and activity of cells taken from individuals of different ages.

□ Both methods described above have disadvantages; suggest one drawback to each method.

■ Tissue culture removes cells from their normal physiological environment and prevents the normal cell-to-cell interactions that would take place in the whole organism. For instance, the effects of hormones and nerves are removed. In comparative studies, it is difficult to know whether the observed differences in cells from donors of different ages are due to intrinsic age-related changes in cell biology or in the donor's behaviour. For example, if the muscle cells of older people differ from those of younger people, is it because of intrinsic ageing processes in the cells, or has lack of activity and a more sedentary lifestyle in the donor brought about changes in their muscle cells?

Despite these and other drawbacks, these methods have identified a number of changes in mammalian cells as they age. The components of cells, the proteins and other molecules as well as the organelles and membranes (Chapter 3), are continuously changing; for example, different amounts of chemicals such as enzymes, hormones and neurotransmitters may be manufactured in response to changing needs. These components are

[4]Tissue culture and other methods of investigating living cells outside the body are considered in *Studying Health and Disease* (revised edition, 1994), Chapter 9.

subsequently broken down into smaller constituents for recycling, but, as the cell ages, the rate of *turnover* of essential components declines.

□ How might this affect the functioning of the cell?

■ Any component that is defective or damaged remains in place longer, and those in short supply are not replenished as quickly as before; this reduces the efficiency of the cell in performing its normal functions and, potentially, also reduces the efficiency of any organ or tissue of which the cell is a part.

The turnover of proteins in normal cells and body fluids produces a 'marker' of ageing. Proteins are broken down by enzymes into their constituent amino acids (the process is similar to that by which proteins in the diet are digested, as described in Chapter 7), and the amino acids are 'recycled' in the synthesis of new proteins. The efficiency of this recycling decreases with age. A by-product of inefficient protein recycling is granules of a yellow, fatty pigment called *lipofuscin* (pronounced 'ly-poh-few-sin'), which start to accumulate in the cell. Lipofuscin is a universal marker of old cells (Figure 8.1). When it is 'fed' to cells in culture it slows their *metabolic activity* (the 'sum total' of chemical interactions taking place in the cell).

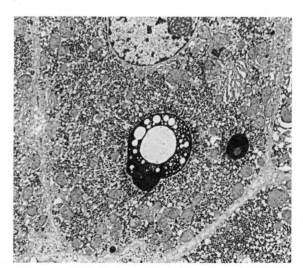

The dark lipofuscin granules are clearly visible in this photograph of a liver cell (magnified 1 300 times) from a person aged 62 years; notice the proportion of the cell volume that has been converted to lipofuscin. (Photo: Photographic Unit, Department of Histopathology, John Radcliffe Hospital, Oxford)

□ If lipofuscin also has this effect on living cells in the body, what are the consequences for cell function?

■ As lipofuscin accumulates, the rate of manufacture and recycling of proteins will further decrease, and there will be a consequent slowing of cell metabolism.

Another noticeable age-related change in mammalian cells is an increase in the number of *lysosomes*, the small intracellular packets of enzymes and other destructive chemicals in the cytoplasm (Chapter 3). It has been suggested that accumulation of lipofuscin and of lysosomes leads to cell death. There is, however, no good evidence that these are harmful to cells and their appearance could be related to some unknown event, unconnected with age. But some of these 'aged' cells die before the organism dies and, in tissues where cells are not replaced, this leads to diminished functioning of organs. For instance, 50 per cent of nephrons (the filtration units in the kidney) are lost between the ages of 30 and 90 years. There is considerable interest in an emerging theory that cells are genetically programmed to die *unless* continuously stimulated by chemical signals from other cells; it may

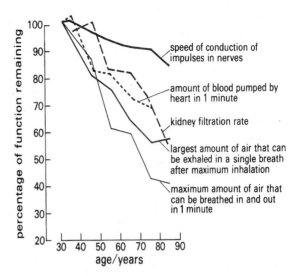

Figure 8.2 *Reserve capacity of some organs in humans with increasing age. (Source: Passmore, R. and Robson, J. S., 1980,* A Companion to Medical Studies, Volume 2, Pharmacology, Microbiology, General Pathology and Related Subjects, *2nd edn, Blackwells Scientific Publishing, Oxford; based on data from Shock, N. W. et al., 1957,* Geriatrics, *12(40).)*

turn out to be the failure of these signals in old age that lead to cells 'committing suicide'.[5]

The major organs in the human body have considerable **reserve capacity** (potential to increase activity in times of need); for example, you could live with only half a kidney functioning instead of two. But there is a marked loss of reserve capacity with age in many organs (see Figure 8.2), which means that an older person may not be able to compensate adequately for some physiological stresses. Notice that the reserve declines at very different rates in different organs.

Bodily signs of ageing

The loss of reserves to call upon in times of physiological stress was identified in the biological definition of ageing given earlier (by Kirkwood). As we get older, our lean body mass reduces and there is also a progressive reduction in the water content of the body. This represents loss from, and consequent decline in functioning of, a variety of organ systems. As you read on, you

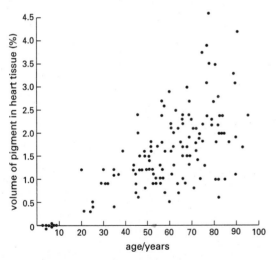

Figure 8.1 *Scatter diagram showing the relationship between age in humans and the concentration of lipofuscin in heart muscle cells; notice that the relationship becomes quite weak (the points are more scattered) among the 'oldest old', some of whom have lipofuscin levels similar to those of 20–30 year olds, while others have levels more than 100 times as great. (Adapted from Strehler, B. L., Mark, D. D., Milchran, A. S. and Gee, M. V., 1959, Rate and magnitude of age pigment accumulation in the human myocardium,* Journal of Gerontology, *14, Figure 2, p. 434)*

[5]The technical term for programmed cell death is *apoptosis* (pronounced 'appoh-toe-sis'), a name that you do not have to remember. For a review of apoptosis, see Raff, 1992.

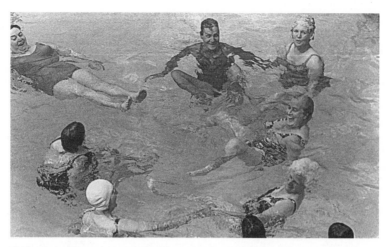

The majority of people remain healthy and active as they age. (Photo: Mike Levers)

might like to consider whether all these age-related changes are inevitable.

☐ What reductions in the efficient functioning of the body are often associated with old age? (You should be able to answer from general knowledge.)

■ The following list is not exhaustive.

1   Structural problems become more common: for example, muscles are weaker, joints move less freely, bones break more easily and repair less reliably.

2   Sensory impairments are often reported, such as poorer sight, hearing, sense of balance, smell and taste.

3   Reduced ability to recall recent and generally trivial events, or to remember 'what I meant to do next' is a problem for some older people.

4   An increased susceptibility to infectious diseases suggests that there has been some reduction in the efficiency of the immune system (Chapter 6).

5   Homeostatic mechanisms, such as the ability to maintain a constant temperature in a cold environment, may become less efficient.

6   After menopause, women lose their ability to conceive a baby without medical intervention.

☐ Are these changes inevitable? (Think about several elderly people whom you know well.)

■ A striking fact about this list is that (with the exception of menopause) none of these functional losses are inevitable; every old person does not experience all these changes. Nor does an individual who suffers from one impairment necessarily suffer from another.

☐ What kinds of diseases are characteristically found in elderly people?[6]

■ Cancers, arthritis, and diseases of the cardio-vascular and cerebrovascular systems (such as heart attacks and strokes) are all more common in older people than in young people, but none of them are exclusively associated with old age.

Later in this chapter we will consider whether any of the bodily signs of ageing listed above can be explained by our knowledge of how cells change with age. But first, we must ask what is different about the changes that occur at menopause. Why is menopause inevitable? This takes us back into the realm of evolutionary theory.

Menopause

Human females are unique among mammals in that they lose the ability to reproduce at menopause, a long time before they die (recall Chapter 2). Various arguments have been put forward to explain the evolution of menopause. Fundamental to these is the fact that, for women, giving birth and feeding babies involves considerable physiological stress that can result in death. Menopause,

---

[6] *World Health and Disease*, Figure 9.2, is useful in answering this question.

by 'switching off' reproductive capacity, removes older women from the risks that attend reproduction.

☐ Why should this be adaptive?

■ Human infants are dependent on their mothers for food, warmth and protection for a large part of their lives. If their mothers did not stop reproducing they would eventually undertake a birth that was so stressful that they would die or would be so severely weakened that they could not continue to care adequately for their existing offspring. Thus menopause favours the survival of existing children, at the expense of potential future children.

Another argument in support of menopause as an adaptive characteristic is that post-menopausal women have a valuable contribution to make to the reproduction of their kin. In many primates (monkeys and apes), infants are cared for not only by their mothers, but also by a variety of relatives, including their siblings, cousins, aunts, uncles and grandparents. There is some evidence that, the larger this extended family of care-givers, the higher is the rate of survival of infants born into it. Post-reproductive females may be of special value to the reproductive success of genetically-related family members because of their experience. A number of studies of birds and mammals have shown that breeding success increases with age; parents get better at rearing their young at each successive breeding episode.

These arguments are based on an extension of the theory of natural selection called *kin selection*. According to this hypothesis, genes that cause a female's reproductive activity to be switched off at a certain age will be favoured by natural selection if, as a result of her post-reproductive behaviour, her progeny and those of other close relatives are more likely to survive. Her kin will tend to carry the same genes by descent, so the loss of reproductive potential by post-menopausal females is offset by their contribution to preserving the genes they share with their kin. Thus, the biological changes at menopause are believed to be adaptive, unlike the other age-related changes described above, which are generally accepted to be non-adaptive.[7]

We turn now to take a closer look at some of the reductions in bodily function which commonly (though not inevitably) occur in old age, and investigate whether they are the result of underlying cellular changes.

[7]A sociological perspective on the menopause appears in *Birth to Old Age: Health in Transition* (1985, and revised edition 1995).

Muscles, cartilage and bones

Loss of muscle strength is an irritation to older people, particularly as some deterioration starts to be noticeable from about 45 years of age. Studies indicate that the problem is caused by a loss of muscle *fibres*, rather than by the atrophy (or wasting) that is experienced when muscles are immobilised, in a plaster cast for example. This loss of muscle fibres can probably be explained by a parallel loss of *motor neurons* (the nerves that activate muscles). Muscle fibres that are not activated eventually die. Studies show that between the ages of 30 and 80 years of age, there may be a loss of 30 per cent of muscle fibres. The functional consequence of this loss of strength is that older individuals may become unable to perform some quite ordinary tasks.

☐ Can you suggest some examples?

■ Opening screw-top bottles and jars; opening heavy swing doors; carrying heavy packages.

Many studies show that these changes are not inevitable or irreversible; muscle performance can be improved through exercise at any age.

☐ Look at Figure 8.3 and suggest what else should be done to ensure the full use of available muscle power.

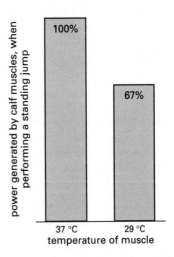

Figure 8.3 *Output of human calf muscles at different temperatures. (Data derived from: Davies, C. T. M. and Young, K., 1983, Effect of temperature on the contractile properties and muscle power of* triceps sorae *in humans,* Journal of Applied Physiology, **55**, pp. 191–5)

■ Keep warm!

Another sign of advancing age due to reduced muscle power is a deterioration in *gait*, the efficiency with which a person walks or runs. However, factors other than reduced muscle power can contribute to a poor gait.

☐ Can you suggest other factors?

■ You may have thought of aching joints and stooping posture, the effects of an injury or an illness that affects muscular coordination.

Not all old people develop these characteristics, but there are changes in cartilage and connective tissue such as tendons that make age an important risk factor in a variety of diseases of the joints and skeleton.

In a young, healthy joint where two bones touch, each surface has a covering of *cartilage*, a tissue that is smoother and softer than bone (see Figure 8.4). Cartilage gives the joint the ability to articulate (slide one bone over the other) without 'grinding' the bones together, and it absorbs jarring forces. Joints are held together by tough bands of connective tissue called tendons, which are also attached to muscles that bend and flex the joint.[8] The space between the bones is filled with a lubricating fluid (synovial fluid) and the whole joint is encased in a capsule. Joints are not static mechanical structures: cartilage undergoes constant wear and repair; tendons under stress are strengthened by proteins; the fluid within the joint drains and is replenished.

The ability to maintain tissues in the joint alters with age, but it is often difficult to distinguish between intrinsic age-related biological changes, the results of repair following minor injuries, and reactions to persistent mechanical stresses such as poor posture or repetitive actions. The thinning of joint cartilage that occurs with age may be due in part to wear and tear, rather than to any underlying age-related changes in the cells that produce new cartilage. However, one extremely common age-related trait is the appearance of bone cells in cartilage. This is not necessarily associated with any observable disability, but it can make joints less mobile. The deposition of bone in the costal cartilage (which joins the ribs to the breast bone) makes this joint more rigid and restricts movements of the rib cage during breathing. Loss of water from the fibrous cartilage of the shock-absorbing

---

[8]You may remember from Chapter 2 that a rigid distinction used to be made between tendons and ligaments (tendons connect muscle to bone and ligaments connect bones together); the composition and mechanical properties of these connective tissues are, in fact, almost identical and so, for simplicity, both are now often referred to as 'tendons'.

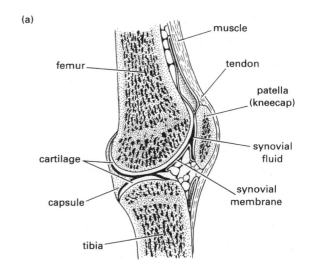

(a)

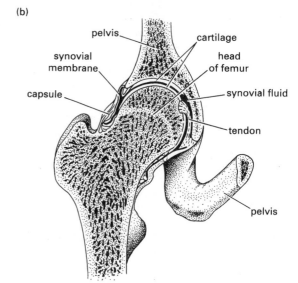

(b)

Figure 8.4 *Diagram of 'side-on' sections through joints that frequently give problems in elderly people: (a) hinge joint in the knee, and (b) ball-and-socket joint in the hip (part of the pelvis is also shown).*

discs between the vertebrae of the backbone is another problem, which can lead to a reduced ability to bear or lift weight.

It has already been observed that the proportion of proteins within cells changes with age, and the same is true for proteins secreted by cells. The amount of a protein called *collagen* in tendons increases with age, making them less elastic. (Incidentally, this change to the proportion of collagen in the skin also makes it wrinkle.)

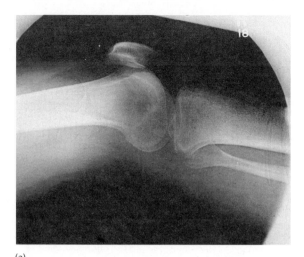

(a)

Figure 8.5 *X-ray photographs of human thigh bones: (a) a healthy young bone has a high density of calcium, which obstructs the transmission of X-rays through the bone so it appears white on the film; (b) this bone from an elderly person with advanced osteoporosis has lost so much calcium that it is almost transparent to X-rays and is prone to fracture. (Sources: (a) Hemel Hempstead General Hospital, Radiography Department; (b) Milton Keynes General Hospital, Radiography Department)*

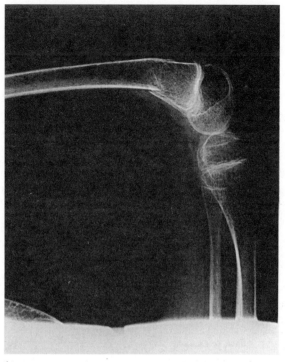

(b)

The collagen itself also alters its structure as it ages, becoming more rigid.

None of these changes represent a disability in themselves, but they make the individual more susceptible to diseases of the muscles, joints and skeleton (including arthritis) and less able to recover from accidents and injury. A report by the Office of Population Censuses and Surveys (OPCS), published in 1988, showed that disorders of the muscles and bones were responsible for approximately 40 per cent of all physical disability in British adults.[9]

Although bones are very tough, they are not rigid non-living structures. In healthy bone, new bone is continually being generated to replace old bone which is being broken down; the construction and destruction processes are in equilibrium. However, older bones can become fragile as a consequence of a loss of calcium from them (a condition known as *osteoporosis*, see Figure 8.5) because old bone is being destroyed faster than it can be replaced. The change is observed in all individuals although, as with all other ageing processes, the onset and severity of the loss shows enormous individual variation. The underlying factor seems to be age-associated

[9]*World Health and Disease*, Figure 9.7, includes these data.

changes in calcium metabolism (chemical activity involving calcium in the body). Older people absorb less of the calcium that they take in with their diet, due to age-associated changes in the cells lining the gut.

☐ Gut lining cells, like skin cells, are continuously replaced. What happens to such cells as they get older?

■ As described earlier in this chapter, these cells change gradually in form and function and are eventually shed. Additionally, they divide less frequently as they age, and so they are replaced less often.

In the gut, cells that are replaced every 30 days in young adults are only replaced every 40 days in elderly people. This slowing up of cell division is reflected in how the cells function; the cells lining the gut secrete less mucus and enzymes in old age, which means that the body may digest food less efficiently. As you already know from Chapter 7, vitamin D promotes the absorption of calcium from the food across the gut lining as well as the uptake of calcium in bone. Vitamin D is absorbed by the gut and is converted to an active form in the liver and kidneys. The active form of vitamin D can only be produced if liver and kidney function are intact. As mentioned earlier, nephrons (the filtration units of the kidney) are progressively lost from the age of 30 years as cells die and are not replaced; in addition, average liver volume falls by over 30 per cent between the ages of about 25 and 90 years.

☐ Why might this be a problem in older people?

■ Reduced function in the kidneys and liver as people age results in a reduction in the amount of vitamin D converted to the active form. This in turn contributes to a reduction in calcium uptake from the diet and its deposition in bone, and hence to the slowing down of new bone growth to replace old bone as it is destroyed.

Changes in calcium metabolism are more pronounced in post-menopausal women than they are in men of the same age. Women in older age groups excrete more calcium in their urine than they take in from their diet. This appears to be a result of calcium being withdrawn from bones as a result of disturbance in the various hormones involved in the normal formation of bone. In some research studies, treatment with oestrogen has had a beneficial effect on calcium balance, and has reduced the rate at which bone density was lost in older women, but the results are contradicted by other studies and so remain controversial. And, unless it is given with another female hormone, progesterone, oestrogen replacement therapy increases the incidence of cancer of the uterus (womb).[10]

The foregoing account should have convinced you that it is because of age-related changes in *cells* that muscles and bones weaken and joints can 'seize up' as we get older, and that these cellular changes are themselves influenced by complex biochemical processes with widespread effects throughout the body. You should also remember that there are a variety of means, principally involving exercise and diet, to reduce the potentially damaging effects of cellular changes in old age.

The senses

There are many age-associated changes in the eye; perhaps best known is the loss of the ability to change focus. This occurs because the lens grows throughout life, adding fibres of proteins known as *crystallins*. By the time it is 50 to 60 years old it is almost impossible to change the shape of the lens and, although distant objects may be in sharp focus, near objects are usually blurred. There may

[10]Hormone replacement therapy (HRT) for women during and after menopause is discussed in *Birth to Old Age: Health in Transition* (1985, and revised edition 1995) and in *Dilemmas in Health Care*, Chapter 9.

also be changes in the structure of some crystallins, which can result in the formation of a cataract, an opaque covering of the lens causing blindness.

The sensory cells of the eye (called rods and cones) manufacture pigments involved in registering the patterns of light that fall on the eye. Proteins are major constituents of these visual pigments. Lipofuscin can be detected in the rods and cones of children as young as 10 years old; by the age of 24 lipofuscin occupies about 8 per cent of the volume of these cells, rising to over 20 per cent by 80 years of age.

☐ What might be the possible functional consequences of this accumulation of lipofuscin?

■ As lipofuscin accumulates, the rate of manufacture and recycling of the visual pigments decreases. Any defective or damaged pigment will remain in place longer, making the rods and cones more susceptible to the effects of cumulative damage. This contributes to the deterioration of vision in old age.

Slowing of other metabolic processes will also occur in the presence of high concentrations of lipofuscin, including those that prevent or repair damage from radiation. Our eyes are exposed to the physical effects of sunlight; damage from this source of radiation slowly accumulates as we age.

Hearing loss in old age is associated with degeneration of sensory cells in the inner ear and/or the nerves involved in sensitivity to sounds. Some types of hearing loss have a familial tendency and hence probably have a genetic basis.

☐ Is there an alternative explanation?

■ There could be an environmental effect on hearing that is common to family members, such as living close to a major road or working in the same (noisy) industry such as coal mining or cotton mills.

It is easy to show that hearing is damaged by persistent exposure to loud noises such as artillery fire and certain kinds of music, but less obvious that everyday noises, from traffic for example, slowly destroy sensory cells. Comparative studies of people who live in non-industrial societies suggests that high-tone hearing loss (a universal feature of Western societies) is mostly due to the level of 'general background' noise. It is difficult to know whether the hearing loss commonly measured in elderly people is the outcome of age-associated changes in sensory cells or the effect of living for a long time in a noisy environment.

This brief look at some of the changes that can occur as people grow older has revealed some common features. Cells do change with age and so do their protein products. Some cells die before the organism dies. All age-related deficits can be traced back to changed cellular activity, so the next stage in our investigation of the ageing process is to enquire about the mechanisms that bring about cellular ageing.

Biological mechanisms of cellular ageing

Most biologists view ageing as a non-adaptive evolutionary process, as described earlier in this chapter. The tremendous variation in the ways and extent to which different individuals age suggests that numerous mechanisms leading to cellular ageing may be at work simultaneously within the population. These mechanisms range from the effects of lifestyle and environment to the action of genes; we will very briefly review the most important of them. Much of the research into cellular ageing has been carried out on species with very short lifespans, such as fruit-flies and small rodents, in preference to waiting 70–80 years to observe the mechanisms involved in this process in humans.

Lifestyle and cellular ageing

There is evidence that lifestyle can have a considerable effect on lifespan but very little evidence that it causes cells to age.

□ Suggest a number of ways in which lifestyle might affect lifespan, from general knowledge.

■ You might have thought of excessive alcohol consumption, participation in dangerous sports, or smoking tobacco products as possible ways of decreasing lifespans, and that a 'balanced' diet and a moderate amount of regular exercise might increase one's chances of living to a 'ripe old age'.

Diet

Diet is of particular interest because of evidence from a study on rats: those fed on reduced-calorie diets lived significantly longer than those allowed to eat as much as they chose, and who consumed almost twice as much as those on restricted diets (Masoro, Shimokawa and Wu, 1991).

□ Can you think of any reasons why the rat experiments might be of no relevance to humans?

■ Apart from the fact that rats are rats and humans are humans, it is also possible that the laboratory rats that eat as much as they wish are the 'abnormal' group and that a low calorie diet is nearer to the 'normal' diet of a wild rat.

Scientists in the United States are studying the effect of a reduced-calorie diet on non-human primates (Warner *et al.*, 1992), but at present there is no evidence that a reduced-calorie diet would lengthen the life of a person who is not already obese. It would still be useful to know more about whether and in what ways diet might interact with individual genotypes to affect the ageing process.

Wear and tear on cells

There are structures, such as teeth, and cartilage at the ends of bones, that generally wear out with time. But they out-last many individuals' needs and, with care, they may last a lifetime with almost no signs of wear and tear. Although, as mentioned earlier, some cells, such as neurons, cannot be replaced when they die, plenty remain. So mechanical wear and tear resulting from common lifestyles is not a major cause of cellular ageing.

Accumulation of toxins in cells

As we get older, the cells of our bodies accumulate toxins that are not excreted. The liver is particularly vulnerable as it is the organ with the major role in detoxification (as described in Chapter 7) and it stores toxins that cannot be excreted. Despite the fact that average liver volume falls by over a third during the lifespan, and that old liver cells have increased lipofuscin and other inactive proteins, there is no evidence that liver function is impaired in old livers unless they are damaged by excessive long-term alcohol consumption. It seems unlikely that cell ageing is a result of the accumulation of toxins.

Decline in the rates of protein synthesis and protein turnover

Evidence from a number of species points to a decline in protein synthesis and turnover being a universal characteristic of ageing cells. The accumulation of protein past its 'sell-by' date within the cell may inhibit the production of new protein, while the 'old' protein may be subtly altered and less effective. A reduced-calorie diet *may* lessen these age-associated changes, as well as decreasing the number of proteins that are damaged by reacting with particular sugars. As protein turnover declines, so lipofuscin begins to accumulate, further reducing protein turnover. These processes may be fundamental to ageing, but the cause of this slowing down of cellular metabolism in the first place is unknown.

Genes and cellular ageing

Comparative studies of fruit-flies which have been carefully bred to produce strains with either long or short lifespans demonstrate that many genes act together to influence the length of life (Luckinbill *et al.*, 1988). There is evidence that this is also true for humans, from studies of a rare and very distressing condition called *progeria*. Infants with this condition develop a senile appearance and seldom live beyond five years of age. The study of progeroid human cells indicates that several thousand genes can influence the development of the senile phenotype (Martin, 1978). This does not rule out the possibility that, in some individuals, it could be the activity of just one gene that is responsible for major age-related changes. In the roundworm, for example, a single recessive mutation has been found that markedly enhances the lifespan of individuals possessing it. The gene containing this mutation has been given the name *age-1* (Friedman and Johnson, 1988).

Somatic mutation theory

There are changes to the DNA of many body cells over time, called *somatic mutations* (described in Chapters 3 and 4; 'somatic' denotes that the mutation does not affect the germline DNA and so is not passed on to the next generation). Most alterations to the sequence of nucleotides in the DNA strand are repaired by special enzymes, but despite this there is an accumulation of somatic mutations as cells divide and divide again throughout life. However, various experiments suggest that these changes are not responsible for the onset of ageing, but they *are* important causes of age-associated diseases, particularly cancers.

Free radical theory

The structure of DNA and proteins can also be altered by the activity of *free radicals*. These are groups of highly reactive atoms, the by-products of normal cellular activity, which are usually very short-lived. They are 'mopped up' by special enzymes, but if they escape de-activation they have the potential to do enormous damage. Free radicals can react with molecules in the cell (the particular chemical process involved is called *oxidation* and was mentioned in Chapter 7), changing the structure of the molecule. The changes in long-lasting proteins, like the crystallins of the eye, may be a direct result of free radical damage to the protein, rather than an indirect result of damage to the gene that codes for that protein.

There are a number of pieces of evidence that fit the notion that free radicals have an important role in ageing. First, human post-mortems show that the brains of older people have more oxidised proteins than are found in younger human brains (Young, 1993).

Second, experiments performed by John M. Carney of the University of Kentucky Medical Centre in 1991, established that a chemical that de-activates free radicals improves the performance of old gerbils in memory tests

and also lowers the levels of oxidised proteins in their brains (quoted in Rusting, 1992).

Third, rodents that had exercised to exhaustion had at least trebled levels of free radicals as well as damaged mitochondria in their cells (Davies *et al.*, 1982). Mitochondria are the cell's 'power houses' (Chapter 3); a process takes place in the mitochondria that releases energy by the oxidation of glucose. Prolonged exercise requires an increase in the amount of energy generated in the mitochondria by oxidation; this in turn generates more free radicals (the agents of oxidation), which damage cell function. Excessive exercise could seriously damage your health!

The free radical theory of ageing is probably the most widely accepted candidate for a *core mechanism* of ageing, that is, one which is of universal importance in all animal species. Less than perfect defences against free radical activity would allow wide variation in the damage that ensued, dependent upon the type of molecules attacked and the types of cell that sustained the damage. Other processes, as yet unknown, are also likely to be important agents of ageing; individual variation strongly suggests that ageing is a *multifactorial* process, that is, one in which several different factors interact.

Ageing and death

In this book, we are concentrating on a biological and evolutionary interpretation of human health and disease, which includes ageing and death. The sociological, personal and ethical aspects of these important subjects are discussed in another book in this series.[11]

The changes in cells and functional abilities described so far in this chapter are not, in themselves, *proximal* causes of death.[12] 'Old age' is no longer entered as a cause of death on medical certificates; most deaths among elderly people are attributed to a specific disease, or combination of diseases. Loss of physiological reserves may make older people more susceptible to disease and hence death, but that doesn't explain why certain diseases are so much more prevalent in old age than they are in youth.

[11] *Birth to Old Age: Health in Transition* (1985, and revised edition 1995).

[12] A proximal cause is the 'last step' in the chain of causality; contributing factors that act earlier in the chain are called *distal* causes. See *Studying Health and Disease* (revised edition, 1994), Chapter 10.

A partial answer may be that most of the diseases with a high incidence in old age, such as heart disease, strokes, and cancers, have multifactorial causes. Several different factors must interact before the disease develops, and it may take many years before all these factors have coincided in the necessary sequence to produce a disease that leads ultimately to death. We can illustrate this general point by considering cancers, a highly varied group of diseases affecting most parts of the body, which increase in incidence very sharply in old age.

Cancers: a major cause of death in old age

In the 1990s, approximately one in five people in industrialised countries dies of a **cancer**, the majority after the age of 65.[13] Medical scientists are beginning to unravel the factors underlying the onset of certain cancers and this increases the chance of future medical control of the disease.

In cancers, cells that would normally have all the characteristics of a particular cell type (a liver cell, for example), lose their specialised structure and functions and become *undifferentiated*. An undifferentiated cancer cell resembles the unspecialised cells that existed in the early embryo, before cells differentiated into liver cells, nerve cells, etc. Cancer cells divide repeatedly, the daughter cells are similarly unspecialised and are repeatedly dividing; they can 'break away' from the original mass (the primary tumour), and travel around the body in the bloodstream and lymphatic circulation (Chapters 3 and 6), eventually settling in a distant site to multiply into secondary tumours.

□ In what ways do you think cancer cells might damage the body?

■ Primary or secondary tumours in organs (such as the liver), use nutrients and oxygen, but do not contribute to the organ function. As cell numbers increase, they may hinder normal functioning of other cells and organs by, for instance, exerting pressure on nearby tissues, distorting them or blocking their blood supply, or interfering with the nerves controlling their function.

Cancer cells may also produce chemicals that disrupt the normal working of the body, or weaken bones by infiltrating them; tumours set off inflammatory reactions (Chapter

---

[13]*World Health and Disease*, Figure 3.1, compares the proportion of deaths in industrial countries with those in Third World countries from different causes, including cancers.

6) and can cause severe pain. Cancers are extremely variable in their progress and in their effects, because the original cancer may have arisen in almost any part of the body and the secondary tumours can be highly variable in their location. Thus, lung cancer is a very different condition from (say) breast cancer or leukaemia (cancer of the white cells in the bloodstream). If a cancer leads to death, it may be from multiple organ failures and generalised breakdown of the body's biochemistry and ability to maintain homeostasis. Many cancers are now medically treatable, but the incidence of some cancers is steadily rising (for example, lung cancer among women).

What triggers the transformation of a normal cell into a cancerous one? It is known that cells change from normal cells to cancer cells in response to signals from specific genes. Genes that send such messages are termed *oncogenes* (*onco* comes from the Greek word meaning 'a lump'). Most of the known oncogenes seem to be variants of the genes that code for proteins involved in normal cell division. When a cell becomes cancerous, the normal gene is altered in some way, becoming constantly active. Over 30 oncogenes have been identified, and several must be activated before they cause a normal cell to become cancerous.

Active oncogenes promote rapid increase in cell numbers, but so-called *anti-oncogenes* or tumour suppressor genes send signals to reduce the rate of cell division and to promote differentiation into the appropriate cell type. (It should be noted that their role is crucial in the *normal* development of cells; anti-oncogenes are activated repeatedly throughout the life of the cell, not only when oncogenes are expressed.) In addition, there are mechanisms that cause damaged cells to 'commit suicide'.

Thus, a cancer cell is one that has both been affected by the activity of oncogenes and has escaped the biological control mechanisms that have evolved to eliminate it. An ability to detect precisely which oncogenes and failed control mechanisms are involved in a particular individual's disease may lead to improved therapy and even prevention of some cancers. But an underlying question remains: what activates the oncogenes? Could it be accumulated damage to the DNA from free radicals, radiation or chemical toxins in the environment, or part of a genetically-programmed process of ageing? The English cancer epidemiologists, Sir Richard Doll and Richard Peto reject the latter explanation:

> Turning finally to the role of age itself, it is sometimes suggested that because cancer is ten or a hundred times more likely to arise in the coming year in old people than in young people, ageing *per se* should be thought of as an

important determinant of cancer. We rather doubt whether this viewpoint is a scientifically fruitful one. (Doll and Peto, 1981b, p. 1205)

Doll and Peto have estimated that about 70 per cent of cancers are potentially avoidable in that they are due to exposure to carcinogens (cancer-causing substances) in the environment, rather than to intrinsic ageing. Their painstaking research over several decades has identified the smoking of tobacco as the major environmental carcinogen, accounting for an estimated 30 per cent of cancer deaths; they attribute less than 4 per cent of cancers to carcinogens derived from industrial chemical pollutants. (We consider the impact of chemical pollution on human health in Chapter 10.) However, the ability to correct 'errors' in DNA caused by chemical carcinogens or radiation appears to decline with age. Moreover, small errors in the replication of DNA occur each time a cell divides and a new set of DNA molecules is synthesised (Chapter 4) so, as a person ages, more cell divisions will have occurred and more uncorrected errors will have accumulated. The chance of damaged DNA leading to activated oncogenes and inactivated anti-oncogenes, and hence to cancer, is therefore likely to increase with increasing age.

Is there a maximum human lifespan?

The events prior to death are clearly a great deal more varied than the events prior to birth. Humans age relatively slowly and the variation between individuals, both in the rate of ageing and the age at death, is huge. But the question remains, if we are not killed by accident or disease, does our life then inevitably terminate after some allotted span?

Stanford rheumatologist James Fries believes that 'it is frailty rather than disease' that kills people at very old age (quoted in Barinaga, 1991). He also believes that there are inborn limits to the human lifespan that start to operate at about 85 years of age. This is disputed by another American researcher, James Vaupel (whose theories are also discussed in Barinaga, 1991). Vaupel went to Sweden where the Lutheran church has kept very accurate records of births and deaths. This has provided evidence that the mortality rates for 85 year-old Swedes has 'dropped dramatically' in the past 50 years. He also used the Danish twin registry to collect data on 4 000

twins born between 1870 and 1890 and then used a computer model to determine whether the pattern of their deaths suggested a genetically-programmed maximum lifespan (McGue, Vaupel, Holm and Harvald, 1993). His conclusion was that deaths below 110 years are 'premature'. Experimental work on insect populations that Vaupel carried out in collaboration with other scientists (Carey et al. 1992), further challenges the notion that all species have absolute lifespan limits.

> The best of men cannot suspend their fate:
> The good die early and the bad die late.
> (Daniel Defoe, 1661–1731, from 'Character of
> the late Dr S. Annesley', written in 1697)

The debate about the upper limit on human age does not deny that death is inevitable and cannot be prevented by evolution (as Chapter 5 explained), so the first line of Daniel Defoe's assertion is clearly correct. Vaupel intends to explore next whether the oldest old who 'die late' are also 'fitter' in evolutionary terms, that is, an elite of biologically adapted individuals.

☐ How can this be done?

■ It requires the investigation of family pedigrees to discover whether individuals who had long lifespans also left more progeny who themselves survived, reproduced and had long life.

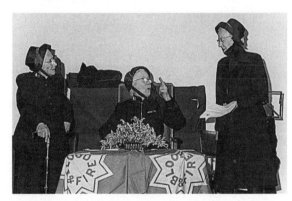

Catherine Branwell-Booth, on her 100th birthday with her two sisters, both in their nineties. All three were officers in the Salvation Army. Is their longevity the result of female biology, of the inheritance of genes that increase lifespan, of companionship and mutual support, or of an abstemious life? (Photo: courtesy of the Salvation Army)

Conclusion

Death is inevitable, but in prosperous, industrialised human societies ageing presents a formidable challenge to health services because the proportion of the population in the oldest age groups is rising.[14] In evolutionary terms, the manifestations of ageing (with the exception of menopause) are not adaptive processes. Currently, we do not understand the underlying mechanisms sufficiently to enable medical science to alter the progress of biological ageing in individuals; doctors can treat the diseases of old age, but they cannot stop people from getting old. If such knowledge becomes available through biomedical research, it will raise important ethical questions about the extent to which humans are justified in 'tinkering with nature'.

But we do not have to wait for a breakthrough in research into ageing before addressing the ethics of altering human biology in profound ways; this is already being hotly debated in the 1990s as a result of progress in other areas of medical science. The next chapter will describe some ways in which medical science is, or may soon become, able to change the quantity and quality of individuals' lives, which have far-reaching ethical and social consequences.

OBJECTIVES FOR CHAPTER 8

When you have studied this chapter, you should be able to:

8.1 Discuss alternative hypotheses about the evolution of ageing, distinguishing between views of ageing as adaptive or non-adaptive.

8.2 Describe some of the age-related changes in the human body and the cellular changes that underlie them.

8.3 Describe biological mechanisms that may be involved in causing the cellular changes associated with ageing, and discuss ageing and death as multifactorial processes.

QUESTIONS FOR CHAPTER 8

Question 1 (*Objective 8.1*)

It has been suggested that ageing and death are adaptive because they prevent overcrowding and consequent depletion of resources. What is the fundamental flaw in this argument?

Question 2 (*Objective 8.2*)

Collagen is a fibrous protein that is an important constituent of tendons and hence joints. It is also found in many other tissues including the lens of the eye, skin and arteries. In all these tissues collagen becomes more rigid with age. Briefly summarise the age-related changes in these tissues and consequent effects on health in old age.

Question 3 (*Objective 8.3*)

Which of the biological mechanisms of cellular ageing described in this chapter could account for the observed change in the rigidity of collagen with age?

---

[14]Data on the 'ageing population' of the United Kingdom and the effect of this demographic trend on the community care policies of the 1990s are discussed in *Dilemmas in Health Care*, Chapter 8. Health and disease in old age are a major topic in *Birth to Old Age: Health in Transition* (1985, and revised edition 1995).

9 Tinkering with nature

This chapter builds on the discussion of the evolutionary significance of DNA and the structure and function of cell membranes (Chapter 3), the contribution of human genes to disease (Chapter 4) and the functioning of the immune system (Chapter 6). You will also find several footnote references to other books in this series, where topics that are merely touched on here receive a more thorough discussion.

During your study of this chapter you will be asked to read a short article, 'The shadow of genetic injustice' by Benno Müller-Hill, which appears in the Reader.[1] There is also an audio-tape, called 'Tinkering with nature', associated with this chapter, in which a British geneticist, Steve Jones, considers the ethical aspects of genetic research. The television programme 'Blood lines' is also relevant.

Introduction

At this point in the book, our focus shifts gradually from the present to the near future, as we speculate about the possible impact of medical science on human biology and even on the evolution of the human species in generations to come. In biological terms, the human species has become hugely successful in the last 300 years, increasing with breathtaking speed from a global population of about 600 million in 1700 to well over 6 billion (6 thousand million) by the end of the twentieth century.[2] The reasons underlying this population explosion are

discussed elsewhere, but the central point is that the contribution of cultural evolution, such as the advent of agriculture, industrial practices and sanitation, have far outweighed the contribution of medical science to the dramatic increase in human survival.[3]

But the balance is tilting as we approach the next century. The power of cultural change to improve human health may be diminishing, as industrial development and urbanisation reach more and more of the globe; indeed, some would claim that 'modern culture' is having the reverse effect by inflicting new diseases and exacerbating old ones, a view we debate in the last two chapters of this book. Medical science rather than cultural change is now expected to provide solutions to many hitherto intractable human diseases, particularly in Western industrialised nations. The significant increase in life expectancy in the developed world has brought with it an epidemic of degenerative diseases, which reduce the quality of the 'added' years and put severe pressure on the ability of health services to meet demand.[4] Chronic conditions affecting children and young adults, such as diabetes, cystic fibrosis, AIDS and multiple sclerosis, have achieved heightened public attention because they have defied all attempts at cure. As we approach the twenty-first century, the opportunities for medical science to affect the future health not only of individuals, but of the human species, are expanding at a seemingly unstoppable pace. News of 'breakthroughs' is reported daily, generating not only hope that suffering may be alleviated and lives saved, but also anxiety about the ethical and practical implications of 'tinkering with nature'.

☐ Think about recent media coverage of medical breakthroughs. Which have caused controversy about the ethics of 'tinkering with nature'?

[1] Health and Disease: A Reader (Open University Press, revised edition 1994).

[2] See World Health and Disease, Figure 5.2, for global population estimates from 40 000 BC to AD 2025.

[3] See World Health and Disease, Chapters 5 and 6, and Caring for Health: History and Diversity, Chapters 3 and 4.

[4] The 'ageing society' in the United Kingdom and its impact on health and social service provision are discussed in Dilemmas in Health Care, especially Chapters 3 and 8.

■ As we finalised this chapter in spring 1994, the major news stories in this category in the preceding six months fell into six groups (others may well have arisen by the time you read this):

(i) methods of overcoming infertility involving donated eggs or surrogate mothers, or restoring fertility to women after the menopause;

(ii) the medical use of living cells from recently aborted fetuses;

(iii) multiple-organ transplants and other highly invasive methods of keeping people alive;

(iv) genetic screening of individuals, including fetuses, for an ever-increasing list of genetic characteristics;

(v) gene therapy, i.e. the insertion of normal human genes into people with genetic diseases;

(vi) genetic engineering, i.e. the insertion of human genes into other organisms, such as bacteria, as a means of producing medically-useful human proteins and drugs.

In this chapter, we will at least touch on all of these groups of medical dilemmas (the intervention of medical science in human fertility is a major topic in another book in this series[5]); our main focus here will be on techniques that involve manipulating human genes, as you might expect in a book with an evolutionary perspective on human health and disease. By altering human genes, medical science can alter human evolution. The potential benefits are enormous and yet many scientists as well as many lay people question where we should draw the line.

It is difficult, even for biologists who work outside the rapidly-advancing field of genetics, to discriminate between genuine scientific potential and 'media hype'. The extraordinary pace at which new knowledge about human genes is being acquired in the 1990s (largely as a consequence of the Human Genome Project[6]), means that even the scientific 'elite' is struggling to grasp the implications for human health and human ethics. Although the main focus of this chapter is on the 'new genetics', the very newness of the biology involved in that story carries with it the shock of the unexpected, so we

have chosen to start with a brief look at a more familiar example of 'tinkering with nature': medical techniques involving the exchange of tissues and organs from the dead to the living. Here, you are on biologically familiar ground prepared in preceding chapters, which nonetheless sharply illustrates the debate about where to draw the line between legitimate medical science and unacceptable interference with human biology; notice that 'the line' shifts as a technique becomes more widespread.

Transfusions, transplants and implants

The transfusion of blood from person to person has become so commonplace in scientific medicine that for most people in the industrialised world it would not be considered as interfering with natural biology. We have forgotten the controversy that blood transfusion caused when experiments began in the seventeenth century, and few but Jehovah's Witnesses today believe it is forbidden by God.[7] The willingness of the majority of the population to accept several pints of another person's blood into their circulation on the advice of a doctor seems a little strange in the context of heated debates about some other types of transplant. Blood may be viewed more like a 'medicinal fluid' which is freely given by one living person to another, whereas the removal of organs from recently-dead people for transplantation into a living body has aroused much anxiety about the ethics of 'spare-part surgery'.

The ethical debate began in December 1967, with the news that a South African surgeon, Christiaan Barnard, had transplanted the first human heart from a recently-dead person into a man with chronic heart disease, Lewis Washkansky, who died 18 days later. The failure of so many of the pioneering heart transplants in the next few years led to the practice being abandoned for about a decade but, in the 1980s, advances in medical science led to **organ transplantation** programmes being established in most industrialised countries, with relatively high rates of success. The breakthrough was due to a combination of progress in different fields: advances in surgical techniques and intensive post-operative care; the development of new drugs that suppress the recipient's immune system so that it does not 'reject' the graft (as described in Chapter 6); and techniques for 'tissue-typing' organ-donors and matching them with suitable recipients.

[5]*Birth to Old Age: Health in Transition* (Open University Press, 1985 and revised edition, 1995).

[6]The Human Genome Project is introduced in *Studying Health and Disease* (revised edition, 1994), Chapter 9, and will be discussed later in the present chapter.

[7]The medical history of blood, including transfusion, is discussed in *Medical Knowledge: Doubt and Certainty*, Chapter 5.

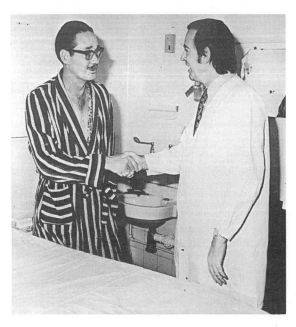

Christiaan Barnard says goodbye to one of his pioneering heart-transplant patients before discharging him from hospital in Cape Town in 1974. (Photo: Camera Press)

□ Why is 'matching' necessary? (Think back to Chapter 6.)

■ The donor and the recipient are genetically different (except in the rare case of identical twins), so the pattern of proteins and carbohydrates on the surface membrane of their cells differs. Unless it is totally suppressed with drugs, the immune system of the recipient will respond to these non-self molecules by attacking the cells of the graft as though they were a mass of invading organisms. Matching the donor and recipient to minimise the degree of genetic difference between them reduces the severity of the 'host-versus-graft' immune response and hence increases the chance of graft survival. It also reduces the need to suppress the immune system with drugs, which leaves the patient prone to infection. You may also have thought about matching for size: an adult heart is not suitable for transplanting into a baby and vice versa.

Single-organ transplants are now routine practice in industrialised countries: among the most numerous and successful are kidney grafts, of which about 1 500 are performed in the United Kingdom annually, and over 2 000 mainly elderly Britons have their sight restored each year by a simple operation to transplant

a healthy cornea (lens) into the eye. (The cornea has no blood supply and is beyond the reach of the immune system, so there is no need to match donor and recipient.) Yet the frequency and success of these operations has not eliminated ethical concerns: for example, whole organs such as a heart or a kidney are mainly given to children and adults who are below retirement age.

□ What *medical* reasons might there be for the majority of organ transplants to be performed on this age group? What *non*-medical considerations might also be taken into account when selecting suitable candidates for transplantation?

■ Very young or very old patients might not withstand major surgery. Social reasons may also influence selection of recipients: the shortage of organs donated for transplantation and the high cost of major surgery may tilt the choice towards children and adults who could expect a significant number of extra years of life from the operation, many of whom are also likely to have dependants.[8]

Concern that some patients are being passed over in the competition for organs has been less of an issue than the fear that pressure may be put on the relatives of a dying person to donate his or her organs, so that someone else can live. There have also been a very few cases of kidneys being sold for cash by healthy but impoverished donors. And as transplant technology improves, there is growing anxiety about the extent of a person's body that can be replaced.

Since the 1980s, multiple-organ transplants are increasingly performed in which more than one organ from a single donor is transplanted into the same recipient. In 1993, a chronically-ill British child (Laura Davies) received, for the second time, an almost complete set of abdominal organs, including the liver, pancreas, spleen, kidneys, stomach, small intestine and colon. If you look back at Figure 7.1 you will see just how extensive a transplant this is. An intense debate about the ethics of such extensive surgery was carried out in the news media, first while Laura Davies waited in America

[8]The rationing of scarce health services and the influence of the age of the patient on the decision to provide expensive procedures are discussed in *Dilemmas in Health Care*, Chapter 3.

for a suitable donor to die, and later when she also died some weeks after the transplant operation. The child's parents received hate mail from people accusing them of letting doctors perform grotesque experiments on their daughter, while thousands of others donated money to the appeal fund set up to support the treatment.

The most forceful argument put forward by surgeons in defence of highly-invasive transplant surgery is that only practice and perseverance will increase the success rate of these techniques, just as the pioneering heart transplants 'failed' but paved the way for today's successful operations. But this was not the case with Laura Davies, according to Professor Thomas Starzl, director of the Pittsburg Transplant Institute where the 15-hour operation was performed:

> Absolutely nothing of any consequence is going to be learned scientifically. To say the operation was done for that purpose is preposterous. There is only one issue with that child, and that is to try to get her to live… It may turn out to be the case that in retrospect it would have been kinder to let her die, but the answer to that question turns on whether she lives or not. If she lives it makes people who take that view [that she should have been allowed to die] look pretty silly. (Quoted by Chris Mihill, *Guardian*, 28 September 1993, p. 3)

The *origin* of transplanted organs and tissues is yet another area of contention. Most people would sanction the properly-negotiated use of an adult human donor, but some would draw the line at giving a person the heart and lungs of a pig; yet the shortage of human donors means that many potential transplant-recipients will die waiting, *unless* doctors develop ways of using the organs of other species. Organs for transplantation have been removed soon after the death of very young babies without much comment, but there is a furore when the origin of the donated tissue is an aborted fetus. (Cells can be kept alive for a time after removal from a recently-aborted fetus, just as an organ can be kept alive temporarily after removal from a person soon after death.)

In 1988, reports were first published in medical journals that relief from some of the symptoms of Parkinson's disease (a progressive deterioration of coordinated muscle movements, caused by the loss of certain cells from a particular region of the brain) could be achieved by implanting fetal tissue into the brains of patients. Cells taken from the corresponding region in the fetal brain were able to grow and multiply in the patient's brain because the immune system of the recipient does not recognise fetal cells as 'foreign'. The fetal brain cells produced chemicals that were depleted in people with Parkinson's disease, although the extent to which the implants actually produce worthwhile improvements is highly variable (Gage, 1993, gives an overview).

In the United States, the outcry was so great against a possible trade in fetal tissue, supplied by women who became pregnant with the intention of aborting for cash, that in 1988 President Bush prohibited the use of living cells from aborted fetuses for any research purpose. The ban was swiftly reversed when President Clinton took office in January 1993.

The medical benefits of **fetal cell implants** in non-related individuals to compensate for cellular deficiencies are very wide-ranging and depend on the very immaturity of the fetal cells. By the time a baby is born, the so-called *stem cells* in its bone marrow are dividing repeatedly to provide all the red blood cells and the white cells of the baby's immune system (as described in Chapter 6). At birth, the white cells have already undergone a complex 'education' in which they become tolerant to (do not attack) the baby's own tissues and organs, but would attack any 'foreign' cells they encounter. The best hope of cure for certain diseases (such as some types of leukaemia) includes a bone marrow transplant from a closely-related donor, containing stem cells that divide and repopulate the recipient's body with healthy red and white cells. The recipient's immune system is first suppressed or destroyed, so the transplanted stem cells are safe from attack. The snag is that the transplanted stem cells *develop into* a functioning immune system, which attacks the body of the person who receives the graft, because the patient's tissues and organs are recognised as chemically 'foreign' by the donated cells (this is known as graft-versus-host disease). However, if the donated stem cells are taken from a fetus, *before* they learn to distinguish between 'self' and 'non-self', then the grafted cells become tolerant to their new host and both graft and host survive.

Fetal stem cells have been successfully transferred to babies still in the womb, who would otherwise have been born with severe deficiencies in their blood (Crombleholme *et al.*, 1991). This opens the door to fetal cells being used to repopulate the blood and immune system of adults whose own blood cells have been destroyed, for example by accidental radiation or during medical treatment of leukaemia and some other cancers. In the future, some individuals will perhaps be a 'biological mosaic' containing cells derived from several different donors.

Since the mid-1980s in the United Kingdom, somatic (body) cells taken from fetal brain, liver and pancreas have been sanctioned by a 'code of practice' for the treatment of certain conditions. However, the growing complexity of the ethical issues raised by scientific progress in fetal research led to a regulatory body being created by government in 1990, the Human Fertilisation and Embryology Authority (HFEA), a panel of 21 experts in human physiology, medicine, ethics, religion and the law. Several members of this authority expressed profound disquiet when it was announced that significant progress had been made in research in mice (Spears *et al.*, 1994) which might, in time, enable the recovery of immature eggs from aborted human fetuses for subsequent transplantation into infertile women. The ovaries develop quite early in fetal life and contain millions of immature eggs; if they could be recovered from aborted fetuses and 'matured' in laboratory cultures, this would solve the considerable shortage of donated eggs for infertility treatment.

□ What ethical issues does the use of fetal eggs raise, over and above those already discussed in relation to fetal somatic cells?

■ There are two main issues. First, there is the question of consent: in removing the egg from a fetus to use in infertility treatment the germline is being 'donated' from an individual who cannot consent to this use of her eggs; the fetal egg contains germline DNA from the man and woman who created that fetus (Chapter 4), so should *they* have some say in what use is made of their genes? Second, what psychological consequences might there be for a child who discovers that its biological 'mother' was an aborted fetus?

Similar issues are raised by the potential use of eggs taken from women and girls soon after death, although in theory an adult female could carry a donor card which allowed this use of her eggs, just as she can currently sanction the donation of certain organs after her death. The potential biological, social and psychological consequences of overcoming infertility with eggs from fetal or dead donors were addressed in a public consultation document issued by the HFEA in January 1994:

...eggs from an aborted fetus have not been subjected to the pressures which govern survival and normal development to adulthood.

This raises questions about the degree of risk of abnormality, at present unquantifiable, in embryos produced using such tissue. This might be seen as breaking a natural law of biology. A further consideration is that miscarriage is frequently due to chromosomal defects in the fetus. Unless it is possible to test a fetus which is the result of miscarriage for such abnormalities, it may seem inadvisable to consider using ovarian tissue from miscarried fetuses for subsequent fertilisation and treatment because of the risk of transmitting genetic abnormality… In the case of children born from cadavers or fetal ovarian tissue, the particular implications of finding out that their genetic mother had died before they were conceived, or was an aborted fetus, are unknown. It would be necessary to consider further how to assess the likely effects on children and their wider family relationships of knowing they were born from donated material from these sources. (Human Fertilisation and Embryology Authority, 1994, p. 6)

In April 1994, an amendment to the Criminal Justice Act was passed which made it a criminal offence in the United Kingdom to use eggs from an aborted fetus for subsequent transplantation into infertile women.

This snapshot of a few key issues in the debate about transplantation of biological material from person to person illustrates the extent to which cultural and social factors influence whether we consider a procedure to be 'standard medical practice' or 'tinkering with nature'. Concerns have focused on the *extent* of the interference with human biology, the *origins* of the material transferred, the issue of informed consent, psychological damage to those concerned, and the wider ethical implications of actions which either threaten or 'unnaturally' prolong life. All these concerns are evident in the rest of this chapter, where we discuss the medical potential and ethical consequences of research on human genes. New techniques for intervening in genetic diseases, such as mass genetic screening, gene therapy and genetic engineering, are among the most fraught areas of debate in modern biology and medical science. Such revolutionary techniques bring with them moral, social and ethical issues. Are these procedures the ultimate way of tinkering with nature in that they open up the possibility of directing our future evolution?

Family decisions in genetic diseases

We begin with the most familiar aspect of medical genetics by looking at diseases with a known genetic predisposition from the perspective of affected families. What are the choices available to families where there is either a known history of predisposition to a genetic disorder, or alternatively a child is born with a genetic disease of which there is no previous family history?

Human pedigrees (described in Chapter 4), have been produced for centuries, although their original purpose was not the same as that of today. In the past, family history, particularly the financial aspects, often played an important role in marriage contracts. Today family histories serve different purposes, as shown below.

Jo began to develop chest pains typical of angina at the age of 25 years, but the diagnosis of coronary heart disease (CHD) was missed because of his youth. Five years later, Jo had his first heart attack, but the diagnosis was again missed because it was thought that at 30 years of age he was too young to have a heart attack. Only when he experienced his second heart attack three years later, and the physician obtained Jo's family history of early CHD in his father and uncle, did it lead to the correct diagnosis of *familial hypercholesterolaemia* as the underlying cause of the heart disease, and to the start of appropriate therapy.

Jo's story emphasises the importance of family history for reaching a correct diagnosis and prescribing appropriate treatment. Another important use of a family history is to diagnose genetic disease *before* the symptoms are manifest (*pre-symptomatic diagnosis*), leading to the prevention or reduction of the disease. For example, once familial hypercholesterolaemia had been diagnosed in Jo, all of his living relatives, and in particular his brother, sister and children, could be given pre-symptomatic testing. Since familial hypercholesterolaemia is a dominant disorder (that is, it is due to the inheritance of a single dominant allele, as described in Chapter 4), the probability of Jo's children inheriting that allele from Jo and being affected is 1 in 2 (on average, half of his children would inherit the disorder). All three of Jo's children were healthy, but two had above average blood cholesterol levels. The family history is shown in Figure 9.1. The affected children were given dietary and drug therapies as preventative measures, in the hope that early intervention would slow the progress of the disease.

Genetic counselling and pre-natal diagnosis

Human pedigrees reveal whether a disease is genetically inherited and from this the probability of a future child of the family being affected can be determined. Figure 9.2 shows the family history of an imaginary family affected

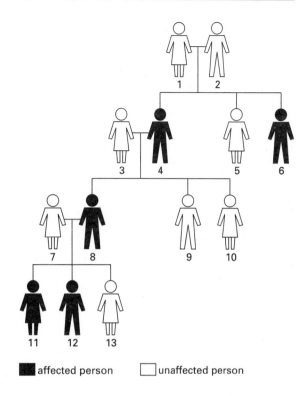

Figure 9.1 *Jo's family history of familial hypercholesterolaemia. Jo is number 8.*

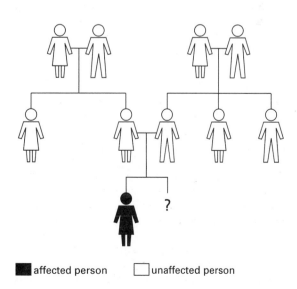

Figure 9.2 *A family history of cystic fibrosis.*

by cystic fibrosis. The mother is pregnant and the couple are concerned about the health of the second child, since the first has cystic fibrosis. At present, the only 'therapy' such couples can be offered is genetic counselling and pre-natal diagnosis of the fetus to see if it carries two copies of the recessive disease allele involved in cystic fibrosis. If it does, then abortion of the affected fetus is the only currently available alternative (in 1994) to proceeding with the pregnancy and raising a second affected child.

☐ Since cystic fibrosis is an inherited disease caused by two copies of a recessive allele, what is the risk of the unborn child indicated by a question mark in Figure 9.2 being affected? (Hint: Both parents are carriers. You may need to refer back to the text and Figure 4.16 on page 85, where a similar situation is considered.)

■ The risk is one quarter or 1 in 4.

Genetic counselling can assist couples facing the consequences of genetic risks such as this. It involves communicating information about the disease, the risks of occurrence and the psychological impact of coping with an affected child. Many European countries and the United States have evolved a system of regional genetic counselling centres to provide a specialist service; in the United Kingdom this service is within the framework of the NHS. The role of the counsellor is not to be *directive*, but rather to ensure that couples have sufficient information on which to base a decision. This is because individuals vary greatly in their responses to genetic risk and wish to make their own reproductive decisions. (Harris, 1988, gives a review of the issues involved in genetic counselling.)

An important point to bear in mind when assessing risks is that the outcome of any fertilisation is *independent* of any other. So even though the first child of the partners shown in Figure 9.2 is affected by cystic fibrosis, the chance of the second child being affected is not reduced; it is still a quarter. You might like to reflect on what risk you might be prepared to take in these circumstances, and what decision you might make if the risk seemed unacceptably high.

Genetic counsellors can also offer information on the options available to couples who find the risk of having an affected child too high, such as contraception, adoption, artificial insemination by donor (which ensures that the affected allele is not transmitted by the father), and pre-natal diagnosis with the option of abortion.

Pre-natal diagnosis has removed from genetic counselling much of the uncertainty about the risks of some genetic diseases. It allows the conversion of a *probable* risk of a specific disease affecting an unborn child to nearer a certainty that it will or will not be affected. However, it must be stressed that pre-natal diagnosis cannot be used to rule out all possible birth defects, nor all genetic disorders, because suitable tests do not yet exist to detect them. Nor is it foolproof even for those diseases that it can generally detect (a point we return to later). A number of techniques are available for diagnosing an affected fetus early in pregnancy. These techniques are listed in Table 9.1 (and are described in more detail in the text), with some indications of the conditions they can be used to detect.

Table 9.1 Techniques for pre-natal diagnosis of fetal abnormalities

Technique	Abnormalities detected
ultrasonography	organ abnormalities of nervous system, kidneys, heart, gut and limbs
fetoscopy	organ and limb abnormalities, skin disorders, blood disorders
amniocentesis—cells	chromosomal disorders (e.g. Down's syndrome)
	metabolic disorders (e.g. PKU)
	DNA studies (many genetic diseases)
amniocentesis—fluid	certain fetal protein levels (which may indicate spina bifida, for example)
chorionic villi sampling, or chorion biopsy	chromosomal disorders (e.g. Down's syndrome)
	metabolic disorders (e.g. PKU)
	DNA studies (many genetic diseases)

Only *ultrasonography* is non-invasive with no known risk to the mother or fetus; it involves 'bouncing' very high frequency sound waves off the fetus, which are reflected back into a receiver and converted into visual images. It can reveal the outline of fetal organs and bones, and detect important 'spaces' such as the chambers in the heart and the fluid in the bladder. *Fetoscopy* has the advantage that the fetus can be visualised directly by

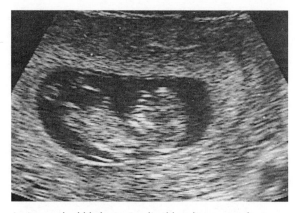

A nine-week old baby is visualised by ultrasonography to check that it is the correct 'size for date'; this technique is also essential to guide the devices used in amniocentesis and chorionic villi sampling to collect samples of fetal cells and fluids safely. (Photo: Milton Keynes Hospital)

inserting a very fine optic telescope (fetoscope) through the abdominal wall into the uterine cavity. Using this method it is also possible to insert a needle into the umbilical cord and obtain blood and skin samples for analysis.

Amniocentesis (Figure 9.3) involves the removal of a small amount of amniotic fluid with a hypodermic syringe. The fluid bathes the developing fetus during pregnancy and contains cells sloughed from the fetus. The fluid can be analysed for its protein content, which may be abnormal in spina bifida and other neural-tube defects;[9] the cells can be grown as a cell culture in the laboratory, which (after several weeks) can be examined with a microscope (e.g. to count the number of chromosomes), or subjected to biochemical tests, or the DNA can be analysed for certain genetic abnormalities. It is mainly offered to women over the age of 35 years, who are at increased risk of having a child affected by Down's syndrome (look back at Figure 4.20), or women with a family history of a genetic disorder or a neural-tube defect.

A less common approach is chorionic villi sampling (or CVS) (Figure 9.4, overleaf), also known as chorion biopsy. Most of the placenta is fetal tissue, derived by cell division from the original fertilised egg, so it is genetically

[9]Neural-tube defects are discussed extensively in Studying Health and Disease and are the subject of a collection of research articles and correspondence in medical journals entitled 'Ethical dilemmas in evaluation', which can be found in Health and Disease: A Reader (1984 and revised edition 1994).

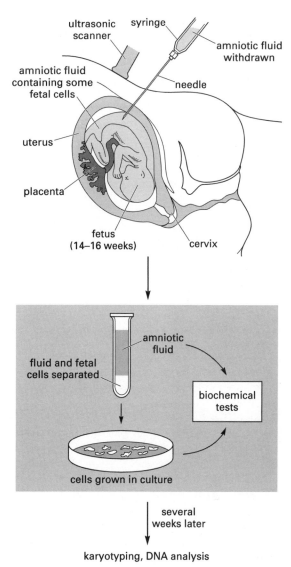

Figure 9.3 Diagram illustrating the technique of amniocentesis used for pre-natal diagnosis.

identical to the cells of the fetus; small samples of the highly-frilled surface of the placenta (called the chorionic villi, rather like the gut villi you saw in Figure 7.2) are removed via a small tube inserted through the vagina of the mother. This technique has the advantage of yielding a greater amount of DNA than is obtainable by culturing the relatively few cells in a sample of amniotic fluid.

These sampling techniques for pre-natal diagnosis are associated with a small increase in the risk of

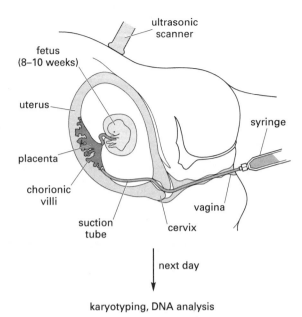

next day

↓

karyotyping, DNA analysis

Figure 9.4 *Diagram illustrating the technique of chorionic villi sampling used for pre-natal diagnosis.* (Remember to turn back to finish reading page 195.)

spontaneous abortion, compared with the risk in pregnancies not screened by these methods, so they raise the acute personal dilemma of whether or not to have a test and, if it detects an abnormality, whether or not to have an induced abortion. We return to the ethical considerations later in the chapter; the use of pre-natal diagnosis as a routine part of antenatal care is discussed elsewhere in this series.[10] Here we focus on the analysis of DNA obtained by these methods.

The importance of DNA analysis to pre-natal diagnosis

Following the extraction of DNA from the fetal cells in the laboratory, powerful techniques can enable the detection of certain mutations involved in genetic disorders, often involving only a single nucleotide change. The methods of detecting mutations are expanding rapidly, with the result that the number of disorders that can be diagnosed pre-nataly is increasing almost weekly. However, for each disease a number of technical problems have to be overcome.

[10]See *Birth to Old Age: Health in Transition* (1985 and revised edition 1995).

First, the techniques of DNA analysis rely on the ability to identify the gene involved in the disorder as a specific piece of DNA. It is no easy task to find one particular gene in the DNA amongst the six billion nucleotides in the human genotype. Not only is it necessary to know which of the 23 chromosome pairs is involved, but also precisely where on a particular chromosome the gene occurs. Nevertheless, the exact location of many genes involved in genetic diseases has now been determined, including those implicated in cystic fibrosis, sickle-cell disease and Tay–Sachs disease.

The second problem to overcome is identifying the presence of a mutation in the gene (that is, the disease allele). DNA analysis may fail to detect the mutation because the test is not yet perfect. Therefore, everyone seeking pre-natal diagnosis is given the degree of certainty of the diagnosis, which further complicates the decision about whether to continue with the pregnancy.

□ If a mutation is detected in the fetus in *both* alleles of the gene associated with cystic fibrosis, would the fetus necessarily be affected?

■ In this case, providing the test is accurate, the fetus would be diagnosed as certainly affected by this recessively inherited disorder.

□ If a mutation is detected in only *one* allele of the gene associated with cystic fibrosis, would the fetus necessarily be affected?

■ No, the fetus could be a heterozygote (a 'carrier'), in which case it would not develop cystic fibrosis. But there is a chance that there could be a mutation in the second allele which had been *undetected*, in which case the fetus would develop the disease.

Newer techniques are expanding the ability to detect novel mutations that cause disease, so in time the degree of certainty of pre-natal diagnosis from DNA analysis will be near to 100 per cent for each genetic disease. So, as we learn more about human genes, difficult choices will become commoner for families and individuals. However, supporters of pre-natal diagnosis point out that as the accuracy of the tests improve, it will lead to a *reduction* in the number of abortions; at present, they argue, a substantial proportion of *normal* pregnancies are terminated because the *estimated risk* of the fetus being affected is higher than the parents can endure. With accurate diagnosis, these fetuses could be saved.

So far we have considered the implications of examining relatives within an affected family for the presence or absence of particular alleles, and discussed the role of the genetic counsellor. Next we broaden the focus to discuss the implications of searching for disease alleles within whole populations.

Population screening for genetic disease

Genetic counselling and pre-natal DNA analysis are available for those families with a *known* risk of having a child with a genetic disease. This is quite distinct from **population genetic screening**, the search in a population of previously unaffected individuals for persons with certain genotypes that are associated with a particular disease. More specifically its purpose is to identify one of two groups: individuals with treatable conditions who do not yet know that they have an increased risk of developing a disease, and individuals or couples at increased risk of having children affected with severe genetic diseases. Some see genetic screening of the population as an important public health activity because the incidence of certain genetic disorders could be reduced, but others believe that the outcomes may have more sinister implications.

Any screening programme must have certain important provisos: the disorder must be an important health problem, it must either be treatable or detection must generate information that could prevent others from being affected, and the test must be inexpensive, acceptable and reliable.[11] Inherited diseases meet the first proviso in that they are considered to be important health problems; for example, they account for over a third of all deaths in infancy (Williamson, 1993). Some of these conditions (like PKU) are treatable if detected early enough. Genetic screening could be defended, even when the condition itself is untreatable, on the grounds that early identification leads to prompt genetic counselling and prevention of the birth of more affected children. A number of programmes have been set up for specific genetic diseases in order to achieve these aims.

Genetic screening began uncontroversially in the 1970s with population screening of newborn babies, to identify infants with genetic diseases for which early treatment could prevent, or alleviate the symptoms. Phenylketonuria (PKU, discussed in Chapter 4) was the first genetic disease for which mass screening was conducted, by analysing blood samples taken from a needle-prick in the baby's heel. An inexpensive and definitive test is available and, if dietary control for those affected begins soon after birth and is maintained, growth and development proceed normally and mental impairment is prevented. PKU is a recessive disorder occurring in Northern European populations in about 1 in 15 000 live births. Before the introduction of screening in the 1960s, it was estimated that the disorder accounted for about one per cent of severe mental retardation; screening has virtually eliminated this. However, the 'heel-prick' test only detects the presence of the PKU alleles *indirectly*; it detects raised levels of the amino acid phenylalanine in the baby's blood, which occur as a result of the defective alleles. There are six known causes for raised phenylalanine in the blood, only one of which is due to PKU.

□ What does this suggest about the detection of PKU by this test?

■ A baby born with raised phenylalanine may in fact not have inherited the alleles involved in PKU, and hence may be wrongly diagnosed. (Such a baby would be a *false positive*, i.e. falsely identified as being positive for the screened defect.)

For example, many babies have moderately raised phenylalanine which does not lead to clinical symptoms. Another group has high blood levels of phenylalanine which persists for only a short time and then spontaneously returns to normal. Thus, babies identified as having raised phenylalanine are given more detailed tests to ensure that treatment for PKU is only administered when necessary, since a phenylalanine-restricted diet may be harmful. The screening programmes for detection of babies with raised phenylalanine have provided interesting information on the general frequency of other genes involved in this phenotype. However, in contrast to PKU, there are other treatable enzyme defects in which similar phenotypes detected by screening tests cannot readily be distinguished from the disease phenotype.

Uncertainties about the reliability of the screening test raise doubts about the advantages of population screening, which are illustrated even more clearly by another example, in which the defective alleles are directly tested for. Direct genetic tests do not produce false positives. Several different mutations can be involved in cystic fibrosis, all affecting the same gene, but

[11]The criteria governing screening programmes in general, not just those aimed at detecting genetic disorders, and the pros and cons of screening, are discussed in detail in *Dilemmas in Health Care*, Chapter 9.

varying from person to person. Once the gene was identified in 1989 (it took ten years and cost millions of pounds to find it), mass screening for these mutations in European populations could be seriously considered. The samples of DNA for screening are simple to extract from cells collected from a 'rinse and spit' mouthwash, a non-invasive procedure that most people would find acceptable. Detection of the relevant mutations would enable a man and a woman, who each know that they are carriers (each has one mutant allele), to recognise their risk of having an affected child together, and to seek counselling.

However, some mutations involved in cystic fibrosis escape detection at present, due to imperfections in the screening test, so only about 70 per cent of such at-risk couples would be identified, even if *everyone* were screened (Williamson, 1993). The *undetected* cases of the carrier state are *false negatives*, since these individuals have the mutant allele but would be falsely reassured by the negative test result. Problems with the accuracy of the screening test, as well as ethical considerations (discussed later), maintain the medical consensus that it would be premature to start mass population genetic screening for cystic fibrosis, but a number of pilot programmes have been set up (for example, over 3 000 women attending antenatal clinics in Edinburgh were screened in 1990–2; Mennie *et al.*, 1992).

As newer and more sensitive techniques are developed to detect *every* mutation, so the number of genetic diseases subjected to population screening is likely to increase. Discussions and decisions on the issues surrounding population screening for certain genes may involve us all in the near future. They raise lots of questions and no easy answers. We look first at the economic aspects of population genetic screening and its effect on disease frequencies, before discussing the ethical aspects.

Economic analysis of genetic screening

Consider the uncontroversial example of population screening for PKU. Is screening all newborn babies financially 'worthwhile' or, put in the jargon of market economics, is it cost-effective compared with *not* screening?

☐ What cost factors need to be taken into account in comparing screening and not screening?

■ The cost of the screening test for all babies and the dietary treatment of those found to have raised levels of phenylalanine, versus the cost of treating and caring for individuals who were not detected early and who suffered brain damage and other defects during infancy.

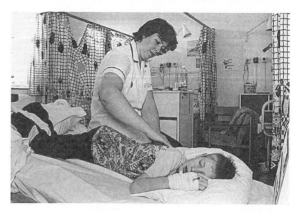

The economic cost to the health service of treating a child with cystic fibrosis was estimated to be £125 000 in 1989; the additional financial cost to affected families has never been estimated. Neither has the contribution to society of people with the disease. (Photo: Mike Levers)

In 1979, it was estimated that the detection and subsequent dietary treatment of one baby with PKU cost about £20 000 (remember, you have to screen 15 000 babies to detect this one). Lifelong treatment is not necessary because the adult brain seems to be resistant to the abnormal level of phenylalanine found in someone with PKU. But failure to detect that baby means that it will almost certainly have to be institutionalised for the rest of its life (about 45 years, on average); at 1979 prices, this was estimated to cost about £126 000 (Komrower, 1984).[12] So, when reduced to economic values, the question could be asked 'Is it better to spend the equivalent of that £20 000 now, or five times that sum later?'. The figures for cystic fibrosis show a much smaller 'saving' from screening and selective abortion compared with lifelong treatment: a report by the Royal College of Physicians in 1989 estimated a cost of £125 000 for the average lifetime (25 years) treatment of a child with cystic fibrosis, versus £80 000 for screening the 2 000 fetuses necessary to detect and abort one fetus with two mutant alleles. These are two examples of genetic screening programmes that have been shown to pay for themselves, in the sense that the cost of screening is more than offset by the savings in lifetime care.

[12]Economic calculations comparing two strategies, as in the PKU example, are rarely performed, which explains why these data are costed in 1979 prices; the point to note is the cost difference between screening and not screening.

It is important to note that these cost-effectiveness calculations are solely based on *medical* costs. They ignore the financial and personal cost to affected families, and the financial and personal *contribution* to society made by a person who has a genetic disease, some of whom are able to work and generate direct income for the state, as well as contribute in many other ways. However:

> ...there are many measurable non-financial costs and benefits which reflect the true objective of the service. Outstanding benefits are an informed population, informed choice for couples at risk, the birth of healthy infants or of accepted affected ones, and the replacement of aborted fetuses with healthy infants. (Royal College of Physicians, 1989, p. 40)

But what if the unmeasured humanitarian benefits, such as the 'saving' in personal anguish, are large relative to the saving in financial costs? Would you cancel a screening programme (for example, to detect cystic fibrosis) that cost £25 000, but saved in total only £15 000 in medical expenditure? Should health-care decision-making also take account of the humanitarian benefits?

Population screening would inevitably result in an increase in abortion of affected fetuses and a decrease in the number of affected people in the population. Society has to consider what it would lose by such a strategy as well as what it might gain. In December 1993, the Nuffield Council on Bioethics published a report, *Genetic Screening: Ethical Issues,* in which the authors expressed concern that cost-effectiveness calculations might carry too much weight in decisions to implement population genetic screening:

> The public health definition of 'success' or 'failure' of a programme may be in danger of turning on too narrow a calculation of costs and benefits. Benefits must not be calculated in purely financial terms of preventing the birth of individuals who may have higher than average health care needs and costs. The benefits should be seen as enabling individuals to take account of the information for their own lives and empowering prospective parents to make informed choices about having children. (Nuffield Council on Bioethics, 1993, p. 80)

The effect of genetic screening on the incidence of disease

A number of crucially important questions arise from the procedure of genetic screening, if the practice is going to increase in the future. For those genetic diseases where a reliable test already exists, what is the effect on the frequency of the disease and on the frequency of the abnormal allele in the population, and what are the social consequences of screening?

The impact of genetic screening (together with counselling and selective abortion) in lowering the incidence of diseases can be dramatic, as the following examples demonstrate. Children with Tay–Sachs disease have paralysis, dementia and blindness and usually die before their third birthday. There is no known cure. Population screening has been carried out on a massive scale in North America since 1969 in the Ashkenazi Jewish populations, in which between 3 and 5 per cent carry the gene, compared with 0.5 per cent in non-Jewish populations. (Ashkenazi Jews are mainly of Central and Eastern European descent, including some who migrated to North and South America, South Africa and Australia.) Screening followed by pre-natal diagnosis of fetuses where both parents are carriers, has already lowered the incidence of the disease by about 80 per cent in the Ashkenazi populations in North America. Prevention of *thalassaemia* by carrier detection and pre-natal diagnosis has brought about a similar drop in the incidence of the disease in heavily-affected areas such as Cyprus, Greece and parts of Italy (see Figure 9.5).

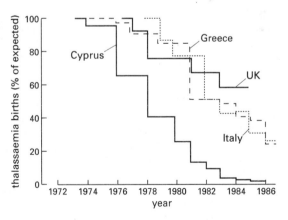

Figure 9.5 *Results of thalassaemia control programmes in Europe. In Cyprus, the fall in affected births approaches 100 per cent. (Data from Modell, B., Kuliev, A. M. and Wagner, M., 1992,* Community Genetics Services in Europe, WHO Regional Publications, European series no. 38, WHO Regional Office for Europe, Copenhagen)*

Thalassaemia, similar in many respects to sickle-cell disease, is a disease of haemoglobin synthesis which affects the functioning of the red cells, thus causing anaemia. Like sickle-cell disease, it confers resistance to malaria. The results of genetic screening on the incidence of thalassaemia are particularly revealing, since it is found in predominantly Catholic communities where abortion is against religious beliefs. Nevertheless, the WHO report by Modell, Kuliev and Wagner, 1992, noted that 98 per cent of pregnant Cypriot at-risk couples requested fetal diagnosis and selective abortion of affected fetuses. Couples who had stopped having children because they were afraid of having a further child with thalassaemia, resumed reproduction, and those about to begin reproduction used fetal diagnosis and selective abortion to ensure a thalassaemia-free family. The wide acceptance of genetic screening in these communities is an indication that the majority of the population is anxious to see this severe disease eliminated.

However, different communities respond differently to the availability of genetic screening. Similar population screening of Cypriots in the United Kingdom reduced the incidence of thalassaemia by only about 40 per cent over an eight-year period (see Figure 9.5). What is the reason for this much lower result? An earlier study by Bernadette Modell, published in 1983, suggested that such cases are due to the inherent problem of offering a medical service to high-risk communities who are scattered among a host community at low risk. Few of those at high risk realise that they might be screened. Prevention of thalassaemia by carrier detection and pre-natal diagnosis in Asian communities in the United Kingdom reduced the incidence of the disease by only 2 per cent, even though about 60 per cent of Asian at-risk couples accepted fetal diagnosis (Modell, 1993).

However, even if pre-natal diagnosis and selective abortion were widely practised, would the frequency of a disease *allele* in the population (as distinct from the frequency of the *disease*) be reduced? For diseases due to inheritance of a single *dominant* allele, mass pre-natal detection of the allele followed by selective abortion would gradually eliminate the allele from the population. But most genetic diseases are due to inheritance of two *recessive* alleles.

☐ In recessive disorders, what effect might pre-natal diagnosis and selective abortion have on the frequency of the allele in the population?

■ Very little effect, since only *homozygous* fetuses will be aborted because only they will develop the disease. Heterozygote fetuses (carriers of a single disease allele) would survive.

Indeed, couples in which both partners carry the recessive allele may have *more* heterozygous children to replace the affected homozygous fetuses lost through abortion, so the number of disease alleles in the population could potentially increase. However, a primary goal of screening and counselling is to prevent disease, not to reduce the number of carriers. Prior to the availability of genetic screening, such couples might have limited their family after the birth of the first affected child. So the overall outcome of genetic screening on the frequency of the allele will depend on how many children carrier-couples choose to have.

Acceptability of genetic risk and abortion varies greatly between ethnic groups; this is but one of several important features which must be taken into account when planning a screening programme. The screening programmes for Tay–Sachs disease and thalassaemia were well planned, provided genetic counselling, and neither were compulsory; both succeeded in reducing the incidence of the disease. The importance of these features can be seen in the comparison carried out by Modell (1983) between these two programmes and the detection of carriers of sickle-cell disease in the black community of the United States, where the programme has had little effect on the incidence of the disease. The aim of the American screening programme was to identify partners at risk of having children with sickle-cell disease, but there is no successful treatment for the condition and pre-natal diagnosis was not offered, so the only preventive measure was for carriers not to partner other carriers, or for high-risk couples not to have children. In addition, there was a lack of community consultation and education, and a number of mandatory screening programmes were set up, which created bad feeling.

In summary, genetic screening programmes aimed at large populations require public education, community support, the consent of those screened, results given through genetic counsellors, confidentiality of results, and assessment of the effectiveness of the programme in terms of disease reduction, and cost savings and benefits to society. Even if the programme achieves all these criteria, the ethical dilemmas remain. They become more acute when the prospect of extending genetic screening to an ever-widening range of conditions is considered.

Preventive medicine of the future

The area of medical genetics concerned with the interaction between environmental factors and different human genotypes, is likely to become one of increasing importance. Many examples are now known of specific genotypes that have an increased risk of certain diseases when exposed to a particular environmental factor. An understanding of the link between particular genotypes and the causative agents in the development of many diseases opens up the possibility of a new strategy for preventive medicine.

□ How could prevention of these diseases be achieved?

■ Population genetic screening could be used to detect people with particular genotypes and inform them of the environmental and toxic agents they should avoid.

For example, dietary restriction helps individuals with PKU; restriction of dietary cholesterol and fats is helpful in lowering cholesterol levels in individuals with familial hypercholesterolaemia.[13] An important and striking example of the effect that environmental factors may have on the phenotype of a genetic disease is α_1-antitrypsin[14] deficiency, a recessive condition that leads to chronic lung and liver disease. The progression of the disease, particularly the destruction of lung tissue, is accelerated by cigarette smoking (we shall look at the underlying reasons for this in Chapter 10). Individuals who are homozygous for α_1-antitrypsin deficiency could be advised of the additional risks of smoking, they could try to find work places where smoking by others was restricted, avoid pubs and shops where smoking was allowed and generally change their lifestyle. Other individuals with a known metabolic deficiency could be advised of particular diets to avoid and yet others of the hazards of potentially toxic substances.

Coronary heart disease and lung disease are both examples of chronic disorders that account for much of the morbidity and mortality in adult life in developed countries. As the techniques of genetic screening develop, should we extend screening to include more subtle genetic effects that might predispose people to common forms of lung cancer or heart disease if they smoke tobacco, for example? Which is the preferable course: to live in ignorance of one's likely fate, or to have the chance to reduce the risk by never smoking?[15]

Population genetic screening clearly demonstrates how modern-day 'high-tech' medicine has the potential to interact with modern culture to affect the frequency of genetic diseases and diseases which have a genetic component. Is preventative medicine that relies on population screening medically sound? Would it make economic sense? Who and how many would benefit? Would it be seen as an invasion of privacy? Would individuals run the risk of possible stigmatisation or discrimination on the basis of having a genotype sensitive to particular environmental factors? These questions and others need to be considered carefully in the context of a preventive disease programme for the future.

Ethical considerations of pre-natal diagnosis and genetic screening

We have already touched on several ethical considerations arising from genetic screening and pre-natal diagnosis, but there are many others. (The report by the Nuffield Council on Bioethics, 1993, discusses them all; see the Further Reading list at the end of this book.) The issues can be divided into those primarily affecting individuals and those with wider implications for society.

At the personal level, the major ethical issue raised by pre-natal diagnosis is that related to abortion. Should a pregnant woman who agrees to pre-natal diagnosis have made a *prior* commitment to terminate the pregnancy if she is carrying a fetus with a genetic (or other serious) disorder? What are the rights of the male partner in such a situation, and will health professionals bring undue pressure to bear on the parents' decision? Professor Robert Williamson, a medical geneticist at St Mary's Hospital Medical School in London, expresses this fear:

While many professional geneticists regard the provision of information as important in its own right so as to facilitate choice, those concerned with the economics of health care may regard this as a frivolous luxury if the majority of those offered the information choose not to act upon it. (Williamson, 1993, p. 199)

---

[13]See Chapter 4 of this book and *Dilemmas in Health Care*, Chapter 10. Note that dietary restriction for treatment of high cholesterol *not* caused by familial hypercholesterolaemia does not work.

[14]Pronounced 'alpha-one-anti-trip-sin'.

[15]This choice is discussed (along with several other aspects of the 'new genetics') in an audiotape that OU students will listen to later in this chapter.

Fewer than 5 per cent of fetuses examined by pre-natal diagnosis techniques are, in fact, affected with the disease being screened for. Therefore, for the vast majority of prospective parents, pre-natal diagnosis serves ultimately to reassure them that the unborn baby is *not* affected by the disease in question. However, a *Lancet* editorial pointed to the anxiety inherent in screening; the editor reviewed two pilot studies of genetic screening for cystic fibrosis, both published in 1992, which (among other aspects) assessed the psychological impact of screening:

> Testing inevitably results in some anxiety—during the process, after notification of a positive result, and before the first counselling session. Longer-term follow-up of screening in primary care revealed that, for most individuals, anxiety levels return to normal after 6 months. This is a short period of follow-up for an event that may have lifelong implications. Screening in antenatal clinics likewise induces anxiety, which seems to revert to normal when a negative test result is obtained for the partner. There is no knowing whether similar anxiety would be experienced in subsequent pregnancies, or what happens to those couples where both are found to be carriers. (*Lancet*, 1992, p. 210)

Many pregnancies end naturally in early miscarriage before the woman realises she is pregnant; this is often because the fetus has a genetic defect. By diagnosing abnormal genes before birth, medical science can shift the boundaries of the natural process of abortion to reduce the number of children born with genetic diseases. But a decision to go ahead with an abortion, or to continue the pregnancy, brings with it an often agonising personal decision and a degree of moral and social responsibility. If the disease detected by pre-natal diagnosis is treatable, as in the case of PKU, then the question of abortion is quite different from what it would be if treatment were not available. Where a disease is life-threatening, with the child having little chance of reaching adulthood, then for some parents there may be little doubt as to what to do. But what about diseases that in the main do not develop until adulthood, such as α_1-antitrypsin deficiency? Here the affected people are destined to become incapacitated and generate a substantial cost to the state in terms of care and medical resource; yet before they become ill, they will contribute to society in many ways, including financially. Should prospective parents take into account this social interest when deciding whether to proceed with an affected pregnancy?

In these late-acting genetic diseases, prior knowledge of one's fate is a heavy burden to carry, without hope of cure. At the time of writing early in 1994, there is no effective treatment for Huntington's disease, a degenerative disorder of the nervous system due to the inheritance of a single dominant allele. The majority of individuals do not show any signs of having the disease until their fourth decade, after they have had children and hence have passed on the mutant allele. Pre-natal screening of fetuses for the alleles leading to Huntington's disease will thus also reveal whether one or other parent has the mutation and is therefore destined to develop the disease themselves. This is something that the parent may prefer not to know.

Disclosure of information revealed by genetic screening is another major concern. For example, should the parents be told that an unborn baby, although unaffected with the disease they agreed to be screened for, has, for example, the abnormal chromosome pattern associated with Down's syndrome? Most genetic counsellors think that full disclosure should be given. Disclosure and confidentiality are two aspects of population genetic screening that may have consequences not only for individuals and families, but also for society 'at large'. Genetic screening of the population would identify the carriers of certain inherited characteristics and so has the potential for creating and supporting social bias and subsequent hardship among those identified. This is especially worrying in diseases that occur more frequently in an ethnic group that already suffers discrimination, as in the case of sickle-cell disease in blacks in the United States and Tay–Sachs disease in Jewish populations outside Israel.

Who controls the genetic information about individuals who are likely to develop crippling and debilitating diseases while they are still part of the work-force? Will prospective employers and insurance companies begin to demand genetic screening of individuals *before* offering a job or agreeing to underwrite a policy?

> The United Kingdom insurance industry does not intend to ask proposers for life insurance to undergo screening for genetic information within the foreseeable future, but where individuals have had a specific genetic test as part of their medical assessment these tests will fall into the same category as other medical tests and will need to be declared on proposal forms. (Submission to the Nuffield Council on Bioethics, 1993, p. 70, by the Association of British Insurers)

Genetic screening tests are increasing in frequency. In Sweden, for example, thousands of newborn babies have already been screened for α_1-antitrypsin deficiency, so their medical condition is on record. The issues here are similar to those raised when insurance companies began asking life insurance applicants whether they had ever been tested for HIV (the virus that causes AIDS), even though the test proved negative. (These issues have been reviewed in two articles on insurance and genetic testing: Harper, 1992 and 1993.)

It is obviously uneconomical to screen everybody for everything, but since the number of genetic diseases or predispositions that can be identified in carriers is rapidly increasing, these are questions of immediate concern to everyone. Concern has been voiced about the possible invasion of privacy, stigmatisation on the basis of an abnormal finding, the failure to obtain informed consent to screening, and the lack of confidentiality of results. What characteristics should be screened for? Who decides who can be screened and who has access to the results? How much counselling needs to be given to affected people? Society needs to demarcate those things which will be permitted and those which should be forbidden.

Concern that genetic screening might damage individual freedoms emerged first in the United States, where most people depend on private insurance for health care and around 15 per cent of the population are either uninsured or under-insured.[16] In the United Kingdom, the issue received little attention until 1991, when it was raised at the International Workshop on Human Gene Mapping in London. Since then there has been wide professional discussion, but there is a need for considered agreements to be reached on how society should apply the science of genetic screening and what legislation should back it up.

You should now be in a good position to understand the ethical concerns raised by the German geneticist, Benno Müller-Hill, in an article, 'The shadow of genetic injustice' (first published in 1993), which you can find in the Reader.[17] He considers the potential effects on future societies (especially the United States) of discoveries

emerging in the 1990s from the **Human Genome Project**.[18] The primary aim of the project is to determine the locations, DNA nucleotide sequences and functions of the 100 000 or so human genes. It is the largest medical project in history, involving 265 laboratories in 6 countries (including the United Kingdom). The result will be a working map of the entire human genotype by the turn of the century, at an estimated cost of $3 billion.

□ What does Müller-Hill predict might be the main *social advantage* to arise in the United States from precise knowledge of each person's individual genotype, and hence the ability to diagnose their predisposition to genetic disorders affecting the *body*?

■ The relatively few people with such a genetic disorder may be helped in that general health insurance cover for everyone in the United States and tough anti-discrimination laws may become a reality.

□ How, in the view of Müller-Hill, could *social disadvantage* result from knowledge about genetic disorders affecting mental health, and the genetic contribution to intelligence?

■ Almost everyone in the population will be affected in some way: if a genetic component to mental ability is confirmed, then it will be possible to make predictions about a person's intellectual 'limitations', which could be self-fulfilling and lead to 'inaction and despair'. People will be stratified according to their genetic superiority or inferiority and discrimination will flourish. The contribution of environmental factors to mental illness or intelligence will be forgotten. If the population believes that mental ability is pre-determined by genes, then why 'waste' resources trying to improve social conditions, education, etc.?

□ How does Müller-Hill suggest that society should prepare for the potential onslaught of results from the Human Genome Project?

■ The right to privacy should be acknowledged and legislated for; the rights of people who he refers to as 'genetically disadvantaged' should have legally-enforced protection; and everyone should change their attitudes to a full 'appreciation of equal human rights'.

[16]A comparison of different methods of funding health services in industrialised nations and in Third World countries, and the consequences for the provision of health care, can be found in *Caring for Health: History and Diversity* (revised edition, 1993), Chapter 9.

[17]*Health and Disease: A Reader* (Open University Press, revised edition 1994).

[18]The Human Genome Project is discussed briefly in *Studying Health and Disease* (revised edition 1994), Chapter 9, in the context of biological determinism.

At the end of this chapter, you will listen to an audiotape in which a British geneticist, Steve Jones, argues that the impact of the 'new' genetics on future societies will be far less damaging than Müller-Hill predicts. But first, we address the most far-reaching of all the aspects of modern medical genetics: the latest techniques for treating genetic diseases.

Treating genetic diseases

We begin with a brief overview of standard therapies in the treatment of genetic diseases, and then introduce the revolutionary new strategy of gene therapy which is likely to be used increasingly in the future. The powerful DNA techniques currently being developed have the potential to make a dramatic impact on the treatment of genetic diseases. Our emphasis will be on those therapies that use the genetic approach.

Genetic diseases can often be treated by intervening at various stages in the complex pathway between the defective gene and the *clinical phenotype* of the individual (i.e. the 'signs and symptoms' of the diseases, as diagnosed by a doctor). These levels of intervention are summarised in Table 9.2. But in many cases effective therapy is not available because insufficient is known about the pathology of the disease.

Table 9.2 The various levels of intervention in genetic diseases, with the corresponding treatment strategies involved at each level. (The terms used are discussed further in the text below.)

Level of intervention	Treatment strategy
the family	genetic counselling, carrier screening, pre-natal diagnosis, presymptomatic screening
clinical phenotype (i.e. signs and symptoms of the patient)	medical or surgical intervention, education of the patient
metabolic or other biochemical abnormalities	disease-specific treatment (e.g. with diet or drugs)
mutant protein	protein replacement, including genetically engineered proteins
mutant gene	modification of the genotype by gene therapy

Earlier in this chapter, we discussed interventions at the level of the family; here we briefly discuss techniques aimed at the intermediate levels in Table 9.2, before focusing extensively on the level of the mutant gene.

Treating the phenotype

Intervention at the level of the *clinical phenotype* with surgery, drugs or education, are all forms of *phenotype modification*, so-called because the patient's phenotype is altered by the treatment, without affecting the underlying genotype. For example, *surgical repair* can successfully modify the clinical phenotype of some genetic disorders, including the commonest multifactorial conditions in newborn babies, such as cleft lip and palate, congenital heart defects and pyloric stenosis (constriction of the valve controlling emptying of the stomach). Tissue and organ *transplants* were discussed in general terms at the beginning of the chapter. Using transplants to treat genetic diseases is difficult: the mortality following transplants is high, morbidity is high because of graft rejection, and there is a shortage of suitable organs and tissues. Nevertheless, there have been very good outcomes in the treatment of thalassaemia with bone marrow transplants.

Intervention at the level of *metabolic abnormalities* is another form of phenotype modification. To date, the genetic diseases which are most successfully treated are those with a metabolic abnormality, such as PKU and familial hypercholesterolaemia, which have been mentioned several times in this book.

Intervention at the level of the *mutant protein* involves *protein replacement*, which is part of the routine therapy for only a few diseases. A prime example is the infusion of blood enriched with the deficient blood protein, Factor VIII, to prevent bleeding in people with haemophilia. The protein α_1-antitrypsin can be infused into people with α_1-antitrypsin-deficiency in doses large enough to maintain the correct protein concentration in the lungs.

Advances in protein biology in the last decade have led to the production of large quantities of purified human proteins in laboratory cultures of bacteria and other micro-organisms. Until recently, the only source of insulin to treat diabetes mellitus (Chapter 7), was from the pancreas of cattle and pigs slaughtered for meat; Factor VIII to treat haemophilia was extracted from human blood donated by blood donors. Both proteins can now also be manufactured using the technique of **genetic engineering.** The basic procedure is shown in Figure 9.6.

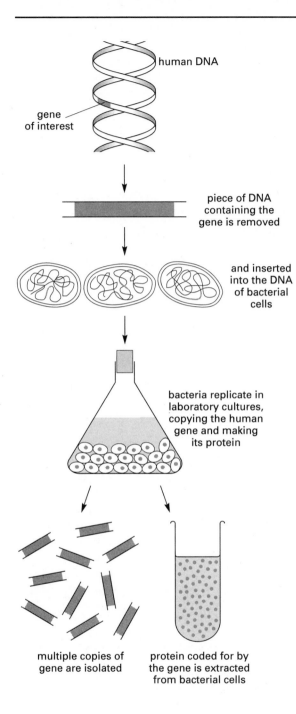

human DNA

gene of interest

piece of DNA containing the gene is removed

and inserted into the DNA of bacterial cells

bacteria replicate in laboratory cultures, copying the human gene and making its protein

multiple copies of gene are isolated

protein coded for by the gene is extracted from bacterial cells

Figure 9.6 *Genetic engineering using bacteria to clone a human gene; the process enables large quantities of the human protein encoded by the gene to be extracted for medical use, and also yields multiple copies of the human gene.*

Once the human gene that codes for the protein of interest has been identified and separated from other DNA sequences, it is inserted into bacteria. Bacterial cells can divide every 20 minutes (their rapid *generation time* was discussed in Chapter 5). Every time they divide, the bacterial DNA replicates so that the two new bacterial cells each get a full set of genes; during this process, the human gene is also reproduced, along with the rest, so that it is present in all the bacterial progeny cells. This method of producing a large number of identical copies of the gene is called *cloning* the gene, or **gene cloning**. The human gene is activated in each bacterial cell, so that the bacteria behave like 'living factories', manufacturing large quantities of the human protein encoded by that gene. This can then be extracted and purified from the bacterial cultures, ready to be injected into humans. Note that this intervention is still a form of *phenotype* modification, because the *patient's* genes are not altered; patients are simply given the normal protein produced (in bacteria) by the normal human gene which they lack.

The amino acid sequence of a human protein and its equivalent found in another species of mammal is likely to differ in small but significant ways. Protein replacement with a genetically-engineered human protein (for example, a hormone or an enzyme) may be more effective than therapy which uses a protein derived from other mammals, because the molecular structure of the human protein makes a 'better fit' with the correct target cell or molecule in the human body. However, genetically-engineered human proteins are not always perfect copies of the human 'original'; some insulin is still extracted from cattle and pigs because some diabetics report that, in practice, genetically-engineered human insulin does not control their blood sugar level satisfactorily.

Genetic engineering has enabled unlimited quantities of certain human proteins to be produced more easily and less expensively than was previously possible. This technique has led to the growth of a huge number of biotechnology companies that produce a range of human proteins commercially, by cloning human genes in bacteria and in yeasts. Some of these companies have also inserted human genes into mammals, such as mice and sheep, a development that has raised far more concerns about 'tinkering with nature' than were ever expressed about putting human genes into micro-organisms. For example, the gene containing the code for human α_1-antitrypsin has been inserted into the DNA of a sheep embryo, which developed into an adult ewe (named Tracy by Pharmaceutical Proteins, the company that owns her); she, in turn, gave birth to twin lambs, one of which inherited the human gene. These animals are the basis of a breeding flock of sheep, which synthesise human α_1-antitrypsin worth $100 million a year.[19] Critics say that geneticists are 'colonising' other species with human genes and distorting their biology; supporters of the new genetics retort that taking a medically-useful product from a sheep is no different than taking its flesh to make Irish stew.

Treating the genotype

The final level of intervention in genetic disease discussed here (and see bottom line of Table 9.2) concerns the powerful techniques for manipulating human DNA, called **gene therapy**. These techniques have raised the possibility of intervening in genetic diseases by *genotype modification*, that is correcting a mutant gene by replacing it with the normal allele. The idea is to insert a normal gene into the appropriate tissues of an individual affected with a genetic disease, thereby permanently correcting the disorder. Unlike genetic engineering, where human genes are used *indirectly* to combat genetic disorders, gene therapy involves *direct* intervention in the patient's DNA.

It is very important to distinguish between *somatic* gene therapy and *germline* gene therapy. In Chapters 3 and 4, we made the distinction between somatic DNA (the DNA found in all the cells in the body *except* the gametes and the cells that give rise to them), and germline DNA (the DNA found in egg- and sperm-producing cells and in the gametes themselves). **Somatic gene therapy**, which involves cells other than the reproductive cells, is considered first since it is currently being tried out in a few pilot studies, and involves no new ethical concerns beyond those already raised in this chapter. It refers to the transfer of normal human genes into the *body* cells of the patient in such a way that the transferred DNA does *not* enter the DNA of the person's eggs or sperm.

☐ Will somatic gene therapy prevent the treated person from passing on the defective gene to their children?

■ No, because the normal human gene they receive in somatic gene therapy does not enter their gametes, and hence cannot be transferred to the next generation.

[19] The marketing of Tracy and other medical innovations is discussed in *Dilemmas in Health Care*, Chapter 7.

Germline gene therapy would (if it were allowed) result in the insertion of a normal human gene into the affected person's gametes, so that their offspring could inherit a normal allele. It carries a risk for future generations through the accidental introduction of new and harmful mutations, and is currently banned in humans in many countries. (However, it is legal to insert genes into the germline of other species, as the case of Tracy illustrated.)

Figure 9.7 outlines the most common method of inserting genes into the patient's cells. You should recall from earlier chapters that viruses insert their genetic material into the cells they infect and this property has been exploited in gene therapy; a detailed understanding of the procedure is not so important as an appreciation of the basic principles. You will need to keep referring to Figure 9.7 as we discuss three of the major scientific hurdles that need to be overcome before the technique of somatic gene therapy can become generally available.

Scientific hurdles in the path of somatic gene therapy

1   The gene of interest must first be identified from among the 100 000 or so human genes, so that it can be separated from all other DNA sequences in the genotype. This area of genetic research is very active. By the end of 1993, several genes involved in genetic diseases had been precisely located and their DNA sequence determined; they include those involved in PKU, cystic fibrosis, sickle-cell disease, thalassaemia, familial hypercholesterolaemia, Huntington's disease and Duchenne muscular dystrophy. In addition, a very large number of genes involved in multifactorial diseases (which are caused by the interaction of genetic and environmental factors) were well on the way to identification; these diseases include the familial types of breast and bowel cancer, heart disease, rheumatoid arthritis, diabetes, multiple sclerosis and Alzheimer's disease.

2   Transferring the normal gene into the patient's cells requires a carrier or **gene vector**. Most ways of getting genes into human cells are not very efficient, but the easiest methods use viruses (as in Figure 9.7). Normally such viruses reproduce extensively, killing the target cell. However, some viruses have been engineered to contain the corrective human gene, but are unable to reproduce and therefore do not kill the target cells.

3   Inserting the gene into target cells has to be done in the laboratory under controlled conditions. Cells from the patient have to be removed and maintained alive in cultures while the corrective gene is transferred; this step must be carried out under totally sterile conditions, because if 'wild' viruses or bacteria get into the cultures some of their genes could be inserted into the human

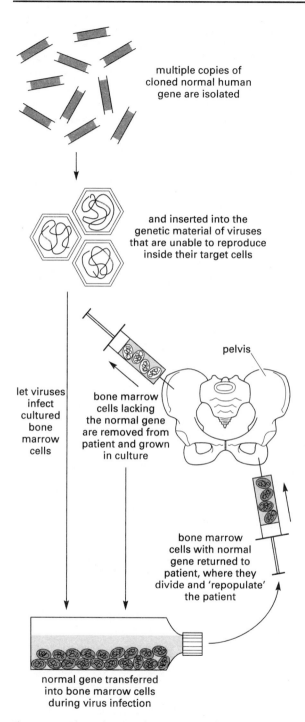

multiple copies of cloned normal human gene are isolated

and inserted into the genetic material of viruses that are unable to reproduce inside their target cells

pelvis

let viruses infect cultured bone marrow cells

bone marrow cells lacking the normal gene are removed from patient and grown in culture

bone marrow cells with normal gene returned to patient, where they divide and 'repopulate' the patient

normal gene transferred into bone marrow cells during virus infection

Figure 9.7 *The technique of somatic gene therapy. A virus is used to 'carry' the normal human gene into the patient's own bone marrow cells in tissue culture, and insert the gene into the patient's DNA. The bone marrow cells are then returned to the patient.*

cells, with unpredictable but possibly very damaging results. The target cells have to be able to divide after reimplantation to ensure the corrective gene is maintained in the patient's body and is not lost when the treated cells die. Only a few human cell types fit this requirement: bone marrow stem cells are ideal as a target tissue for gene therapy because they survive long enough in tissue culture and go on dividing once reimplanted in the patient.

Candidate diseases for gene therapy

A number of genetic disorders are potential candidates for correction by gene therapy, in particular blood conditions, such as thalassaemia (described in the TV programme 'Blood lines') and sickle-cell disease and various forms of immunodeficiency diseases; this is because the defective cells originate in the bone marrow (the tissue most suited for gene therapy). However, gene transfer into bone marrow cells may also be an effective treatment for diseases that do not affect bone marrow directly, such as PKU, familial hypercholesterolaemia and α_1-antitrypsin deficiency. The idea is that the normal protein produced by the gene inserted into the bone marrow cells would be transported in the bloodstream to wherever it was needed in the body.

The first candidate gene for somatic gene transfer in humans was the gene associated with *adenosine deaminase deficiency* (ADD). The gene codes for an enzyme (adenosine deaminase), which is normally present in high levels in white cells in the immune system; its absence causes severe immunodeficiency disease. The first transfers of the gene to correct the lack of the enzyme were successfully achieved in two girls in 1990 in the United States (Rosenberg, 1990; Cournoyer and Caskey, 1990). The gene was transferred to the girls' bone marrow cells in the laboratory, which were then reimplanted in their bodies; there they divided and gave rise to some white cells that could synthesise the enzyme. Both girls were still alive in 1993, but since they were both receiving the standard forms of medical treatment as well it is difficult to draw conclusions about the success of gene therapy in this instance. By the end of 1993, the regulatory body in the United States that restricts gene therapy research had approved 50 different gene therapy trials, involving over 150 patients, and many more were in the pipeline.

One of the most promising candidate diseases for gene therapy is cystic fibrosis. The reasons for optimism can be summarised as follows. The lungs and gut are normal at birth, so the early insertion of a normal gene could correct the biochemical defect *before* damage is caused by the accumulation of mucus (a major feature of the disease). The lungs are very accessible, so gene transfer may be feasible without the need to remove the patients' cells to a laboratory culture; an aerosol containing viruses with the DNA sequence of the normal human gene can be sprayed at high pressure into the lungs. The gut lining is also reasonably accessible to agents given 'by mouth', if a way can be found to deliver gene vectors that survive digestion (the problems should be evident from Chapter 7). Gene delivery systems are being tested in several inbred strains of mice, which carry mutations that give rise to a condition resembling cystic fibrosis in humans; normal genes have been successfully transferred by direct application to the walls of arteries in their lungs. Animal tests have shown that if the normal gene can be transferred to only 5 per cent of cells in the lungs, this is sufficient to restore normal functioning. And finally, there exists a large number of young adults with cystic fibrosis whose informed consent for experimental gene therapy could be obtained. Three separate trials of gene therapy for cystic fibrosis in human patients began in the United States in 1993 (Coutelle *et al.*, 1993). The results are eagerly awaited.

Ethics of gene transfer therapy

With any new therapy, there are concerns about risks versus benefits. The ethics of somatic gene transfer therapy do not pose any new issues as long as the germline is not involved. Some regard replacing a damaged gene as not much different from replacing a damaged organ such as a kidney, and as much less invasive than performing multiple transplants. Nevertheless, the World Health Organisation and the Council for International Organisation of Medical Sciences have formally resolved to consider the moral and social issues arising from the new DNA technologies. Some of the consequences may be far-reaching.

☐ Initial trials of somatic gene therapy are likely to involve disorders that are currently untreatable by other methods and have, until now, generally prevented the affected person from having children through illness or premature death. What are the likely consequences for the frequency of the disease allele in the population if somatic gene therapy successfully treats the disease?

■ Recipients of gene therapy, although phenotypically normal, still carry the disease alleles in their germline DNA and could transmit them to their children. Somatic gene therapy could increase the frequencies of these alleles in the population because the treated person lives to reproduce.

Thus, somatic gene transfer therapy is a procedure that has the potential to change the frequencies of disease alleles in the population. Note that *all* the treatment strategies listed in Table 9.2 (earlier) have the potential to increase the frequency of disease alleles, to the extent that affected individuals are enabled to survive and reproduce. These examples illustrate how modern culture may affect human biological evolution in the future. However, other cultural forces are at work to counteract this tendency, making it unlikely that the frequency of genetic *diseases* will rise, even though the frequency of disease *alleles* may increase. (This is discussed further in the final chapter of this book.)

The period from 1980 onwards may be viewed a few generations hence as the golden age of gene therapy, a time when diseases with a genetic predisposition could be overcome. Genetic medicine—screening, counselling and therapy—offer prospects that are both promising and disturbing. By tinkering with DNA we have the potential to influence our evolution and we need to consider the options carefully.

The 'new' genetics in context

It is easy to get carried away with the potential that genetic engineering, genetic screening and gene therapy have to offer, and just as easy to view them with deep alarm. These techniques need to be put into perspective by considering them in the total context of health and disease. To help you do this, listen to the audiotape entitled 'Tinkering with nature', in which a British geneticist, Steve Jones (Professor of Genetics at University College, London) reflects on the history of genetic research and its potential impact on human health in the future.[20] You should listen to it now and then answer the questions below.

☐ Why does Steve Jones claim that modern genetic techniques like gene therapy can only alter the course of human evolution 'in the most trivial way'?

■ Because such a tiny percentage of the population is affected by the 'single gene' defects that gene therapy may be able to cure. (Genetic diseases associated with a *single* gene account for only two per cent of total live births with any kind of disorder.)

[20]This audiotape has been specially recorded for Open University students; consult the Audiocassette Notes before playing the tape.

By far the most important diseases of the Western world, in terms of quantity, are the multifactorial diseases, such as coronary heart disease and other cardiovascular problems, cancers, diabetes, hypertension, stroke, schizophrenia, manic–depressive psychosis and certain forms of obesity. These complex disease phenotypes depend on a large number of genes and environmental factors, and on critical interactions between the two.

☐ Why is gene therapy an unrealistic option for multifactorial diseases? (Think back to Chapter 4.)

■ A number of different genes are involved in these conditions and each gene has only a small effect, so multiple gene therapy may be required; even if this were feasible, the effects of environmental factors on disease development could not be taken into account.

☐ What alternative approach to reducing the burden of multifactorial diseases does Jones advocate?

■ A more effective approach would be to tackle the hostile environmental factors that are associated with the development of these diseases. We need to make the environment safe for our particular genotypes, rather than attempt to alter our genotypes to survive in unhealthy social conditions.

Jones argues that detecting the genes associated with multifactorial diseases would enable individuals to make informed choices about their lives (for example, by weighing up a known personal risk from smoking or obesity). However, he also believes that a nationwide programme of genetic screening is highly unlikely as a form of preventive health care, because of its enormous cost. Discrimination (as envisaged by Benno Müller-Hill) could not be supported by genetic evidence if a genetic 'profile' of every citizen would be too costly to obtain.

☐ Jones points to an inherent dilemma in the decision to allow limited trials of somatic gene therapy, but to ban germline gene therapy. What is it?

■ Somatic gene therapy will enable people (who would otherwise have died young) to survive and have children, some of whom will inherit their affected parent's disease allele. Germline gene therapy could prevent these children from inheriting the disease allele.

Other developments in gene technology are on the horizon, raising other ethical and practical problems. For example, drugs that alter the activity of human genes are being actively researched; the pharmacist of the future may be able to reach into our DNA with a chemical 'spanner' and turn parts of the central mechanism of life on or off. One of the most active areas is cancer research, where methods for switching off inappropriately activated oncogenes or for switching on anti-oncogenes (Chapter 8) in tumour cells are already being tested in animals, with promising results. The practical problems are considerable but most biologists would agree they are not insuperable, given enough time and research resources. Ethical objections, however, may ultimately keep the spanner out of the works.

This ethical debate is about the *intentional* use of chemicals we call 'drugs' simply because they have been designed to alleviate or prevent disease. As the next chapter shows, the *unintentional* use of chemicals we call 'pollutants' has been affecting the activity of human genes, cells and body fluids for over a century, with little concern being raised until recently about the consequences for the future health of the human species. We move on in Chapter 10 to examine human biology in the context of the chemical industrial environment.

OBJECTIVES FOR CHAPTER 9

When you have studied this chapter, you should be able to:

9.1 Summarise the principal areas of public concern about the ethical aspects of organ and tissue transplants and implants of fetal tissue, and comment on the biological mechanisms that either support or undermine graft survival.

9.2 Discuss the practical and ethical issues raised by genetic screening and pre-natal diagnosis (a) for individuals and families, and (b) at the level of populations, and the impact that these techniques might have on human health and disease.

9.3 Distinguish between somatic and germline gene therapy and discuss the practical and ethical issues raised by these techniques. Evaluate their potential to affect the future evolution of human biology.

QUESTIONS FOR CHAPTER 9

Question 1 (*Objective 9.1*)

A commentary in the leading scientific journal *Nature* by three American paediatricians who support the use of fetal tissue in research, argued for the following ethical framework:

> ...the use of discarded fetal tissue for research and/or therapy should be to increase knowledge of human development and/or improvement of the human condition. Acknowledgement of the unique and non-trivial nature of the material should be mandatory. The review panels now assembling must ensure that human material is essential, and animal or substitute models should be used for preference when possible. (Bianchi, Bernfield and Nathan, 1993, p. 12)

(a) What criticisms could be made of this framework by opponents of the use of fetal tissue, and what safeguards does it refer to?

(b) What is the principal biological rationale for using fetal cells rather than their adult equivalents?

Question 2 (*Objective 9.2*)

Imagine that you are addressing the Huntington's Disease Association. The disease, caused by a dominant mutation, is associated with degeneration of the nervous system and is usually first manifested in mid-life. A severely affected man, 40 years old, comments that he is not at risk of passing on the disorder because his parents are not affected with Huntington's disease and so his condition must be due to a new mutation. Evaluate this claim.

Question 3 (*Objective 9.2*)

A new life-threatening disease called 'degeneration' is known to be inherited as a genetically recessive disease. It affects significant numbers of people living in small communities. Careful studies of DNA from normal and affected individuals identifies the gene associated with this disease. What factors should be considered before a programme of population screening for the defective allele is begun? (Give your answer in note form, as a list of numbered points.)

Question 4 (*Objective 9.3*)

Describe the central aim of somatic gene therapy and explain how this example of modern culture might affect the future evolution of human biology.

10

Living with the chemical industrial evironment

Early in this chapter you will be asked to study a Reader article by Alexander Leaf entitled 'Potential health effects of global climatic and environmental changes', first published in 1989.[1] This chapter draws extensively on material in earlier chapters of this book.

In Chapter 2, you saw something of how cultural evolution affected patterns of health and disease in early human settlements. Since the Industrial Revolution, which began in England in the middle of the eighteenth century,[2] we have undergone rapid cultural change; this has affected our environment in all its aspects, physical, chemical, biological and social, with profound impacts on human health. In this chapter, we are going to focus on ways of evaluating the effects on health of changes in the chemical environment, both through the production of synthetic chemicals for domestic, agricultural and industrial use, and through the linked production of waste. As you will see, it is extremely difficult to obtain reliable evidence about the long-term consequences for human health, even in the case of a well-documented chemical accident and its effects on the local community. This puts into context the far greater problems in estimating the impact of the industrial chemical environment on health at the global level.

[1]In *Health and Disease: A Reader* (revised edition 1994).

[2]See *World Health and Disease*, Chapter 5, and *Caring for Health: History and Diversity* (revised edition, 1993), Chapter 3, for a full discussion of the health effects of the Industrial Revolution.

Direct and indirect health effects of the chemical industrial environment

For most of the twentieth century, concern about **environmental exposure** has centred on the *direct* toxic effects on human biology of physical agents (such as radiation) and chemical agents released into the environment by industrial development. We shall spend most of this chapter discussing such direct toxicity. However, awareness has been increasing since the 1980s that *indirect* effects on human health, through disturbance of the ecosystem and food sources, can potentially have an even greater impact on human health. These indirect effects may become the driving forces behind urgent changes in environmental regulation in the 1990s. These concerns were reviewed in 1989 in an article by Alexander Leaf, an American doctor and a member of the Department of Preventive Medicine at Harvard Medical School; you will find an edited extract from this article, called 'Potential health effects of global climatic and environmental changes' in the Reader. You should read it now.

□ According to Leaf, the industrial chemical environment is affecting the ecosystem and food sources in major ways. What *indirect* consequences for human health does he predict?

■ Global warming, leading to drought and the creation of deserts in some parts of the world, and floods and rising sea levels in other parts; acid rain and its toxic effects on forests, crops and lakes; and destruction of the ozone layer leading to damage to living organisms from ultraviolet radiation in all parts of the global food web.

Global warming or the 'greenhouse effect' refers to the effects that the accumulation of carbon dioxide (produced in all combustion processes whether industrial or in motor vehicles) and other gases such as methane and nitrous oxide have on the temperature of the Earth's atmosphere. If the worst predictions of climatic change due to global warming hold true, then we can ultimately expect a redistribution of people and food sources on this planet, as well as a redistribution of tropical parasitic diseases. The consequences for human health in the transitional period, for example due to refugee movements, would depend on the speed of change.

The ozone layer in the outer atmosphere protects the earth from the sun's ultraviolet (UV) rays. Reduced ozone protection would increase the risk of skin cancer and cataracts in humans, and cause suppression of the immune system. Suppression of the immune system could potentially be the most important consequence of UV exposure, because of its consequences for the whole spectrum of human infectious disease. However, not enough is known at present about the immuno-suppressive effects of UV radiation to make reliable predictions. In addition, greater exposure to UV radiation would destroy phytoplankton, which are particularly vulnerable to UV damage, in the oceans. Phytoplankton are the basis of the food web for all marine creatures and also produce significant amounts of oxygen. (You can find an example of a food web involving phytoplankton in Figure 5.14.)

These *global* effects of the chemical industrial environment are extremely difficult to predict accurately and they provoke heated debate between those who (like Alexander Leaf) foresee disastrous consequences for life on Earth, and those who calculate the risks to be far smaller. Such calculations must combine predictions about the likely levels of environmental pollution (in the face of uncertain changes in human activity), the effect of pollution on the ecosystem and climate, and the effect of these changes on human health. It should be much easier to demonstrate the existence of *local* effects of industrialisation, which are manifest all over the world. The indirect effects of local chemical pollution on health, via its effects on food sources, are of particular concern in communities that depend on subsistence farming, fishing or hunting, or whose economy depends on the sale of these products. In newly-industrialising countries, such as those of Asia and Latin America, the coexistence of small rural communities and industry, which is often inadequately subjected to pollution control, is a particularly difficult problem. For example, local communities can be devastated when chemical pollution depletes fish in rivers.

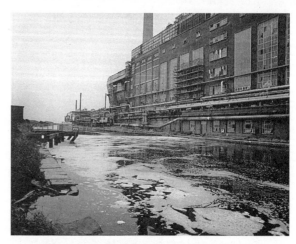

A heavily-polluted river flows past a chemical plant in Merseyside in 1989. Pollution such as this is likely to provoke concern about the direct effects of the chemicals on health in the locality, but less attention is given to possible indirect effects of pollution on health at the local and global level. (Photo: Greenpeace)

In countries such as the United Kingdom, attention to local pollution often focuses on direct toxicity. The rest of this chapter focuses on direct toxicity, illustrated primarily through a case study of the health effects of the industrial chemical dioxin. But, before we examine the effects of chemical exposure on health, we will refresh your memory about the body's capacity for defence against toxic chemicals and its ability to repair damage. We also consider why some people may be more affected by a chemical exposure than others.

Defence and repair

The study of evolution leads us to expect that the human body would have a wide range of defences against potentially harmful external influences, whether biological, physical or chemical. You have already learned a great deal about some of them in earlier chapters of this book. In Chapter 6 you saw how the body defends itself against harmful micro-organisms and larger parasites.

☐ Can you give examples of some of the body's defence mechanisms against pathogenic organisms?

■ Defences range from simple barriers such as a relatively impermeable skin covering, to mucus protecting the respiratory lining, to the complex mechanisms of the innate and adaptive immune systems including phagocytic cells and antibodies.

As Chapter 7 described, the liver contains a variety of enzymes that detoxify chemicals, although sometimes these metabolic changes actually result in the conversion of a harmless chemical to a toxic form. This special role of the liver makes it particularly vulnerable to the action of many toxins, because such high concentrations are found there, and because the toxins may damage the liver before (or during) detoxification, i.e. the process of breaking them down by further chemical reactions.

As well as defence mechanisms, there are repair mechanisms. If there is a lot of cell damage or death in a localised area, then the body can repair itself by cell division and the formation of scar tissue, made up from collagen fibres. Not all cells retain the capacity to divide that they had during fetal life; nerve cells, for example, cannot divide after the fetal brain has formed. Repair in the nervous system must then be carried out entirely by the deposition of collagen. By contrast, bone can heal almost entirely by the formation of new cells. Skin comes between these two extremes. Damage to the outer layer (the *epidermis*) is repaired perfectly by new cells growing up from the deeper layers (the *dermis*), which divide continuously throughout life. If the damage penetrates right through to the dermis then, although cells migrate in from the edges, collagen is laid down and, as a consequence, the repair leaves a scar.

□ Why do you think that elderly people with a poor circulation in the skin on their legs frequently have a diminished capacity to heal skin lesions such as leg ulcers? (Think back to Chapter 8.)

■ The process of cellular repair depends on a good blood supply, because it needs energy and nutrients. (Note that it is implied therefore that the body is making an energy investment in repair.)

Maintenance and repair within cells involves a constant process of checking and eliminating mutations in the DNA and faulty proteins. Repair of DNA, either after spontaneous errors in replication or damage caused by radiation or chemicals, is a remarkable process, whereby mismatches in base pairs are checked for and replaced, or more extensive damage is repaired by enzyme systems. If the damage is too extensive to repair, the cell may die. The natural turnover (breakdown and replacement) of proteins and lipids is another method by which damaged molecules can be disposed of, as you learned in Chapters 7 and 8.

So how can an environmental exposure to toxic chemicals or radiation overcome this elaborate system of defence and repair? First, the system might quite simply be overwhelmed by an exposure that is so high or so prolonged that the body cannot compensate. Second, the body may be challenged by new toxins to which evolution has not had time to produce appropriate defences. Third, the repair process itself can prevent *acute* (short-term) damage, but ultimately lead to *chronic* (long-term) disease. For example, the mucus in the respiratory tract produced after inhalation of harmful substances, eventually contributes to chronic bronchitis if it persists because of long-term exposure. Scar tissue is also a response to acute damage, but has disadvantages compared to normal tissue. Scar tissue in the brain can provoke neurological disorders. Scar tissue in the liver, characteristic of cirrhosis of the liver produced by excessive alcohol intake, is laid down following cell damage. Eventually, it compresses the liver cells and interferes with their function. Moreover, DNA repair itself, while protecting the integrity of the DNA molecule, can sometimes introduce new and harmful mutations.

□ Why have we not evolved defence and repair mechanisms that also protect against long-term damage?

■ In evolution, the importance of maintenance and repair of the body has been balanced against investing the body's resources in growth and reproduction (recall the discussion on the evolution of ageing in Chapter 8).

Sensitivity and hypersensitivity

An important principle in the study of the relationship between the environment and health is the identification of sensitive or critical groups in the population. This is essential to achieve the aim of *equity* of access to a healthy environment. Equity means that each person has access to an environment that does not harm his or her health, so it is important to identify those individuals who are most at risk in a given environment. The concept of a **critical group** is used here to refer to people who are most likely to be exposed to a chemical. Examples are people in certain occupations, people with particular dietary habits, people who live in or near sites of high exposure, or particular age groups who might have a behaviour which makes them more likely to be exposed, for example children who eat soil.

The concept of a **sensitive group** is used here to refer to people who may or may be more likely to be exposed to a chemical, but once exposed, are more likely than others to develop adverse health effects.[3] The newborn baby is one example: since it lacks or is deficient in several of the enzymes involved in the detoxification of chemicals, it eliminates drugs from the body more slowly, and has an inefficient *blood–brain barrier*. (In adults, the walls of the blood vessels in the brain have a special structure that prevents many molecules getting from the bloodstream into the brain cells, but this is not fully developed in babies.) Another example is people who are genetically more predisposed to develop a particular disease, and react more strongly to environmental exposures.

☐ Can you think of any examples where genetic susceptibility affects the way people react to an environmental exposure?

■ In Chapter 9, you saw that people with inherited α_1-antitrypsin deficiency are highly sensitive to tobacco smoke, which accelerates the progression of liver and lung disease. You may also have thought of the fact that white-skinned people are more susceptible than dark-skinned people to skin cancer caused by exposure to ultraviolet radiation.

People with *xeroderma pigmentosa*, a genetic defect that prevents the repair of UV damage, always get skin cancer, and albino people, who have faulty melanin production (melanin is a protein that absorbs UV light and thereby protects other proteins), commonly get skin cancers. People with α_1-antitrypsin deficiency have a genetic predisposition to *emphysema*, a serious lung condition, because they have a defect in a chemical that normally inactivates an enzyme released by white cells in response to inhaled bacterial or chemical irritants. If the enzyme is not inactivated in a short time, it speeds up the breakdown of protein in the lungs, particularly of elastin, the protein which gives elasticity to structures in the lung. The alveoli (tiny air-filled bags in the lungs where the exchange of oxygen and carbon dioxide takes place) become more rigid and breathing becomes extremely difficult. This type

of emphysema provides a good example of the interaction of environmental with genetic factors in the cause of disease: the environmental irritant means that the destructive enzyme is released and the inherited lack of the normal inactivator means that the destructive enzyme has widespread harmful effects on health.

A commonly encountered sensitive group in the population consists of individuals who are *hypersensitive*, or allergic, to particular industrial chemicals, certain metals, or organic material such as pollen and cat fur. **Hypersensitivity** is said to exist when the immune response to a harmless foreign substance produces harmful effects in the body. In other words, hypersensitivity is an example of the situation in which the body's defence itself leads to disease. Hypersensitivity reactions are of several types. We shall look at only two: one mediated by circulating antibodies and one by T lymphocytes (or T cells; the terms and mechanisms in the following account should already be familiar to you from Chapter 6).

Antibodies circulating in the bloodstream are implicated in acute (rapid, short-term) hypersensitivity reactions, such as hay fever, some types of asthma, and hypersensitive reactions to wasp and bee stings (such reactions are commonly called *allergies*). When the *allergen*, the substance that triggers a hypersensitive reaction (for example, pollen, house dust mites, cat fur or insect venom) enters the body, it elicits the production of antibodies which become attached to a stationary type of white cell, called *mast cells*; subsequent exposure to the allergen causes the mast cells to release an excessive amount of histamine and other irritant chemicals. It is these chemicals that produce the hypersensitivity reaction, which is exactly the same as an acute inflammatory response to pathogens, except that it is triggered inappropriately by harmless proteins in organic sources such as pollen and bee venom. This type of reaction particularly affects mucous membranes (for example, in the nasal passages and inside the eyelids) and skin, where mast cells abound. In asthma, swelling of the mucous membranes and spasm of the muscles in the walls of the lungs causes narrowing of the airways and difficulty in breathing. The type of hypersensitivity found in asthma and hay fever tends to run in families and may, therefore, have some genetic basis.

☐ Look at the data in Figure 10.1 and describe the trends in hospital admissions and deaths from asthma among children in the United Kingdom in recent decades.

---

[3]There is some variation in the precise definitions of critical group and sensitive group in current usage in the field of environmental health, but the general distinction between the two (as described here) is the important point to note.

■ The number of hospital admissions per 10 000 children aged 5–14 years increased steadily from 1958 to about 1966, then flattened out for about 10 years, before starting to climb sharply again. By 1986, hospital admissions for asthma in this age group were about 6 times greater than in 1958. Deaths per million children aged 5–14 years increased sharply until about 1967, and then fell just as sharply to a fairly stable rate from about 1972 to the end of the period.

It is difficult to determine trends in the *prevalence* of asthma from data such as those in Figure 10.1.[4] Hospital admissions constitute only a very small proportion of the total problem of 'wheeze' that could be labelled 'asthma' in the population. A slight tendency among GPs to refer children to hospital more easily could result in a large increase in hospital admissions without any real change in the prevalence of asthma symptoms. Similarly, the declining rate of deaths from asthma may be related to improved medical management rather than to the frequency of asthma attacks. More reliable prevalence data can only be achieved from specially-designed surveys of children, but such studies encounter the difficulty of defining at what point mild wheezing should be counted as asthma; different clinicians disagree about this. Hospital admissions and deaths also reflect the frequency of *severe* asthma attacks, rather than the total proportion of affected children; the severity of attacks could increase, even though the total number of asthmatic children remains the same.

Recently it has been suggested that the apparent increase in recorded asthma attacks is associated with *photochemical smog*. Photochemical smog contains nitrogen oxides, sulphur dioxide and carbon monoxide from vehicles and industry, which react with sunlight to produce 'ground-level' ozone. Ozone at low concentrations in the air we breathe causes coughing,

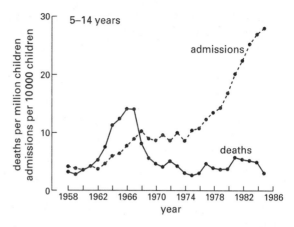

Figure 10.1 *Trends in admissions to hospital (per 10 000 children in the age group) and deaths (per million children in the age group) from asthma in children aged 5–14 years in the United Kingdom, 1958–86. (Adapted from Anderson, H. R., 1989, Is the prevalence of asthma changing? Archives of Disease in Childhood,* **64***, un-numbered Figure, p. 173)*

nausea, irritation of the eyes, nose and throat, and headaches; at higher concentrations, it damages lung structure and function. It is thought that ozone, and/or other components of photochemical smog, may make asthmatics more sensitive to allergens, including other pollutants. (You should not confuse these harmful effects of ozone in the air we breathe with its beneficial effects in the upper atmosphere, where it protects the Earth from ultraviolet rays.)

The second type of hypersensitivity is due to the action of T cells. The *cytotoxic* T cells normally attack the body's own cells only if they become infected with intracellular micro-organisms such as viruses. However, if certain chemicals come into prolonged contact with the skin they can combine with proteins to form allergens, which 'trigger' the cytotoxic T cells to attack otherwise healthy skin cells. The result is skin redness, blistering and weeping, known as contact dermatitis. Common allergens include rubber, tanning agents in leather, and nickel; some people react to components in the jewellery they wear. Initially, the reaction is localised in the region of the skin that has been in contact with the chemical, but later it may spread to other areas. Contact dermatitis is an important occupational health problem, but there is considerable uncertainty as to why some individuals are prone to it while most are not. This form of hypersensitivity is illustrated in photographs overleaf.

[4]The prevalence of a fluctuating, episodic condition (such as asthma) is calculated by counting the total number of people in a population, or section of a population (in this case, children aged 5–14 years in the United Kingdom) who experienced symptoms of asthma in a defined period of time, and dividing this by the number of individuals in the population at risk during that period. Prevalence rates are discussed in *Studying Health and Disease* (revised edition, 1994), Chapter 7.

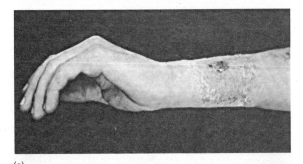

(a)

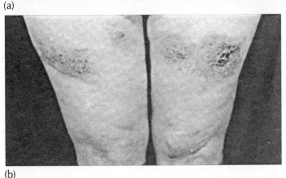

(b)

Contact hypersensitivity in the skin of people who are unusually sensitive to (a) the chemicals in a leather watch strap; (b) the nickel used in suspender clips before plastic clips became widespread; and (c) chemicals in adhesive resin used in this person's occupation. (Photos: (a) courtesy of Dr R. E. Church; (b) courtesy of Dr D. J. Gawkrodger, Royal Hallamshire Hospital, Sheffield; (c) Royal Infirmary, Sheffield.

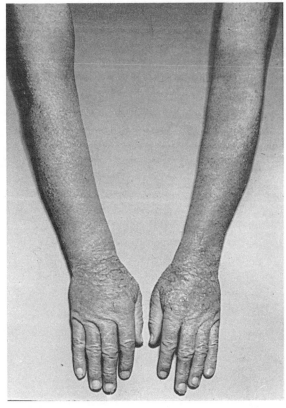

(c)

Chemical toxicity: the case of dioxin

A quick review of public, media and scientific concern in environmental health will reveal many currently unanswered questions about direct toxicity from environmental exposures. We have chosen to focus on one of them: 'What hazards do exposures to dioxin pose to local communities?'. Before investigating that question, we can do no more here than point to several other areas under active consideration, with reference to a few relevant research publications for readers who wish to investigate further. Does electromagnetic radiation, from power lines and electricity substations, for example, cause cancer or depression? (Coleman and Beral, 1988). Does radiation exposure of workers in parts of the nuclear industry lead to increased risk of leukaemia in their children? (Gardner *et al.*, 1990; Beral, Roman and Bobrow,

1993). Are the weakly oestrogenic (hormone-like) qualities of some chemicals, including PCBs (polychlorinated biphenyls), leading to cancer or male reproductive disorders, including falling sperm count? (Sharpe and Skakkebaek, 1993). All these questions are the subject of active research.

We are going to illustrate the subject of 'living with industrial chemicals' by looking at a chemical called *dioxin*.[5] Why is there particular concern about dioxin, when people regularly come into contact with thousands of chemicals? There are at least two scientific reasons for this, both of which are explored here: first, the persistence in the environment and 'bioaccumulation' of the chemical (it becomes more concentrated as it passes up the food chain, a subject we return to later); and, second, evidence of strong toxicity from animal experiments. In addition, the chemical has been associated in the public mind with well-publicised industrial disasters and warfare. For the purposes of this chapter, it is also a good example because of the long research history on the effects of this chemical, and the controversy that remains about its significance for human health at current exposure levels.

[5]Dioxin is a generic name for a number of closely-related compounds, which have the same basic molecular structure but differ in their chlorine composition.

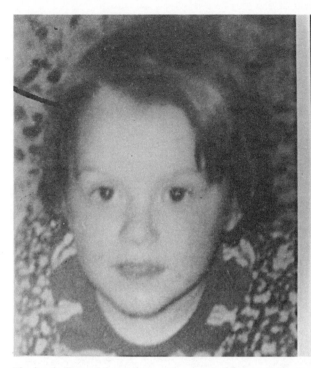
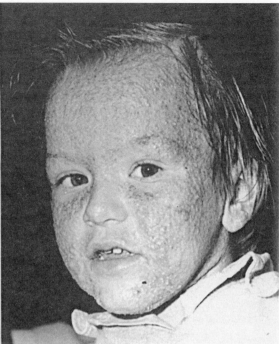

The local effects of the explosion in a chemical factory in Seveso, Northern Italy, which took place on 10 July 1976, are illustrated in the face of four-year old Alice Senno, photographed (left) on 18 June and (right) on 29 October that year. The sores are chloracne, caused by exposure to chlorine-containing compounds. (Photo: AP-Wirephoto)

Dioxin exposures

On 10 July 1976, in Seveso, a quiet industrial town in the province of Milan in northern Italy, an explosion took place at a TCP (trichlorophenol) pesticide manufacturing plant, which released a large quantity of dioxin, a byproduct in the manufacturing process, into the densely populated surroundings. Many domestic animals grazing nearby died; there were no known human fatalities. However, *chloracne* (an acne-like skin disorder that comes from exposure to certain chlorine-containing compounds) started to appear on the fourth day and was reported by nearly 200 residents and workers, some of whom also had liver problems. Those living in the most contaminated area close to the plant were evacuated from their homes for several weeks.

During the Vietnam war, Agent Orange, a herbicide, was sprayed from the air to defoliate jungles and destroy food crops. Agent Orange, like many herbicides and fungicides, is contaminated by dioxin. Vietnamese citizens and US veterans subsequently reported skin rashes, chronic depression, cancer and birth defects. Later in this chapter we shall discuss the difficulties in interpreting such reports.

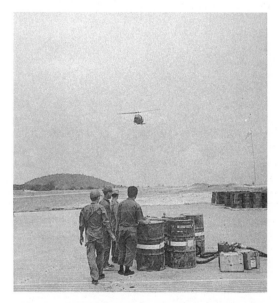

An American helicopter prepares to land and refill its tanks with pesticide at An-Thiot, after a defoliation mission to Phu Quoc island during the Vietnam war, 1968. (Photo: US Army Military History Institute)

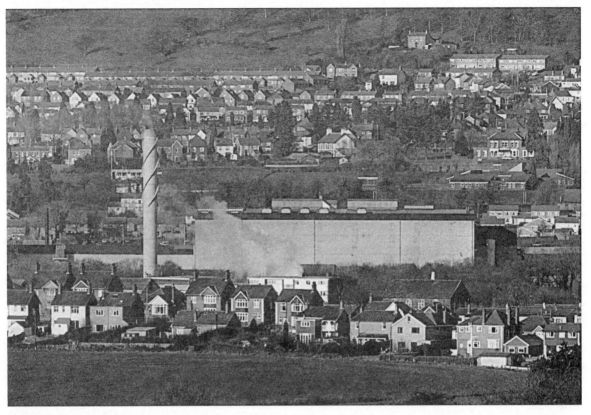

An industrial chemical incinerator disposes of toxic waste in the heart of a residential area in Pontypool, South Wales. (Photo: Hoffman/Greenpeace)

In both these examples, the first effect of dioxin was chloracne. This is an example of **acute toxicity**, an immediate effect of a single exposure to a high dose. Industrial accidents are a typical situation in which acute toxicity occurs. Other situations in which acute toxicity is observed are when chemicals in common external use are accidentally consumed (for example, concentrated pesticides), or when food is contaminated by chemicals.

One notorious example of a food poisoning incident concerns a chemical closely related to dioxin, commonly known as PCB (polychlorinated biphenyl), which contaminated rice oil in Japan in 1968. Over 1 000 individuals were poisoned; they experienced chloracne, pigmentation of the skin, general weakness, numbness of the limbs, respiratory symptoms and impaired immune function.

There are, however, many sources of low-dose dioxin exposure where levels never reach the dose needed for an acute effect like chloracne. Apart from its presence as a contaminant in pesticides, dioxin is produced by combustion (burning) processes in industry and in waste incineration; it is present in cigarette smoke; it occurs in some liquid industrial-waste effluent, and in products of paper and pulp manufacture which involve chlorine-bleaching.

In the 1980s, a Working Group was set up by the Department of the Environment in the United Kingdom to review and assess the available information on dioxin. In their report (1989), the Working Group pointed to municipal incinerators, domestic coal fires, and vehicle exhausts (mainly from engines using leaded petrol) as the most important sources of dioxin in the United Kingdom. The related compounds, PCBs, were formerly used in the capacitors and transformers of electrical equipment and thus reached the environment through the disposal of old equipment. Dioxin can be formed by thermal degradation and incineration of PCBs. The concern is that long-term exposure to low or intermittent doses can also produce adverse effects on health, in other words the concern relates to **chronic toxicity**.

Bioaccumulation and persistence of chemicals in the environment

Dioxin, and the related compounds PCBs, have special properties which cause them to build up in body tissue and in the environment. They are *lipophilic* (literally, 'liking fats'; in biological usage the term means 'readily dissolves in fats'); in practice, this means that they accumulate in body tissue where lipids are found, and are able to cross cell membranes and enter cells.

☐ Why can dioxin cross cell membranes? (Refer back to Chapter 3 if you need to remind yourself of membrane structure.)

■ Lipids form the basic framework of cell membranes, with proteins embedded or attached to them. Dioxin is lipophilic, so it is soluble in cell membranes and easily passes across.

Lipophilic compounds generally are not soluble in water, and thus dioxin tends to stick to soil or to sediment. Dioxin is also resistant to degradation, which means that it does not react easily with other chemicals or with air to form new compounds or breakdown products. Because of these properties, dioxin tends to accumulate in the food chain: a phenomenon known as **bioaccumulation.**

☐ Can you think of some food chains that involve humans? (Refer to Chapter 5 if you need help.) How many 'levels' do your examples contain?

■ You may have thought of these: Human eats cow which eats grass (3 levels); human drinks milk from cow which eats grass (3 levels); human eats fish which eat smaller fish which eat plankton (4 levels); humans eat shellfish which eat plankton (3 levels); humans eat vegetables (2 levels).

Whatever we eat, we eventually excrete most of the material in one form or another, either in faeces, urine, perspiration or exhaled air (Chapter 7). Since dioxin, for example, tends not to be excreted but remains in the fatty tissues, it accumulates in the body. When this happens at an early stage in the food chain, and the animal (along with many others) is eaten by another animal, which is in turn eaten (again along with many others) by another animal, the chemical gets steadily more concentrated at each level of the food chain.

☐ Which of the food chains that end in humans would result in the highest dioxin exposure to humans?

■ Food chains with the most levels, since dioxin becomes more concentrated each time an animal eats another contaminated animal.

It is estimated that if human exposure to dioxin is averaged over the whole population of a country, most exposure is via ingestion of contaminated food. However, there are also other exposure routes, such as inhalation of contaminated air, ingestion of contaminated water (remember that dioxin is not soluble in water but sticks to sediment), and absorption through the skin from soil or pesticide use, or handling other contaminated products. The main routes of exposure and level of exposure for different groups within the population depends on their dietary habits, contamination of their area of residence, and occupation. Thus, it is important to think of critical groups in the population, and not just average population exposure.

It is estimated that once dioxin enters the body, its **biological half-life** is 6–10 years. 'Half-life' refers to the time it takes for the amount of something to reach half its original amount. We most often hear this term in relation to radiation. The half-life of radioactive isotopes gives a good idea of how long the radioactive exposure will persist in the environment. Radioactive iodine, for example, has a half-life of 8 days, whereas some forms of radioactive caesium have a half-life of 32 years. However, the *biological* half-life, or the half-life inside the body, refers not only to properties of the chemical itself, but also to how quickly the body transforms or excretes it. The long half-life of dioxin leads to its accumulation in the body.

Evidence of toxicity from animal experiments

Dioxin has been found to be highly *carcinogenic* (cancer-causing) in rats and mice. Liver cancer is found in both these species, but other cancers seem to depend on species, sex, and the method of administration of the chemical. Dioxin is thought to belong to a small group of compounds that are carcinogenic but not **mutagenic** (dioxin does not cause mutations in the DNA of exposed cells); this finding is based on animal experiments and *in vitro*[6] experiments, which have failed to find a mutagenic effect. The development of a cancer (carcinogenesis) is considered to be a multi-stage process requiring a number of different steps, as Chapter 8 described. These steps may include mutations, but also other events, called

[6]Literally 'in glass', referring to experiments with isolated cells and tissues in laboratory cultures.

'promoting' events, which lead to increased cell division and therefore the growth of the cancerous cells. Increased cell division may, in itself, promote mutation, since it is during cell division that the genetic material is most vulnerable to mutation. Thus carcinogenic agents may be either mutagens, or non-mutagens that promote cell growth.

Dioxin and the related compounds, PCBs, also cause *reproductive anomalies*, or 'adverse reproductive outcomes', in experimental animals: these include cleft palate, renal (kidney) anomalies, decreased fetal weight, increased fetal death rates, and adverse effects on sperm production in males. The effects differ in different species.

☐ From general knowledge, can you give some examples of human reproductive anomalies (however caused)?

■ You may have thought of one or more of the following: congenital malformations (birth defects such as spina bifida); premature birth; intra-uterine growth retardation ('small-for-dates' babies); spontaneous abortion or stillbirth; developmental problems linked to pre-natal factors such as some forms of cerebral palsy (spasticity) and mental retardation; problems after puberty in sperm or ovum production or quality, including those leading to infertility.

☐ From what you know of the effects of dioxin on DNA, what types of congenital effects would you be *less* likely to expect from human exposure to dioxin?

■ Congenital effects due to mutations in the gametes (sperm and ova) of the baby's parents, because dioxin is thought not to be mutagenic.

Dioxin has also been shown in animal experiments to be *immunotoxic,* i.e. it adversely affects the immune system, especially the developing (pre-adult) immune system. This could be expected to reduce resistance to infection.

Extrapolating from animal experiments to human exposures

Inferring human health effects from animal experiments is very difficult.[7] The effect of a chemical depends on how it is absorbed by the body, distributed in the body, broken down by the body (including detoxification in the liver), and excreted. Other animal species can be very different

in these characteristics from humans. For example, thalidomide, a drug prescribed around 1960 to alleviate morning sickness during pregnancy, proved to be highly **teratogenic** in humans, that is, it caused severe congenital limb malformations and other physical defects as the embryo developed. But this effect is not seen in rats, one of the species used for safety-testing of drugs. (A teratogen is an agent that causes congenital malformations if the fetus is exposed to it during pregnancy, usually during the first few months when the main formation of the organs takes place.)[8]

☐ For what evolutionary reasons do we pay attention to the results of animal experiments, but nevertheless expect differences from humans?

■ Humans and primates share a recent (in evolutionary terms) common ancestor, a more distant common ancestor with other mammals, and a yet more distant common ancestor with other vertebrates. The closer the evolutionary relationship between us and the animal species used as a substitute for humans in biomedical research, the more like ourselves biologically we can expect it to be, and the more reliably can the results of the research be applied to humans. However, no matter how close the relationship, an 'animal model' differs from humans in many aspects of its biology and behaviour, and this may crucially affect the outcome of the research, as the thalidomide tragedy illustrates.

Each species of animal has, during the course of evolution, adapted to its habitual environment; this includes adaptation to the various chemicals it encounters in its diet and surroundings. Thus, different species have evolved biological responses to different chemicals, and the responses that evolve to the same chemicals may also differ.

It takes very intensive research on a particular chemical and how it is absorbed, distributed and metabolised in the bodies of different animals, to understand a little better whether it is likely that human exposures will have similar effects. For example, dioxin concentrates particularly in the liver in rats, mice and hamsters, but in fat, muscle and skin in guinea pigs and rhesus monkeys.

---

[7]For a detailed discussion of the reasons underlying this statement, see *Studying Health and Disease*, Chapter 9.

[8]Critical periods in the development of the human fetus are described in *Birth to Old Age: Health in Transition* (1985, and revised edition 1995).

Not only is it difficult to predict the type of effect, it is also not easy to estimate the human equivalent of the dose given to an animal.

Another aspect that needs consideration is *how* the animal has been exposed to dioxin. The same amount of dioxin administered in different ways is treated very differently by the body. Thus, if dioxin were injected straight into the bloodstream of animals, the relevance of the results to human exposures, which do not happen in this way, would be very uncertain. It is known that dioxin is better absorbed when administered in oil, but less well when it is stuck to soil or ash. Similarly, absorption through the skin depends on what the dioxin is mixed with. The general area of biological extrapolation from animal experiments to humans is the job of a *toxicologist*.

Evidence of chronic toxicity in humans

What about evidence from exposed humans? In fact, evidence about chronic toxicity is generally difficult to obtain.

□ Why might it be easier to identify *acute* toxicity than *chronic* toxicity in humans?

■ Toxicity can be readily identified if the exposure and the disease are close together in time, if the disease is unusual without such exposure, or if the disease almost always follows exposure. These conditions tend to apply for acute toxicity, but not for chronic toxicity.

Even studies of acute toxicity can present severe problems. For example, the acute toxicity of Agent Orange during the Vietnam war was not well documented, and we now have to rely on retrospective accounts of health effects, related to very inaccurate estimates of exposure. After industrial accidents also, it is common for the public health response to be concentrated on practical measures to alleviate the immediate effects, but to neglect the gathering of information that might be useful to an epidemiologist.[9]

Epidemiological studies of chronic toxicity tend to focus on high-exposure situations, where the health effects are either more frequent or more severe and therefore easier to study. For dioxin, these include certain occupational groups who use herbicides or work in chemical plants, Vietnam veterans, and people living in a contaminated area like Seveso. (The research evidence

discussed below is reviewed by Lilienfeld and Gallo, 1989, and by Nessell and Gallo, 1992.)

□ What are the problems of relying on studies of high-exposure situations among certain occupations to predict environmental risks to the *general public* from low-dose chemical exposures?

■ It is often difficult to extrapolate reliably from the effects of high doses to the effects of low doses. Also, occupational studies tend to refer to men exposed during their working years, and it may be difficult to extrapolate to the effects on women, children, fetuses, newborns or elderly people, as well as sensitive groups in the population who are under-represented in the workforce.

Some studies of dioxin exposures in humans have shown an increase in certain cancers, but the results are inconsistent and there has been no clear **dose–response relationship**. A dose–response relationship for cancer means (broadly) that more highly exposed people have a higher incidence of cancer than less highly exposed people, and the less highly exposed have a higher incidence than the unexposed.

Interpretation of epidemiological studies needs to be very careful to determine whether an association between an exposure and an outcome exists. Both false-negative and false-positive findings can occur (these terms were defined in Chapter 9). Studies of small numbers of people cannot distinguish between real and chance effects; larger or multiple-site studies which include many types of cancer are likely to find one or two cancers increased in frequency by chance alone. A long period of follow-up is needed after exposure in order to study cancer as a possible outcome. People are often exposed to a mixture of chemicals and it is difficult to know which chemical is the important one, or if the mixture itself is critical. It may also be difficult to assess accurately the exposure of the individual, especially when it was in the past, which makes it particularly hard to find a dose–response relationship. Moreover, there is sometimes a danger of *bias* when the health status of an individual is ascertained by assessors who already know his or her exposure status, or conversely when exposure status is ascertained by assessors who already know the individual's state of health.[10] The best human evidence to

[9]The methodological approach of epidemiology to establishing valid associations between an event and its health consequences are discussed in *Studying Health and Disease* (revised edition, 1994), Chapters 7 and 8.

[10]Issues of bias, confounding, and chance associations in epidemiological studies are discussed in *Studying Health and Disease*, Chapter 8.

date nevertheless suggests that dioxin is not as strong a carcinogen in humans as would be expected from animal experiments.

At the time of writing (early 1994), human studies of teratogenic effects of dioxin have been very few. They include an epidemiological study of pregnant women at Seveso, which found no increase in congenital malformations. One theory is that dioxin is not teratogenic in humans because the doses that would be needed to produce a congenital malformation are also doses that would be clearly toxic to both mother and fetus. Many chemicals would be teratogenic if given in a high enough dose. The important question is whether by protecting the adults (including the mother) from toxicity, we also adequately protect the fetus. If the *teratogenic dose* is as high as the *adult toxic dose*, protection of the fetus is achieved by prevention of toxic exposures in the general population.

There is more evidence about the teratogenicity of the dioxin-related compounds, PCBs, which have been involved in several large-scale food-poisoning disasters where oils or fish were contaminated. Various effects have been reported, including low birthweight, shorter duration of pregnancy, small impairments of the nervous system, and skin defects. Exposure often continued after birth via breast milk and, in most cases, other chemicals were also present along with PCBs.

Threshold effects in toxicity

Human studies are still in progress, but do not so far suggest that dioxin is strongly carcinogenic. Human evidence points to a possible excess risk of cancer among those exposed to high doses (often those who, at the time of exposure, showed acute effects like chloracne). This leaves the question of what the effects might be for those exposed over a long period to very low doses. Extrapolation from observations made at high doses to the low-dose situation means that we must have a model of how much effect on health there is with every 'unit of increase' in dose. This requires a knowledge of **threshold effects**.

Some long-term effects occur only after doses have exceeded a certain *threshold* and, beyond this threshold, the effect may be more severe the greater the dose. For example, high exposure to certain kinds of radiation results in cataracts or sterility. Other effects, such as cancers, occur with an increasing probability the higher the dose, and there may be no threshold at all, nor any relationship between the dose and the severity of the disease. Knowledge of thresholds and the relationship between the dose and the probability or severity of

disease is fundamental to the regulation of chemicals, and is therefore the subject of much research.

When a disease is a consequence of the destruction of tissue and therefore loss of function, it is reasonable to suppose that a considerable amount of destruction is necessary before the body is no longer able to repair it. Many teratogenic effects, for example, are thought to need threshold doses before the fetus is no longer able to compensate, or repair the damage and develop normally; above the threshold, the malformation may be more severe the higher the dose.

Cancers, however, are the result of a number of mainly genetic changes (mutations) within cells, which affect their growth relative to other cells (see Chapter 8). For these effects, we suppose that the lower the dose of exposure, the lower the probability that the mutation will occur (and that genetic repair mechanisms will 'miss' the mutation) but, although the probability becomes smaller and smaller, there is no threshold. On the other hand, dioxin belongs to the group of *non*-mutagenic carcinogens and, without knowing about its exact mechanism of action, it is difficult to know whether a 'no-threshold' model should apply.

Thinking about risks

The example of dioxin leads us to ask to what extent we should minimise the exposure of human populations to aspects of the chemical industrial environment. The United Kingdom 1991 Environmental Protection Act introduced the *BATNEEC principle:* Best Available Technology Not Entailing Excessive Cost. Radiation protection operates on the *ALARA principle*: As Low As Is Reasonably Achievable. But what is 'excessive' or 'reasonable'?

One approach to answering this question is the *prioritisation of risks* to human health. The British epidemiologists Sir Richard Doll and Richard Peto (Doll and Peto, 1981b) studied the causes of cancer deaths in the United States. They estimated (although they also emphasised scientists' ignorance about many possibly carcinogenic exposures) that 30 per cent of all cancer deaths were due to tobacco, 35 per cent to diet-related factors, 3 per cent to alcohol, 7 per cent to reproductive and sexual factors (including hormonal factors), 10 per cent to infection, 4 per cent to occupational exposures to chemicals and radiation, 2 per cent to pollution (of air, food and water), and 3 per cent to geophysical factors (including naturally-occurring radiation and UV light). On this analysis, the chemical industry is a minor contributor to cancers.

A pioneer in the testing of chemicals for mutagenicity, Bruce Ames, has recently (1987) been questioning the focus of regulatory institutions on *synthetic* chemicals for carcinogenicity testing. His argument is that most chemicals that humans are exposed to are 'natural' chemicals in the diet, and that the modes of action of natural and synthetic chemicals in the body are not fundamentally different. Ames claims that the defences evolved against naturally occurring chemicals tend to be *general* defences, rather than specific for certain chemicals, and that gaps in these defences apply as much to 'natural' as to synthetic chemicals. Ames argues that most human genetic damage comes about through the production of free radicals during normal metabolism (as described in Chapter 8). In addition, he cites natural plant pesticides (which plants use to defend themselves), and products formed when food is cooked and burned, as major mutagens.

However, although the information provided by epidemiologists and toxicologists is a very important basis for prioritising the risks from environmental exposures, it does not in itself *constitute* prioritisation. When people are ranking environmental hazards, they are consciously or unconsciously taking account of many other variables. Is the exposure voluntary or involuntary; does the individual have any control over the extent of his/her exposure? Is it a predictable low-level exposure, or an unpredictable exposure with a possibility of disasters such as industrial accidents? Is it new or old and can we be confident that we know the possible consequences? What would we lose in economic, social or personal terms from reduction of the exposure? Is everyone equally at risk or are there certain critical or sensitive groups?

When thinking about risks, it can be useful to divide the subject into 'risk assessment' and 'risk management'. **Risk assessment** is mainly carried out by scientists who seek to characterise the potential adverse health effects of human exposures to environmental hazards. We have already discussed elements of this process, particularly the use of animal and human data, and the establishment of the relationship between dose and effect. Another important part of risk assessment is finding out which parts of the population are exposed, by what route, and by how much. Risk assessments are generally very difficult, since they are almost always based on incomplete data and on assumptions, and finding ways to assess and present the uncertainty in the assessment (without it being no use at all) is essential for its use in risk management.

Risk management is the process of weighing policy alternatives and selecting the most appropriate regulatory action. It involves integrating the results of risk assessment with engineering data and with social, economic and political concerns in order to reach a decision about what actions to take. Risk management must weigh the health costs of the chemical (as revealed by risk assessment) and other costs, against its benefits. There are sometimes question marks over the sustainability of the benefits we gain from some chemicals, for example many insect species are developing resistance to pesticides.

Another increasingly important element in our decisions is that we cannot just look at risks to human health in terms of the *direct* toxicity of chemicals. As we (and Alexander Leaf) mentioned at the beginning of this chapter, much of the impetus for regulation of chemical production and waste emission now comes from the fear of adverse consequences for the *ecosystem*, and *indirect* effects on human health. These are even more difficult to measure or predict than the direct effects, since there is considerable uncertainty about how the ecosystem will be affected by changing industrial practices and patterns of industrial activity.

Finally, international cooperation is essential in looking at these problems. Current practices in shipping waste or dirty industries to economically less-developed regions of the world need scrutiny. For example, the 1992 report of the World Health Organisation's Commission on Health and the Environment, entitled *Our Planet, Our Health*, mentions the case of export of toxic wastes to Thailand. Large quantities of chemical wastes from all over the world are being stored in Bangkok's main port. It is feared that the barrels contain PCBs and dioxin, which can only be destroyed in high temperature incinerators, which Thailand does not possess.

It is clear, therefore, that the world community needs to think carefully about how to live with the chemical products of industrialisation. In the next and final chapter in this book, we will take a broader view of modern industrial culture and its effects on health.

OBJECTIVES FOR CHAPTER 10

When you have studied this chapter, you should be able to:

10.1 Summarise the various ways in which the chemical industrial environment can directly and indirectly affect human health; define the terms carcinogen, mutagen and teratogen, and illustrate them from the case study on exposure to dioxin.

10.2 Give examples of how the body can defend itself against, and repair damage from, environmental toxins and explain why disease sometimes results despite these mechanisms.

10.3 Distinguish between critical group and sensitive group (as defined in this chapter), and describe the mechanisms underlying hypersensitivity to certain chemicals.

10.4 Distinguish between acute and chronic toxicity and explain why knowledge of the chronic effects of environmental pollutants is very incomplete; refer to the difficulties of extrapolating from animal experiments to humans and the problems of risk assessment.

QUESTIONS FOR CHAPTER 10

Question 1 (*Objective 10.1*)

Based on your reading of Chapters 7, 8 and 10, and the Reader article by Alexander Leaf, how might the chemical industrial environment alter the level of ultraviolet (UV) radiation reaching the surface of the Earth, and what health effects might result?

Question 2 (*Objective 10.2*)

Explain how the process of cellular repair involving cell division might lead to disease. (You will also have to think back to Chapters 4 and 8 to answer this question fully.)

Question 3 (*Objective 10.3*)

Distinguish between an acute inflammatory response to an infection in the respiratory tract and an acute hypersensitivity reaction to an inhaled allergen such as pollen. (You will also have to think back to Chapter 6 to answer this question.)

Question 4 (*Objectives 10.3 and 10.4*)

(a) Use the thalidomide tragedy to illustrate the concept of a *sensitive group.*

(b) What features of the thalidomide tragedy helped clinicians and epidemiologists to establish a *causal* relationship between the drug and limb malformations?

(c) Suggest some reasons why toxicity testing of thalidomide in other species might fail to give an accurate assessment of the risk to human fetuses.

11

The impact of modern culture

This short chapter draws the book to a close and speculates about the future in terms of impacts on human health arising from the pace of cultural change. The article by Alexander Leaf, which you studied with Chapter 10, is also relevant here, and you will be asked to read an extract entitled 'The evolution of Utopia' from a book written by the British geneticist Steve Jones; both can be found in the Reader.[1]

Genetic and cultural evolution

In the earlier chapters of this book, we considered how genetic evolution, through natural selection, has made us what we are: multi-celled, sexually reproducing, with long gestation, a complex brain and a complex immune system. We also considered why, despite our long evolutionary past, we are neither disease-free nor immortal.

Chapter 2 introduced the idea that cultural evolution also affects human health and disease, and other chapters have looked at the effects of modern cultural changes, including industrialisation, medical technologies, dietary changes, and the consequences of living longer. What are the essential differences between cultural evolution and genetic evolution?

Genetic evolution, based on the theory of natural selection (as described in Chapters 2 to 4), could be summarised as follows. Through mutation, the reassortment of chromosomes that takes place when eggs and sperm are formed, and the mixing of genes from both parents at fertilisation, *genetic variability* is created in the population. Sometimes a new genetic variant is beneficial, within a specific environment, in the sense that such

an individual is more likely to survive and leave offspring in the next generation. In the 'shorthand' of evolutionary biology, this genetic variant will be *selected for*, that is, the frequency of this genetic variant will increase in the population over time. Conversely, natural selection will *act against* genetic variants that reduce reproductive success, and these will tend to decrease in the population over time.

There are three important features of evolution by natural selection. First, it is based on the reproductive success of the *individual*; you might even state that it is based on the 'reproductive success' of a particular gene. Natural selection will *not* favour a characteristic that is *not* good for the individual or their closest kin (who have genes in common), even though it is good for the wider group or community of which they are a part. Second, reproductive success as a basis for natural selection also means that characteristics that produce benefits for the individual *only* during the post-reproductive years cannot be selected for (if you are unclear about why this is so, look back at the section in Chapter 8 on the evolution of ageing). The third feature of genetic evolution by natural selection is lack of foresight or strategy. A gene will never increase (or decrease) in frequency in *readiness* for a future change in the environment, but only in *response* to a change that has already occurred.

Cultural evolution can be distinguished from genetic evolution by these three (and no doubt other) features. Human societies can choose to change their cultural practices so that they will be of eventual benefit to the whole community, not just to the individual; we could introduce new cultural practices which will favour people in their post-reproductive years; and we can look ahead to the consequences of our actions in future generations and decide to forsake some of our temporary well-being for the sake of the future. (Scientists disagree over the extent to which human cultural development might be 'conditioned' by our genetic evolutionary past. So-called 'sociobiologists' have argued that we are 'programmed' to protect ourselves and our kin at the expense of others, but this view is controversial.)

[1] *Health and Disease: A Reader* (Open University Press, revised edition 1994).

Human health, as defined by the World Health Organisation in its frequently quoted constitution of 1958, is 'a state of complete physical, mental and social wellbeing and not merely the absence of disease and infirmity'. In this sense, much of human endeavour and culture can be seen as an effort to improve health. However, it is not always clear *whose* health. By improving the health of one subgroup of the population, does this damage the health of others, or of future generations? Does society do enough to assess the impact of cultural change on health, and who is included in this impact assessment? Even if assessment of the impact of cultural change on human health becomes a priority, is the relationship between environment and health, and the interrelation between different aspects of human biology well enough understood?

Cultural evolution, itself perhaps inexpertly aimed at promoting health, causes problems to the environment and to human biology, which require further cultural adaptation to combat, not only for the survival of the human species but also for the survival of other species. However, the capacity of both humans and other species to adapt to environmental change, whether through genetic or cultural adaptation, depends not only on the *nature* of the change, but also on its *speed*. It has been the speed of change in industrialised societies that has caused particular concern in recent years.

Genetic adaptation is a very slow process because it cannot begin until new mutations or genetic variants appear that are better adapted to the current environment, and then these have to spread through the population from generation to generation. Probably a sequence of genetic variations, each building on the last, will be necessary before any lasting adaptation occurs. However, maintenance of a high degree of genetic diversity in a population, whether human or otherwise, can speed up this evolutionary 'response time'.

> ☐ Can you explain why?

> ■ It increases the chance of a favourable combination of genes occurring, which can be passed on to subsequent generations.

Cultural adaptation means that human societies must recognise what the problem is, devise a solution, and change the behaviour of the population in order to implement that solution. This might happen extremely quickly (as in the introduction of car seat-belt legislation), or it might take many generations (as in the slow decline of cigarette-smoking among men in the United Kingdom). An important concern is that the speed of cultural change in the twentieth century may *in itself* be psychologically damaging and thus have a direct effect on health.

The impact of modern culture on human genetic evolution

Although cultural evolution is now a predominant force in explaining changes in human health and disease, we can still expect genetic changes to occur. Framed in terms of genetic evolution, a disease could be thought of as a state that lowers individual *fitness* (Chapter 3). However, many 'diseases' no longer affect fitness. For example, infertility treatments have changed the reproductive prospects of infertile couples, and some children born with severe genetic birth defects now survive to reproductive age following treatment of their conditions (Chapters 4 and 9).

Other genetic characteristics may have less influence *now* on explaining differences in reproductive success between individuals than was the case in the past. For example, people who are more genetically susceptible to infection may now be protected from pathogens by antibiotics, effective sanitation and vaccination (Chapter 6). People with visual impairments can have their sight corrected with glasses, or can adopt a lifestyle that prevents their visual impairment from being a major handicap. In future, screening for genetic susceptibility to disease may allow early interventions, whether directed at the genes or the environment of the susceptible person, which will reduce the risk of developing the screened disease (Chapter 9 cites examples of this). Thus, many cultural developments are leading to a relaxation of the *power* of natural selection to act against (reduce the frequency of) formerly disadvantageous genetic characteristics in the population.

This relaxation of natural selection will inevitably lead to *increases* in the frequency of certain defective alleles. On the other hand, we also have the potential to impose stronger selective pressures against those alleles, for example by pre-natal screening and selective abortion, or if we engage in the future in forms of gene therapy that result in heritable changes to the genetic material. So far, as explained in Chapter 9, gene therapy involving germ-line changes to the DNA is not sanctioned. Society is becoming increasingly conscious of the necessity of clarifying and regulating the ways in which we are interfering with our genetic inheritance.

Cultural change may also create strong selective pressures that alter our genetic make-up, as the following example illustrates. Scientists have been speculating about the genetic evolutionary basis of an epidemic of non-insulin-dependent diabetes in the Pacific island of Nauru.[2] Over a short time period, the economy of the island was transformed from one of subsistence farming and fishing, to phosphate mining. The Nauruans quickly became wealthy, and this manifested itself in high calorie intake, obesity and low physical activity: well-known risk factors for this form of diabetes. Diabetes rose to epidemic proportions in young adults after 1950, but since 1975 has been found to decline markedly in prevalence and incidence.

One hypothesis to explain both the rise and decline of diabetes in Nauru is known as 'Neel's thrifty genotype hypothesis' after the American geneticist who formulated it in 1962. (This hypothesis has been discussed more recently in easily accessible British journals by the American evolutionary biologist, Jared Diamond, 1992, and by two epidemiologists, Gary Dowse and Paul Zimmet, working at the International Diabetes Institute in Australia, 1993.) According to Neel's hypothesis, the reason why the genotype associated with non-insulin-dependent diabetes was so frequent before the Nauruans adopted a Western lifestyle is because it (thriftily) favoured fat deposition during periods of plentiful food. This genotype would be advantageous in situations where food sources are unpredictable; the fat stored during 'good times' would be used up quite quickly when food became scarce again and, as a consequence, diabetes did not develop. However, when the Nauruans' lifestyle changed suddenly to one of permanent plenty, they remained obese and became prone to diabetes.

□ Can you suggest a hypothetical explanation for the decline in diabetes among Nauruans after 1975, even though their calorie intake, levels of obesity and inactivity remained as high as before?

■ The decline may be due to natural selection, in that people with diabetes-prone genotypes with a high-calorie, low-activity lifestyle might have *fewer* children than other Nauruans who don't have this genotype. In such a situation, the 'thrifty' genotype would gradually decline in frequency in the population, and so would the incidence of diabetes.

[2]This is a distinct form of diabetes which is not caused by insulin deficiency, in contrast to the insulin-dependent form of diabetes, the condition described in Chapter 7 of this book.

In Western populations, the 'thrifty' genotype may have decreased in frequency over a much longer period of stable food supply, when it was no longer advantageous. There is little hard evidence to support this hypothetical evolutionary explanation of events on Nauru, but we can identify two important general points in this example: the *interdependence* of cultural and genetic evolution, and the potential *speed* of genetic evolution under strong selective pressure from sudden cultural change.

Speculating about the future evolution of human genes is a risky venture, but Steve Jones, a leading British geneticist, has attempted to do this in the final chapter of his book *The Language of the Genes* (published in 1992, based on his Reith Lectures broadcast by the BBC in 1991). An extract from the last chapter, entitled 'The evolution of Utopia', appears in the Reader.[3] You should read it now and then answer the following questions.

□ What effect on the frequency of serious human genetic diseases, such as cystic fibrosis, does Steve Jones predict will occur when medical treatments enable children with previously fatal disease alleles to survive and reproduce, thereby passing on their genes?

■ He thinks it will have little effect for three reasons. First, most serious genetic diseases are caused by *recessive* alleles and disease results only if *two* copies of the disease allele are inherited; most of the copies of these alleles in the population occur in unaffected 'carriers', so increasing the total number of disease survivors in the population will produce little increase in the total number of disease alleles. Second, the increase in the number of disease alleles passed on to the next generation by affected people (who survive to reproduce as a consequence of medical treatment) is likely to be offset by a decrease in the birth of affected babies, as more genetic advice is available to potential parents, who then decide against having affected children. Third, increased population movements and intermarriage between people from different parts of the world greatly *decreases* the chance of two carriers of a disease allele having a child.

□ What cultural change does Jones predict will have a significant effect on the frequency of human genetic diseases arising by new mutations?

[3]*Health and Disease: A Reader* (1994 edition).

■ The falling age at which people now *complete* their families will reduce the mutation rate. (Even though the age at which parents have their *first* child is tending to increase, the age at which they have their *last* child has fallen sharply.) The gametes of younger parents are less likely to carry mutations and hence new disease alleles will arise less often.

□ Jones thinks that the pace of human evolution is slowing down, for three reasons. What are they?

■ First, remember that natural selection acts on genetic variations between individuals, which are partly determined by the rate of new mutations. Jones thinks that industrial sources of radiation and chemicals have a much smaller effect on the mutation rate than do natural sources (such as radon gas leaking from granite) so, even as industrialisation spreads, the effect on mutation rate will be insignificant. At the same time, falling parental age (mentioned above) will tend to reduce the mutation rate. Lower mutation rate means less genetic variability for natural selection to act on and hence the pace of human evolution will slow down.

Second, important genetic differences between individuals in terms of evolution are those affecting their fertility and the survival rates of their offspring. Jones points out that, as people have fewer children, most of whom survive, these evolutionarily significant differences are tending to decrease. Greater longevity and the decline of infectious diseases in many parts of the world mean that genetic differences between individuals will tend to affect susceptibility to the degenerative diseases of the *post-reproductive* years, when natural selection cannot act directly.

Third, he argues that random genetic change will also be less likely as genetically isolated small population groups disappear (a point also made at the end of Chapter 4 of this book).

The impact of modern culture on human health

Since the Industrial Revolution, average life expectancy has increased through the combined effects of improved diet (in quality, quantity and predictability), sanitation and protection from pathogens, protection from physical environmental extremes (e.g. by improved housing) and medical innovation and access to health services.[4] Much of the disease burden in modern culture now occurs in old age. Ageing is associated with the degeneration of many different biological processes and systems, as Chapter 8 described. There is currently much research and debate over the extent to which age-associated disease, as well as its progression to disability, is potentially preventable (or postponable) by social and medical interventions or lifestyle changes during youth, as well as during old age. The evolutionary heritage of 'post-reproductive degeneration' need not be seen as inevitable; as with all biological processes, genes and environment have a complex interaction and we can alter the expression of our genes by changing our environment.

We can consider the 'environment' in three categories: the physical and chemical (usually abbreviated to physico–chemical) environment, the biological environment, and the psycho–social environment.

Cultural change and the physico–chemical environment

Industrialisation has been characterised by a rapid use of resources beyond their capacity for self-renewal, the production of a range of synthetic chemicals, and the production of wastes at a rate too great for their absorption in the environment. The negative impact of these processes on human health via changes in the *physico–chemical environment* (including both the direct and indirect health effects discussed in Chapter 10), depends on society's ability or will to regulate industrial processes.

What factors have limited the regulation of industry and its waste emissions? There are complex economic and political conditions and forces (which are discussed elsewhere in this series[5]), and which are worth thinking about again when you have finished this chapter. In the poorer newly-industrialising countries, the situation is particularly serious, since these communities have the least power to ensure that the negative effects of industrialisation are reduced to a 'reasonable' level.

[4]For a comprehensive discussion of the relative contributions of these factors to changes in the health profile of the United Kingdom during and since the Industrial Revolution, see *World Health and Disease*, Chapters 5 and 6, and *Caring for Health: History and Diversity*, Chapters 3 to 7.

[5]See *World Health and Disease*, Chapters 7, 8 and 11, and *Caring for Health: History and Diversity*, Chapters 8 and 9.

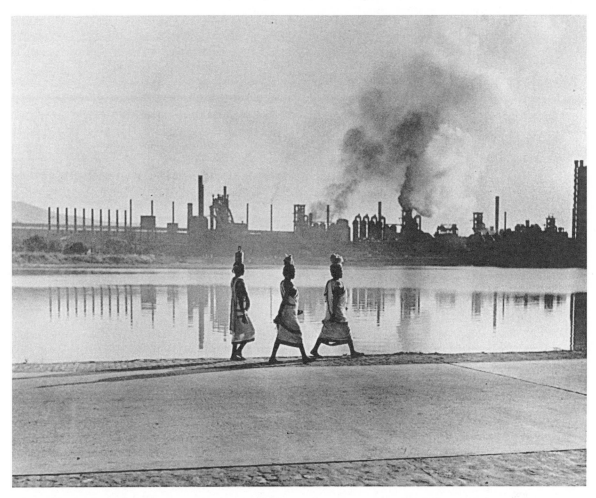

What is the impact of industrialisation on local communities? Local women go about their daily activities next to the Jamshedpur steel works in India. (Photo: Werner Bischof/Magnum)

Unfortunately, we are also limited by our lack of knowledge of the health effects of many environmental contaminants, and this lack of knowledge further limits the ability of citizens to ensure that costs and benefits of industrial activities and processes are properly balanced. Issues such as global warming and ozone depletion are beset with difficulties, not just in understanding the relationship between environmental change and health, but in predicting just what that environmental change will be. (The article by Alexander Leaf which you read with Chapter 10 illustrates this difficulty.)

Cultural change and the biological environment

Human health depends on the *biological environment* for food, for oxygen produced by plants and phytoplankton,

and for recreation. The biological environment in the form of the vast range of pathogens also presents some of the greatest challenges to human health. The biological environment is being affected by changes in the physical and chemical environment: for example, in the use of pesticides to increase crop yields, by the effects of chemical pollution on plants and animals and, on a larger scale, by the possible effects of global warming on the distribution and survival of pathogenic organisms and food sources. It is also subject to direct destruction or manipulation; agricultural practices (such as the chopping down of rainforests for farming in Brazil) may result in direct environmental degradation, as can population pressure and sprawling urbanisation on fragile or marginally fertile areas. Problems of sanitation, particularly in urban areas, outweigh the health effects of industrial pollution in developing countries.

The exploitation of genetic variability in other species has been at the basis of agriculture and drug development, and the reduction of biological diversity (biodiversity) is therefore of great concern, not only for its own sake, but for its implications for human wellbeing. As you saw in Chapter 5, coevolution with pathogens is a driving force in evolutionary change, and may even be the basis of the evolution of sexual reproduction itself. Humans are interfering with this coevolution by introducing very strong and uniform selective pressures on pathogens. One example is the use of antibiotics, which was discussed in Chapter 5.

□ How do bacteria become resistant to antibiotics?

■ Within each population of bacteria, there is a range of resistance to antibiotics. Bacteria have very short generation times, so unless all are destroyed by the drug, the most resistant survivors will rapidly increase in subsequent generations. In addition, in each generation there is an opportunity for a new mutation to arise, which gives the mutant bacterium greater or even total resistance to the antibiotic, greatly increasing its reproductive success and the survival of its genes.

The simplest part for humans to play in the 'coevolutionary race' is to keep changing the antibiotic and so keep one step ahead of the bacteria, but this is very difficult and expensive. Other strategies are: give several different antibiotics at once, so that any bacterium has to have more than one mutation to overcome the effect and survive; to use antibiotics less often and only when absolutely necessary so that bacteria are unlikely to encounter them and become resistant; and to improve hygiene conditions, especially in hospitals, so that bacteria become less of a disease threat, irrespective of the use of antibiotics.

Two examples of humans interfering with coevolution between hosts (in this case, the crops grown by humans) and their pathogens are: first, agricultural *monoculture* (the continuous growing of one type of crop), and second, the use of pesticides. Humans can only exert artificial control over pathogens for so long before they evolve the necessary changes to become resistant to our methods of control. Unless we can continually devise alternative means of control, the pathogens will win! Human ability to devise new methods of affecting the biological environment to reduce the threat of pathogens is endangered by the depletion of the reserves of genetic variability in nature which we could attempt to exploit. The preservation of biodiversity may be in our own interest.

Cultural change and the psycho–social environment

One of the more complex areas of human biology is that of the biological basis of stress and psychological adaptation, or the interaction of mind and body. This is part of what is often termed the *psycho–social environment*. Modern culture is characterised by speed, not only the speed of our communication networks which require constant response, but also the speed of change in the form of technological developments and the structure of society and social support. How this can affect human health via psychological effects is beyond the scope of this book, but is as important a part of human biology as the other factors we have discussed.[6]

We should mention a specific area of social interaction, that of human conflict. While conflict in the rest of the animal kingdom is limited to direct contact between animals, human conflict is distinguished by the sophisticated use of 'tools' of warfare, and modern culture has produced the escalation of these tools of warfare to weapons of potential mass destruction. Health effects are not only those that directly result from use of such weapons, but also those that result from the massive diversion of resources from welfare-related productivity to the arms industry, and the destruction of people's homes and livelihoods. In addition, war can wreak destruction on the physico–chemical and biological environments.

War, however, is not the only means by which one group of humans can cause the destruction of another. The massive reduction in the populations of Native Americans and Aborigines in Australia, for example, has resulted not only from genocide, but from the results of exposure to new diseases (as you read in Chapter 5), economic impoverishment, and the health problems that result from disintegration of cultural identity. Modern Western culture also poses a continuing threat to the health of many populations in the Third World, since its 'success' is currently underpinned by the unequal distribution of resources.

Some of the limitations of human biology can be overcome by cultural developments, but it is notable how

[6]The effect of stress in the workplace on human health is discussed in *Birth to Old Age: Health in Transition* (1985, and revised edition 1995).

inequitable the effects can be for different population groups, and how inadequate is our knowledge of the complexities of human ecology for predicting the consequences of our actions. The future of human life on Earth need not be determined by blind natural selection, but there are many challenges in developing an informed and ethical structure for human cultural evolution, which will lead to an overall improvement of human health in its broadest sense, while preserving biological diversity. Using what you have learnt in this and other books in this series, you may like to reflect on whether 'nature knows best'.

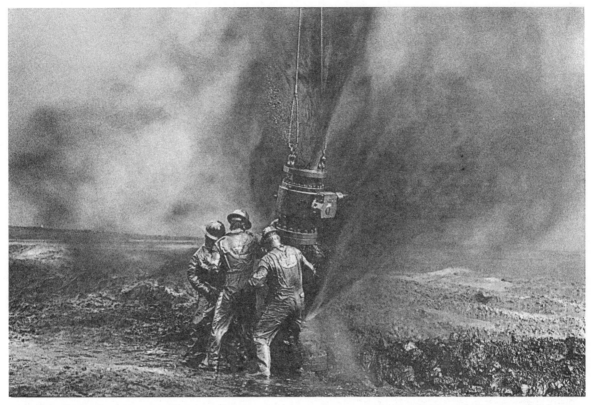

As the army of Iraq retreated from Kuwait at the end of the Gulf War in 1990, more than 500 oil wells were set ablaze, sending millions of tons of burning oil into the atmosphere. It took over a year for all the wells to be capped; the environmental damage is incalculable as are the indirect effects on health, not only of the pollution but of the war itself. (Photo: Sebastiao Salgado/Magnum)

OBJECTIVE FOR CHAPTER 11

When you have studied this chapter, you should be able to:

11.1 Distinguish between genetic and cultural evolution and give examples of ways in which they interact with each other and with the environment in affecting human health and disease; comment on ways in which modern culture may have an impact on human evolution in the future.

QUESTION FOR CHAPTER 11

Question 1 (*Objective 11.1*)

In times of persistent plenty, Nauruans with the diabetes-prone 'thrifty' genotype may be at a reproductive disadvantage compared with others in the population who lack it. Yet in the research article in which J. V. Neel first proposed the thrifty genotype hypothesis to explain the epidemic of diabetes on Nauru, he stated that:

> …efforts to preserve the diabetes genotype through this transient period of plenty are in the interests of mankind. (Neel, 1962)

(a) Justify this statement and use the Nauruan example to illustrate the interaction between genotype, phenotype and environment.

(b) Explain why, in times of persistent plenty, the thrifty genotype cannot be preserved through natural selection. How then might it be preserved?

Appendix

Table of abbreviations used in this book

Abbreviation	What it stands for
A	adenine
ADD	adenosine deaminase deficiency
AIDS	acquired immunodeficiency syndrome
ALARA principle	as low as is reasonably achievable
ATP	adenosine triphosphate
B cell	bone-marrow derived lymphocyte
BATNEEC principle	best available technology not entailing excessive cost
C	carbon
C	cytosine
CHD	coronary heart disease
CO	carbon monoxide
CO_2	carbon dioxide
CVS	chorionic villi sampling
DNA	deoxyribonucleic acid
G	guanine
H_2	hydrogen gas
H_2O	water
HFEA	Human Fertilisation and Embryology Authority
HIV	human immunodeficiency virus
HRT	hormone replacement therapy

Abbreviation	What it stands for
LA	lactose absorption phenotype
LM	lactose malabsorption phenotype
MDR	multi-drug resistant (strains of bacteria)
mRNA	messenger RNA
N_2	nitrogen gas
NHS	National Health Service
NK cell	natural killer cell
O	oxygen
OPCS	Office of Population Censuses and Surveys
PCB	polychlorinated biphenyl
PKU	phenylketonuria
RNA	ribonucleic acid
STD	sexually-transmitted disease
T	thymine
T cell	thymus-derived lymphocyte
TB	tuberculosis
TCP	trichlorophenol
UV	ultraviolet (radiation)
UV(B)	a particular band of UV radiation
WHO	World Health Organisation

References and further reading

References

Ames, B. N., Magow, R. and Gold, L. S. (1987) Ranking possible carcinogenic hazards, *Science*, **236**, pp. 233–364.

Anderson, H. R. (1989) Is the prevalence of asthma changing? *Archives of Disease in Childhood*, **64**, pp. 172–5.

Anderson, R. M. and May, R. M. (1991) *Infectious Diseases of Humans*, Oxford University Press, Oxford.

Barinaga, M. (1991) Research News section: How long is the human life-span? *Science*, **254**, 15 November, pp. 936–8.

Begon, M., Harper, J. L. and Townsend, C. R. (1990) *Ecology: Individuals, Populations and Communities*, 2nd edn (1st edn, 1986), Blackwell Scientific Publications, Oxford.

Beral, V., Roman, E. and Bobrow, M. (eds) (1993) *Childhood Cancer and Nuclear Installations*, BMJ Publishing Group, London.

Bianchi, D. W., Bernfield, M. and Nathan, D. G. (1993) A revived opportunity for fetal research, *Nature*, **363**, 6 May, p. 12.

Bogin, B. (1993) Why must I be a teenager at all? *New Scientist*, 3 March, pp. 34–8; reprinted in Davey, B., Gray, A. and Seale, C. (eds) (1994), *Health and Disease: A Reader*, 2nd edn, Open University Press, Buckingham.

Brundtland, G. H. *et al.* (1980) Height, weight and menarcheal age of Oslo school children during the past 60 years, *Annals of Human Biology*, **7**, pp. 307–22.

Campbell, N. A. (ed.) (1993) *Biology*, 3rd edn, The Benjamin/Cummings Publishing Company, Inc., Redwood City, California and Wokingham, Surrey.

Caren, L. D. (1991) Effects of exercise on the human immune system, *BioScience*, **41**(6), pp. 410–5.

Carey, J. R., Liedo, P., Orozco, D. and Vaupel, J. W. (1992) Slowing of mortality rates at older ages in large Medfly cohorts, *Science*, **258**, pp. 457–61.

Cohen, S. and Williamson, G. M. (1991) Stress and infectious disease in humans, *Psychological Bulletin*, **109**, pp. 5–24.

Coleman, M. and Beral, V. (1988) A review of epidemiological studies of the health effects of living near or working with electricity generation and transmission equipment, *International Journal of Epidemiology*, **17**, pp. 1–13.

Cournoyer, D. and Caskey, C. T. (1990) Gene transfer into humans, *New England Journal of Medicine*, **323**, pp. 601–2.

Coutelle, C., Caplan, N., Hart, S., Huxley, C. and Williamson, R. (1993) Gene therapy for cystic fibrosis, *Archives of Disease in Childhood*, **68**, pp. 437–43.

Crombleholme, T. M., Langer, J. C., Harrison, M. R. and Zanjani, E. D. (1991) Transplantation of fetal cells, *American Journal of Obstetrics and Gynecology*, **164**, pp. 218–30.

Cuatrecasas, P., Lockwood, D. H. and Caldwell, J. R. (1965) Lactase deficiency in the adult, *Lancet*, **7375**, pp. 14–18.

Curtsinger, J. W., Fukui, H. H., Townsend, D. R. and Vaupel, J. W. (1992) Demography of genotypes: failure of the limited lifespan paradigm in *Drosophila melanogaster*, *Science*, **258**, pp. 461–3.

Daintith, J. and Isaacs, A. (1989) *Medical Quotations*, Collins Reference Dictionary, Collins, London and Glasgow.

Davies, C. T. M. and Young, K. (1983) Effect of temperature on the contractile properties and muscle power of *triceps sorae* in humans, *Journal of Applied Physiology*, **55**, pp. 191–5.

Davies, K. J. A., Quintanilha, A. T., Brooks, G. A. and Packer, A. (1982) Free radicals and tissue damage produced by exercise, *Biochemical and Biophysical Research Communications*, **107**, pp. 1198–205.

Dawkins, R. (1976) *The Selfish Gene*, Oxford University Press, Oxford.

Department of the Environment (1989) *Dioxins in the Environment: Report of an Interdepartmental Working Group on PCDDs and PCDFs*, Pollution Paper No. 27, HMSO, London.

Diamond, J. (1992) Diabetes running wild, *Nature*, **357**, pp. 362–3.

Dobson, A. (1992) People and disease, Chapter 10.4 in Jones, S., Martin, R., Pilbeam, D. and Bunney, S. (eds), *The Cambridge Encyclopedia of Human Evolution*, Cambridge University Press, Cambridge.

Doll, R. and Peto, R. (1981a) *The Causes of Cancer*, Blackwell Scientific Publications, Oxford.

Doll, R. and Peto, R. (1981(b)) The causes of cancer: quantitative estimates of avoidable risks of cancer in the United States today, *Journal of the National Cancer Institute*, **66**(6), pp. 1191–308.

Dowse, G. and Zimmet, P. (1993) The thrifty genotype in non-insulin dependent diabetes, *British Medical Journal*, **306**, pp. 532–3.

Durham, W. H. (1991) *Coevolution, Genes, Culture and Human Diversity*, Stanford University Press, Stanford, California.

Ewald, P. W. (1993) The evolution of virulence, *Scientific American*, April, pp. 56–62.

Fiennes, R. N. T. W. (1978) *Zoonoses and the Origins and Ecology of Human Disease*, Academic Press, London.

Følling, A. (1934) Über Ausscheidung von Phenylbrenztraubensaüre in den Harn als Stoffwechselanomalie in Verbidung mit Imbezillität, *Hoppe-Seyler's Z. Physiol. Chem.*, **227**, pp. 169–76.

Friedman, D. B. and Johnson, T. E. (1988) A mutation in the *age-1* gene in *Caenorhabditis elegans* lengthens life and reduces hermaphrodite fertility, *Genetics*, **118**, pp. 75–86.

Gage, F. H. (1993) Fetal implants put to the test, *Nature*, **361**, 4 February, pp. 405–6.

Gardner, M. J., Snee, M. P., Hall, A. J., Powell, C. A., Dounes, S. and Terrell, J. D. (1990) Result of case-control study of leukaemia and lymphoma among young people near Sellafield nuclear plant in West Cumbria, *British Medical Journal*, **300**, pp. 423–9.

Goldstein, J. L. and Brown, M. S. (1989) Familial hyper-cholesterolaemia, in Scriver, C. R., Beaudet, A. L., Sly, W. S. and Valle, D. (eds) *The Metabolic Basis of Disease*, 6th edn, McGraw-Hill, New York.

Hamilton, W. D. and Zuk, M. (1982) Heritable true fitness and bright birds: a role for parasites, *Science*, **218**, pp. 384–7.

Harper, P. S. (1992) Genetic testing and insurance, *Journal of the Royal College of Physicians*, **26**, pp. 184–7.

Harper P. S. (1993) Insurance and genetic testing, *Lancet*, **341**, pp. 224–7.

Harris, R. (1988) Genetic counselling and the new genetics, *Trends in Genetics*, **4**, pp. 52–6.

Hebb, D. O. (1953) Heredity and environment in mammalian behaviour, *British Journal of Animal Behaviour*, **1**, pp. 43–7.

Herzog, V., Sies, H. and Miller, F. (1976) Exocytosis in secretory cells of rat lacrimal gland, *Journal of Cell Biology*, **70**, pp. 692–706.

Human Fertilisation and Embryology Authority (1994) *Donated Ovarian Tissue in Embryo Research and Assisted Conception*, Human Fertilisation and Embryology Authority, London.

Jones, S. (1993) *The Language of the Genes*, HarperCollins, London (hardback) and (1994) Flamingo, London (paperback); extracts from Ch. 16 'The evolution of Utopia', reprinted in Davey, B., Gray, A. and Seale, C. (eds) (1994), *Health and Disease: A Reader*, 2nd edn, Open University Press, Buckingham.

Jones, S., Martin R., Pilbeam, D. and Bunney, S. (eds) (1992) *The Cambridge Encyclopedia of Human Evolution*, Cambridge University Press, Cambridge.

Kirkwood, T. G. L. (1992) Biological origins of ageing, Chapter 2.1 in Evans, J. G. and Williams, T. F. (eds) *Oxford Textbook of Geriatric Medicine*, Oxford University Press, Oxford.

Komrower, G. M. (1984) Phenylketonuria and other inherited metabolic defects, in Wald, N. J. (ed.) *Antenatal and Neonatal Screening*, Oxford University Press, Oxford.

Lancet editorial (1992) Screening for cystic fibrosis, *Lancet*, **340**, June 25th, pp. 209–10.

Leaf, A. (1989) Potential health effects of global climatic and environmental changes, *New England Journal of Medicine*, **321**, pp. 1577–83.

Lerner, I. M. and Libby, W. J. (1976) *Heredity, Evolution and Society*, 2nd edn, W. H. Freeman, San Francisco.

Lilienfeld, D. E. and Gallo, M. A. (1989) 2,4-D, 2,4,5-T, and 2,3,7,8–TCDD: an overview, *Epidemiologic Reviews*, **11**, pp. 28–58.

Lindgren, G. (1976) Height, weight and menarche in Swedish urban school children in relation to socio-economic and regional factors, *Annals of Human Biology*, **3**, pp. 501–28.

Lopez, A. D. (1993) Causes of death in the industrialised and developing countries: estimates for 1985, in Jamison, D. T. and Mosely, H. (eds) *Disease Control Priorities in Developing Countries*, Oxford University Press, New York.

Loudon, I. (1984) The history of pernicious anaemia from 1822 to the present day, in Black, N. *et al.*, (eds) *Health and Disease: A Reader*, 1st edn, and in Davey, B., Gray, A. and Seale, C. (eds) (1994), *Health and Disease: A Reader*, 2nd edn, Open University Press, Buckingham.

Luckinbill, L. S., Graves, J. L., Reed, A. H. and Koetsawang, S. (1988) Localizing genes that defer senescence in *Drosophila melanogaster*, *Heredity*, **60**, pp. 367–74.

Martin, G. M. (1978) Genetic syndromes in man with potential relevance to the pathobiology of aging, *Birth Defects: Original Article Series*, **14**, pp. 5–39.

Martin, R. D. (1992) Primate locomotion and posture, Chapter 2.8 in Jones, S., Martin, R., Pilbeam, D. and Bunney, S. (eds), *The Cambridge Encyclopedia of Human Evolution*, Cambridge University Press, Cambridge.

Masoro, E. J., Shimokawa, I. and Wu, B. P. (1991) Retardation of the ageing process in rats by food restriction, *Annals of the New York Academy of Sciences*, **621**, pp. 337–52.

May, R. M. (1992) How many species inhabit the Earth?, *Scientific American*, **267**(4), pp. 18–24.

McGue, M., Vaupel, J. W., Holm, N. and Harvald, B. (1993) Longevity is moderately heritable in a sample of Danish twins, *Journal of Gerontology*, **48**(6), pp. 237–44.

McKeown, T. (1976) *The Modern Rise of Population*, Edward Arnold, London; edited version of Chapter 5 appears as 'The medical contribution' in Black, N. *et al.*, (eds) *Health and Disease: A Reader*, 1st edn, and in Davey, B., Gray, A. and Seale, C. (eds) (1994), *Health and Disease: A Reader*, 2nd edn, Open University Press, Buckingham.

Meltzer, D. J. (1992) How Columbus sickened the New World, *New Scientist*, October, pp. 38–41.

Mennie, M. E., Gilfillan, A., Compton, M. *et al.* (1992) Prenatal screening for cystic fibrosis, *Lancet*, **340**, July 25th, pp. 214–6.

Mihill, C. (1993) 'Saving life the only issue in Laura Davies case, says doctor', *Guardian*, 28 September, p. 3.

Modell, B. (1983) Screening for carriers of recessive disease, in Carter, C. O. (ed.), *Developments in Human Reproduction and their Eugenic, Ethical Implications*, Academic Press, London.

Modell, B., Kuliev, A. M. and Wagner, M. (1992) *Community Genetics Services in Europe*, WHO Regional Publications, European series no. 38, WHO Regional Office for Europe, Copenhagen.

Moltz, H. (1993) Fever: causes and consequences, *Neuroscience and Behavioural Reviews*, **17**, pp. 237–69.

Müller-Hill, B. (1993) The shadow of genetic injustice, *Nature*, **362**, 8 April, pp. 491–2.

Neel, J. V. (1962) Diabetes mellitus: a thrifty genotype rendered detrimental by 'progress'?, *American Journal of Human Genetics*, **14**, pp. 353–62.

Nessell, C. S. and Gallo, M. A. (1992) Dioxins and related compounds, in Lippman, M. (ed.), *Environmental Toxicants, Human Exposures and their Health Effects*, Van Nostrand Reinhold, New York.

Nuffield Council on Bioethics (1993) *Genetic Screening: Ethical Issues*, Nuffield Council on Bioethics, London.

Office of Population Censuses and Surveys (1988) *The Prevalence of Disability among Adults*, OPCS Report No.1, HMSO, London.

Passmore, R. and Robson, J. S. (1980) *A Companion to Medical Studies, Volume 2, Pharmacology, Microbiology, General Pathology and Related Subjects,* 2nd edn, Blackwells Scientific Publications, Oxford.

Penrose, L. S. and Smith, G. F. (1966) *Down's Anomaly,* 1st edn, Churchill Livingstone, Edinburgh (2nd edn, 1976).

Perry, M. M. and Gilbert, A. B. (1979) Yolk transport in the ovarian follicle of the hen *(Gallus domesticus)*: lipoprotein-like particles at the periphery of the oocyte in the rapid growth phase, *Journal of Cell Science,* **39**, pp. 257–72.

Raff, M. C. (1992) Social controls on cell survival and cell death, *Nature,* **356**, April 2nd, pp. 397–400.

Rietschel, E. T. and Brade, H. (1992) Bacterial endotoxins, *Scientific American,* August, pp. 26–33.

Rosenberg, L. E. (1990) Treating genetic disease: lessons from three children, *Pediatric Research,* **27**, pp. S10–S16.

Royal College of Physicians (1989) *Prenatal Diagnosis and Genetic Screening, Community and Service Implications,* RCP, London.

Rusting, R. L. (1992) Why do we age?, *Scientific American,* December, pp. 86–95.

Sharon, N. and Lis, H. (1993) Carbohydrates in cell recognition, *Scientific American,* January, pp. 74–81.

Sharpe, R. M. and Skakkebaek, N. E. (1993) Are oestrogens involved in falling sperm counts and disorders of the male reproductive tract?, *Lancet,* **341**, pp. 1392–5.

Simoons, F. J. (1978) The geographic hypothesis and lactose malabsorption: a weighting of the evidence, *American Journal of Digestive Diseases,* **23**, pp. 963–80.

Spears, N., Boland, N. I., Murray, A. A. and Gosden, R. G. (1994) Mouse oocytes derived from *in vitro* grown primary ovarian follicles are fertile, *Human Reproduction,* **9**(3), in press.

Stern, C. (1973) *Principles of Human Genetics,* 3rd edn, W. H. Freeman, San Francisco.

Strassburg, M. A. (1982) The global eradication of smallpox, *American Journal of Infection Control,* **19**, pp. 53–9; reprinted in Black, N. *et al.,* (eds) *Health and Disease: A Reader,* 1st edn, and in Davey, B., Gray, A. and Seale, C. (eds) (1994), *Health and Disease: A Reader,* 2nd edn, Open University Press, Buckingham.

Strehler, B. L., Mark, D. D., Mildvan, A. S. and Gee, M. V. (1959) Rate and magnitude of age pigment accumulation in the human myocardium, *Journal of Gerontology,* **14**, pp. 430–9.

Strickberger, M. W. (1990) *Evolution,* Jones and Bartlett, Boston, Massachusetts.

Suzuki, D. T., Griffiths, A. J. F. and Lewontin, R. C. (1981) *An Introduction to Genetic Analysis,* 2nd edn, W. H. Freeman, San Francisco.

Tanner, J. M. (1992) Human growth and development, Chapter 2.13 in Jones, S., Martin, R., Pilbeam, D. and Bunney, S. (eds), *The Cambridge Encyclopedia of Human Evolution,* Cambridge University Press, Cambridge.

Thornton, R. (1987) *American Indian Holocaust and Survival: A Population History since 1492,* University of Oklahoma Press, Norman, Oklahoma and London.

U205 Course Team (1985) *The Biology of Health and Disease,* Open University Press, Milton Keynes.

Voltaire, F. M. A. de, (1759) *Candide,* translated by Lowell Bair (1959 edn), Bantam Books, New York.

Warner, H. J., Campisi, V., Cristafalo, R. *et al.* (1992) Control of cell proliferation in senescent cells, *Journal of Gerontology: Biological Sciences,* **47**(6), pp. B185–9.

Watson, J. D. and Crick, F. H. C. (1953) Molecular structure of nucleic acids: a structure for deoxyribose nucleic acid, *Nature,* **171**, 25 April, pp. 737–8.

Williamson, R. (1993) Universal community carrier screening for cystic fibrosis?, *Nature Genetics,* **3**, March, pp. 195–201.

World Health Organisation (1958) *Constitution of the World Health Organisation,* Annex 1, WHO, Geneva.

World Health Organisation (1992) *Our Planet, Our Health,* Report of the WHO Commission on Health and Environment, Geneva.

Yorke, J. A. and London, W. P. (1973) Recurrent outbreaks of measles, chickenpox and mumps: II, Systematic differences in contact rates and stochastic effects, *American Journal of Epidemiology,* **98**, pp. 469–82.

Young, S. (1993) Against ageing, in 'Mind and Body', *New Scientist* supplement, April 17th, pp. 10–12.

Further reading

General

The following books and articles are highly recommended to anyone who wishes to read very broadly about human evolutionary biology and the interaction with human culture; they are relevant to many of the chapters in *Human Biology and Health: An Evolutionary Approach.* They are followed by further reading of a more specialist nature, linked to specific chapters.

Boyden, S. (1987; reprinted 1992) *Western Civilization in Biological Perspective,* Clarendon Press, Oxford. An exploration of the interplay between biological and cultural processes in human affairs, from the early evolution of *Homo sapiens* to the present day.

Campbell, N. A. (ed.) (1993) *Biology,* 3rd edn, The Benjamin/Cummings Publishing Company, Inc. Redwood City, California and Wokingham, Surrey. A wonderfully illustrated and produced general textbook of biology, at an astonishingly low price for such a weighty hardback. Each main section (for example, on the cell, the gene, animal and plant form and function, and on evolutionary history) is written by leading biologists, including David Suzuki and Stephen Jay Gould. Each section begins with an interview with the author about their life's work and their personal speculations on the future of their subject. The book takes an evolutionary perspective throughout and is highly recommended.

Cohen, M. N. (1989) *Health and the Rise of Civilization,* Yale University Press, New Haven and London. A historian's view of human health through the ages, and of attempts to avoid, eradicate or cure disease.

Diamond, J. (1991) *The Rise and Fall of the Third Chimpanzee,* Vintage, London (paperback). A wide-ranging, popular vision of human evolution with an overview of history and speculation about the future of our species, written by a distinguished physiologist and ornithologist.

Jones, S. (1993) *The Language of the Genes,* HarperCollins (hardback) and (1994) Flamingo (paperback with amendments and additional bibliographic essay). Based on the highly-acclaimed BBC Reith Lectures, broadcast by Steve Jones in 1991, this readable and fascinating book covers the scope of modern genetics from the fine details of individual genes to the broad sweep of human evolution and its interaction with human culture. It is readily accessible to non-biologists and contains a wealth of illuminating examples, anecdotes from history, references to literature and much else besides, written in the author's direct and amusing style which reveals his penetrating insight into human society as well as human biology.

Jones, S., Martin, R., Pilbeam, D. and Bunney, S. (eds) (1992) *The Cambridge Encyclopedia of Human Evolution,* Cambridge University Press, Cambridge. A wide-ranging introduction to the human species that places modern humans in an evolutionary perspective. This definitive text on human evolution, although enormous, is broken down into sections by theme, each subdivided into short and accessible chapters on specific topics contributed by experts in (among others) genetics, functional anatomy, palaeontology, anthropology, archaeology, medicine and agriculture.

McKeown, T. (1988) *The Origins of Human Disease,* Basil Blackwell Ltd., Oxford (paperback). A physician's account of the many causes of disease in humans from primeval to modern society, and of habits and policies that reduce or perpetuate disease.

McMichael, A. J. (1993) *Planetary Overload: Global Environmental Change and the Health of the Human Species,* Cambridge University Press, Cambridge. A discussion of global environmental problems and their consequences for health within an ecological framework.

McNeill, W. H. (1976) *Plagues and Peoples,* Basil Blackwell Ltd, Oxford (paperback). A historian's account of the incidence of disease from prehistory to the beginning of the twentieth century, and its military and political consequences.

Meltzer, D. J. (1992) How Columbus sickened the New World, *New Scientist,* October, pp. 38–41. A readily obtainable article that discusses why early European settlers in the USA passed serious infectious diseases to native Americans, and why this was a largely one-way process. Most central libraries have this journal in their reference section.

Chapter 2

Much of the information in Chapter 2 is derived from texts already listed in the General section above: Cohen, M. N. (1989), Diamond, J. (1991), Jones, S., Martin, R., Pilbeam, D. and Bunney, S. (eds) (1992), McKeown, T. (1988), and McNeill, W. H. (1976), and from the books listed below, which provide far more detail and assume much more background knowledge, than the Open University's *Health and Disease* course requires.

Clutton–Brock, J. (1987) *A Natural History of Domesticated Mammals,* Cambridge University Press, Cambridge (paperback). A popular, profusely illustrated account of the origin and modern biology of domesticated animals.

Fiennes, R. N. T. W. (1978) *Zoonoses and the Origins and Ecology of Human Disease,* Academic Press, London. The definitive study of how and when diseases transfer between people and animals, based upon a lifetime's experience of veterinary medicine in zoo and wild animals.

Heiser, C. B. (1981) *Seeds to Civilization: The Story of Food,* W. H. Freeman and Co., San Francisco (paperback). A botanist's popular account of the wild origins, domestication and modern cultivation of major food crops.

Lewin, R. (1984) *Human Evolution: An Illustrated Introduction,* Blackwell Scientific Publications, Oxford (paperback). The biological mechanisms and palaeontological record of human evolution, as told by an anthropologist.

Chapter 3

Campbell, N. A. (ed.) (1993), already listed in the General section above, is an excellent general textbook of biology.

Chapter 4

The most relevant texts are listed in the General section above: Diamond, J. (1991), Jones, S. (1992), and Jones, S., Martin, R., Pilbeam, D. and Bunney, S. (eds) (1992). In addition, we recommend:

Thompson, M., McInnes, R. R. and Willard, H. F. (eds) (1991) *Genetics in Medicine,* Saunders, Philadelphia. A medical genetics textbook with good broad coverage of the field, which goes beyond the scope of the material in Chapter 4.

Chapter 5

See Meltzer (1992), listed in the General section above, together with the following:

Brown, P. (1992) The return of the big killer, *New Scientist,* October, pp. 30–7. A readily obtainable article that discusses the reasons why tuberculosis is once again becoming a major problem in developed countries, such as the United States, from which it was previously largely eradicated. Most central libraries have this leading journal in their reference section.

Ewald, P. W. (1993) The evolution of virulence, *Scientific American,* April, pp. 56–62. A readily obtainable article that reviews the evidence that pathogenic organisms may become either more or less virulent in response to selection pressures imposed by their environment. Most central libraries have this leading journal in their reference section.

Hamilton, W. D. and Zuk, M. (1982) Heritable true fitness and bright birds: a role for parasites, *Science,* **218**, pp. 384–7. A very significant paper in evolutionary theory, which sets out the theoretical argument that bright plumage in male birds indicates to females that they carry low infestations of parasites. Most central libraries have this leading journal in their reference section.

Hudson, P. J., Dobson, A. P. and Newborn, D. (1992) Do parasites make prey vulnerable to predation? Red grouse and parasites, *Journal of Animal Ecology,* **61**, pp. 681–92. A paper reporting a field study of how parasites affect the behaviour of red grouse in northern England and, in consequence, influence the risk of the grouse being taken by predators; the authors raise general issues about the relationship of parasites to predation.

Lively, C. M. (1987) Evidence from a New Zealand snail for the maintenance of sex by parasitism, *Nature,* **328**, pp. 519–21. The hypothesis that sexual reproduction is an adaptation against the harmful effects of parasites is clearly difficult to investigate, but supportive evidence is reported in this study of New Zealand snails, which use sexual reproduction where parasites are abundant and asexual reproduction where parasites are rare. Most central libraries have this leading journal in their reference section.

Chapter 6

Cohen, S. and Williamson, G. M. (1991) Stress and infectious disease in humans, *Psychological Bulletin,* **109**, pp. 5–24. A comprehensive review of experiments to determine whether or not stress leads to an increase in the incidence of infection. The authors explain the difficulties of investigating this question scientifically, and make clear the all-important distinction between, on the one hand, demonstrating (as many have done) that the immune system changes under stress and, on the other hand, showing that this has any consequences for human health.

Davey, B. (1989) *Immunology: A Foundation Text,* Open University Press, Milton Keynes and Bristol. Written by an Open University lecturer for a third-level OU course, this paperback is aimed at biology undergraduates, nurses, medical students and anyone who requires a general introduction to the theory and practice of immunology. Each chapter has objectives and self-assessment questions.

Roitt, I. (1994) *Essential Immunology,* 8th edn, Blackwell Scientific Publications, Oxford. Probably the most popular and influential textbook of basic immunology. The subject is taught to first degree (and in places to postgraduate) level and yet will be accessible to anyone with a basic grounding in biology; its accessibility rests on a clearly and often amusingly written text, supported by excellent diagrams and photographs. The author regularly updates this highly-recommended textbook, so check if a more recent edition has been published.

Scientific American Special Issue (1993) Life, death and the immune system, September. An excellent collection of articles on a wide range of topics, including the development of the immune system and the nature of its defensive mechanisms; self-tolerance; the immune response to infection; autoimmune diseases and allergies; and the manipulation of the immune system in treatments for cancer and in organ transplant preservation. Well worth ordering from *Scientific American's* back-issue service.

Chapter 7

Vander, A. J., Sherman, J. H. and Luciano, D. S. (1986) *Human Physiology: the Mechanisms of Body Function,* McGraw–Hill Book Company, New York, London, etc., 4th edn (paperback). One of the best modern textbooks of human physiology, written primarily for nurses and other medical workers.

Chapter 8

Dice, J. F. (1993) Cellular and molecular mechanisms of ageing, *Physiological Reviews,* **73**(1), pp. 149–59. A review article that gives more detail of biological mechanisms than was possible in Chapter 8. It will be of particular interest to those with some prior knowledge of biology.

Martin, G. M. (1992) Biological mechanisms of ageing, Chapter 2.2 in Evans, J. G. and Williams, T. G. (eds), *Oxford Textbook of Geriatric Medicine,* Oxford University Press, Oxford. This review will be most relevant to anyone working in geriatric medicine, with a reasonable knowledge of biochemistry.

Olshansky, S. J., Carnes, B. A. and Cassel, C. K. (1993) The ageing of the human species, *Scientific American,* April, pp. 18–24. This is a clear account of demographic trends and evolutionary theories of ageing. This readily obtainable article also considers the social and ethical implications of an ageing human population.

Young, S. (1993) Against ageing, in 'Mind and Body', *New Scientist* supplement, April 17th, pp. 10–12. This article is written for non-biologists and is enjoyable and informative; most central libraries stock this journal.

Chapter 9

Certain of the texts already listed in the General section are also relevant here: Jones, S. (1993), Jones, S., Martin, R., Pilbeam, D. and Bunney, S. (eds) (1992); and from the Chapter 4 list see Thompson, M., McInnes, R. R. and Willard, H. F. (eds) (1991). In addition, we recommend:

Ciba Foundation Symposia 149 (1990) *Human Genetic Information: Science, Law and Ethics,* Wiley and Sons, London. This contains papers written by specialists from the diverse disciplines of molecular biology, medicine, philosophy, theology and law, who discuss the major scientific, legal, ethical, social and economic issues arising out of recent progress in mapping the locations of all the human genes and determining their nucleotide sequences. Although many technical terms are used in this collection, the breadth of coverage is excellent and it expands on a number of areas only mentioned briefly in Chapter 9, such as germline gene therapy, future trends in prenatal diagnosis, the legal implications of human genetic information and issues about who has the right to know the genetic constitution of an individual.

Friedman, T. (1989) Progress towards human gene therapy, *Science*; **244**, pp. 1275–82. A readily obtainable article (most central public libraries stock *Science,* the leading American scientific journal), which discusses the methods and the technical difficulties of human gene therapy in greater detail than was possible in Chapter 9.

Harper, P. S. (1993) *Practical Genetic Counselling,* 4th edn, Butterworth-Heinemann, Oxford. The author outlines the main steps in the process of genetic counselling and, though fairly technical, it is one of the few definitive texts in this area.

Harper, P. S . (1992) Genetic testing and insurance, *Journal of the Royal College of Physicians,* **26**, pp. 184-7, and/or Harper P. S. (1993) Insurance and genetic testing, *Lancet,* **341**, pp. 224–7. Peter Harper is a Professor at the Institute of Medical Genetics, University of Wales Medical School; in these two papers, written in a readily accessible style, he reviews the concerns of insurers, applicants for insurance, and health professionals with regard to genetic screening. The *Lancet* is stocked by most central public libraries.

Nuffield Council on Bioethics (1993) *Genetic Screening: Ethical Issues*, published by (and obtainable from) Nuffield Council on Bioethics, 28 Bedford Square, London WC1B 3EG (send cheque for £6.00). The Council was set up in 1991 to consider ethical issues presented by advances in biomedical and biological research, and chose genetic screening as the subject of its first report. The report includes a review of screening programmes in progress in the United Kingdom in 1993, and considers the ethical aspects of obtaining informed consent to screening, protecting confidentiality, the legal framework relating to employment and insurance, and issues of public policy.

Chapter 10

We recommend McMichael, A. J. (1993), listed in the General section, together with the following:

Lippman, M. (ed.) (1992) *Environmental Toxicants: Human Exposures and their Health Effects*, Van Nostrand Reinhold, New York. A reference book with each chapter reviewing an environmental toxicant, e.g. asbestos, benzene, carbon monoxide, dioxin, lead, electromagnetic fields, ozone and radon.

Elsom, D. M. (1992) *Atmospheric Pollution: A Global Problem*, 2nd edn, Blackwell, Oxford. A textbook looking at the causes, effects, and control of air pollution.

Timbrell, J. A. (1989) *Introduction to Toxicology*, Taylor and Francis, London. A review of toxicological principles, with specific chapters on drugs, industrial chemicals, food additives and contaminants and pesticides.

Chapter 11

See Boyden, S. (1987, reprinted 1992), listed in the General section.

Answers to self-assessment questions

Chapter 2

1 (a) Most primates, including nearly all monkeys, are active by day and live in tall trees where they locate their food, often coloured fruit or flowers, from some distance by sight. They jump across gaps between trees, where scent trails would be useless but good vision is essential. Many species also live in social groups and communicate with each other by means of visual signals such as facial expressions and gestures, as well as by sounds.

(b) The typical primate diet consists of soft, easily digested, fresh food, such as fruit, flowers, leaves and small animals which does not require massive teeth.

(c) Primates move by climbing and leaping, using their opposable fingers and toes to grasp branches, while they swing from their arms or tail. Fingernails and toenails are not used in climbing, but may facilitate delicate handling of small objects.

2 The upper part of the human pelvis became shorter and wider while the lower part became narrower than the pelvis of non-human primates (see Figure 2.1c). The spinal column became more curved, particularly at its lower end, and the sacrum broader. The ilium curved forwards around the contents of the abdomen, supporting larger muscles that stabilise the hip and thigh. These changes permitted humans to take longer, more powerful strides than is possible in apes.

However, the more compact human pelvis is less efficient for birth, particularly that of babies with enlarged heads; limited observational evidence suggests that birth complications are much more common in humans than in apes. The aperture of the human pelvis in females does not reach full size until several years after fertile eggs are first produced (see the article by Barry Bogin in *Health and Disease: A Reader*, entitled 'Why must I be a teenager at all?'), so difficulties in giving birth are commonest among very young mothers.

There are major sex differences in the shape of the human pelvis: that of females is wider relative to the size of the body as a whole, and more rounded, forming a pelvic canal that is more satisfactory for birth than the narrower pelvis of males; as a consequence, most women cannot run as fast as most men of a similar age.

3 (a) Living in caves and shelters over many generations permitted the evolution of a species of flea and a species of louse that breed only in association with humans; these ectoparasites trouble us with their irritating bites and lice can transmit the bacteria that cause typhus. The occupation of caves and shelters may have brought humans into contact with the fleas of wild mammals such as rats, badgers and bats, which 'shared' the same shelters and whose fleas can transmit life-threatening or disabling infectious diseases, including plague and rabies. The later use of fire to protect and heat living areas greatly increased the incidence of burns and damage from the inhalation of smoke.

(b) Humans who settle permanently in one place, in the absence of modern public health measures, remain in close association with their own debris and excrement, thereby promoting the spread of many infectious diseases and parasites. Permanent settlements enabled the development of agriculture and animal husbandry, but the latter practice brought people into close, continual contact with domestic livestock, from which they acquired parasites, many of which were pathogenic. Agricultural crops and domestic livestock form a less diverse diet than wild food, which often led to poorer nutrition. Living permanently in one place also fostered the concept of land ownership, which promoted internecine warfare and diminished the status of women, both of which increased human morbidity and mortality.

4 (a) Blood-sucking insects transmit pathogenic micro-organisms (e.g. those that cause sleeping sickness, malaria, yellow fever) and multicellular parasites (e.g. the nematodes that cause river blindness and elephantiasis), from other species of mammal to humans, and between infected and uninfected people. Examples of such insect vectors include ectoparasites such as lice and fleas, and mosquitoes (e.g. *Anopheles*) and blackflies (*Simulium*) which suck the blood of many different kinds of mammals as well as humans.

(b) Several species of freshwater snails and shrimp-like animals are essential secondary hosts for schistosomes and guinea worm; most mosquitoes, including those that carry the pathogens that cause malaria and yellow fever, breed in fresh water. When fish became an important food many thousands of years ago, people would spend more time standing or swimming in freshwater (and defaecating in or near it) than would have been necessary when they hunted land mammals. More recently, artificial irrigation systems created additional habitats for the snails that serve as the secondary host for schistosomes.

(c) People can contract *Toxocara*, a nematode worm that is normally a parasite of dogs, cats and their rodent prey; the larvae can cause abdominal pain and (rarely) blindness. Measles virus may have arisen from canine distemper virus, and dogs have long been a major route of infection for the virus that causes rabies.

Chapter 3

1   The three mechanisms are: *passive diffusion*, by which small molecules such as oxygen, carbon dioxide and water pass freely through a membrane without expenditure of energy, in response to a concentration gradient across the membrane; *active transport*, in which transport proteins in the membrane bind to molecules outside the cell by lock-and-key interactions, and then carry them through the membrane, using up energy in the process; and *endocytosis* (or *exocytosis*), by which large molecules are carried through the membrane, packaged in bags of membrane called vesicles.

2   The bases (A, T, C or G) in adjacent nucleotides along a length of DNA are arranged in a series of triplets, such as CAG or TTA. A 'meaningful' sequence of triplets is one way of describing a gene. Each triplet in a gene uniquely specifies a particular amino acid. The complete message, encoded in the series of many hundreds of triplets in the gene, corresponds to a series of amino acids, which are joined together in a unique sequence to give a unique protein molecule.

3   Both cells have virtually identical DNA, because they were both derived by cell division from a single fertilised egg, so they have exactly the same genes. This set of genes forms the unique genotype of the individual whose body contains these two cells. However, there are differences in which of these genes are active and which are 'switched off' in the two cells. For example, the gene that carries the instructions for making the protein insulin (the gene product) is active in the cell from the pancreas, but switched off in the skin cell. Conversely, the gene that encodes the structure of the pigment protein is active in the skin cell, but inactive in the pancreatic cell.

4   Within individual cells, homeostasis is maintained primarily by the cell membrane, which selectively takes

in or expels substances when their levels fall below or rise above some optimum level. For example, cells must maintain a certain optimum level of glucose which provides enough energy to fuel chemical reactions, but not so much that it damages the cell. In addition to the sum total of these cellular homeostatic processes being carried out in all the billions of cells in the body, large multicellular animals also regulate their internal environment by adjusting internal bodily mechanisms, under the control of the nervous and hormonal systems, which alter the animal's temperature, respiration, digestion, immune defences, blood supply, etc., within certain limits. Homeostasis can also be assisted by actions, such as moving to another location; in the case of humans, some actions may be consciously willed, e.g. the blood sugar homeostasis can be affected by eating a sugar-rich snack or fasting or even administering an insulin injection.

5   Figure 3.23 gives the correct sketch.

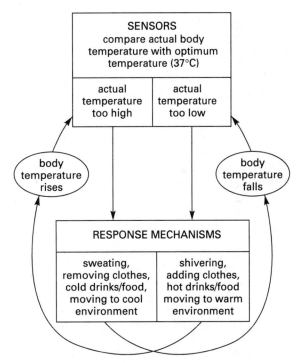

Figure 3.23 *Schematic diagram of a negative feedback circuit to maintain human body temperature by homeostasis.*

6   The 'struggle for existence' arises because, during reproduction, more offspring are produced than can survive, due to a shortage of the resources that support life. Mutation is the source of variation between different versions of DNA and hence between different

individuals. Although many mutations are deleterious and result in an organism which is less well adapted to survive and reproduce in its current environment, some mutations produce advantageous characteristics that enhance the organism's chance of survival and reproduction. Evolution can be defined as all the changes that have transformed life on Earth from its earliest beginnings to the diversity of life forms we see today. Inheritance of mutations is essential for evolution by natural selection because organisms pass on their characteristics to their offspring; those mutations that confer greater fitness increase the chance of those offspring surviving to reproduce in their turn and, over many generations, those adaptive characteristics become established in the population; mutations that decrease fitness tend to disappear from the population under the selective pressure of competition for scarce resources.

Chapter 4

1   The pairs are a–1, b–3, c–4, d–2 and e–5.

   (a)   Since achondroplasia is dominant and neither parent is affected, a new mutation in the gametes of one of the parents must be involved.

   (b)   The incidence of club-foot in *both* members of a twin-pair is much higher among identical twins (who have exactly the same genes) than among non-identical twins (who have only some of their genes in common). This suggests there is some genetic influence on the development of club-foot. However, the fact that in the majority of twin-pairs (whether identical or not), only one twin manifests the characteristic, suggests that environmental factors also play a role.

   (c)   Both parents are presumably heterozygous and the child inherited the two defective alleles, one from each parent. The chance of two new mutations occuring in the same gene in both parents at a similar time is extremely small.

   (d)   The members of a chromosome pair separate during meiosis and end up in different gametes. Because of the random assortment of these chromosomes such a female could produce four kinds of eggs: some with the defective allele for both genes, some with the normal allele for both genes, some with the defective allele for cystic fibrosis and the normal allele for phenylketonuria and, finally (the kind she transmitted to her daughter), some with the defective allele for phenylketonuria and the normal allele for cystic fibrosis.

   (e)   The disorder appeared in the woman's father and in her sons, but neither she nor her daughters were affected. This inheritance pattern is typical of sex-linked recessive alleles, in which female *carriers* do not express

the disease because the defective allele on one of their X chromosomes is masked by a normal allele on the other. Males, however, inherit the defective allele from their mother on the X chromosome she transmits in the egg, but the short Y chromosome inherited in their father's sperm does not include any alleles of the relevant gene and so cannot mask the effect of the single recessive allele.

2   The individual has two X chromosomes and hence would be female.

3   The prevention of skin cancer in people with xeroderma pigmentosa could be brought about by changing their environment, that is by protecting them from exposure to ultraviolet light (principally sunlight).

4   Gametes of two genotypes would be produced, one with a normal allele and the other with the allele associated with cystic fibrosis.

5   In phenylketonuria (PKU), affected individuals fail to make the enzyme that breaks down phenylalanine and converts it to tyrosine (both of which are amino acids, the building blocks of proteins). Since phenylalanine cannot be broken down, it accumulates in the body, and since tyrosine cannot be produced, there is a deficiency of tyrosine. The clinical features of children with the disease are developmental delay and mental retardation, first apparent in infancy, accompanied by seizures, hyperactivity and behavioural disturbances. They also tend to be blond and skin pigmentation is absent.

   The enzyme deficiency is linked to the clinical features as follows. The absence of phenylalanine in individuals with PKU affects the synthesis of myelin in the brain. Myelin is a component of the protective fatty sheath around nerves and is essential for their normal activity; its absence may be responsible for the mental retardation and behavioural changes. Tyrosine is required for pigment formation and its deficiency accounts for the fair complexion and blond hair.

6   The frequency of genetic diseases is determined by a combination of mutation rate, random processes (chance) and natural selection.

   (a)   The high frequency of porphyra in South Africa does not appear to be due to *new* mutations, since we are told that all affected Afrikaners inherited the disease allele from the same couple. Nor does natural selection seem to be involved in increasing the frequency of the allele, since there is no survival advantage to the individual who has it. Thus the high frequency is best explained as being due to chance or random processes preserving the disease allele in an 'isolated' population.

   (b)   The evidence suggests that the allele involved in thalassaemia is maintained by natural selection in certain regions of the world, particularly those in which malaria is, or was, rife. Thalassaemia seems to work in a similar way to sickle-cell disease, conferring an advantage on carriers (who have only one copy of the disease allele and are not anaemic), in that it gives some resistance to malaria; (some experts maintain that it also confers some protection against coronary heart disease). The process of natural selection preserves the thalassaemia gene in populations exposed to malaria because carriers have a reproductive advantage over non-carriers.

(c)   The occurrence of neurofibromatosis, a dominant disorder, in families with no previous history, suggests that affected individuals have inherited a new mutation. (In fact the mutation rate for this disease is as high as 1 per 1 000 gametes, but the reason for this is unknown.)

Chapter 5

1   (a)   A microparasite is a very small organism, typically visible only with the aid of powerful microscopes. Most microparasites are endoparasitic, living within the bodies, often within the cells, of their hosts. The microparasite derives some benefit from this relationship, at a cost to the host. This may simply be by diverting small amounts of food from the host, but some microparasites are *pathogenic,* that is, they cause disease.

(b)   A vector is an organism that carries a pathogen from one host individual to another. For example, mosquitoes are the vector of malaria.

(c)   Virulence is a measure of how severely a pathogen affects its host. It is expressed as the percentage of infected host individuals that die from an infection.

2   Coevolution refers to intimate relationships between species, such as pathogens and hosts, over extremely long periods of time, in which an adaptation in one species leads to an appropriate adaptation in the other. For example, the evolution of increased virulence in a pathogen leads to the evolution of greater resistance to that pathogen in the host.

3   Three important defences against pathogens are:

(i)   Possession of an effective and flexible immune system, which can protect the host from significant harm, including reduction of reproductive success, and counter any new strains that emerge as a result of mutation within a species of pathogen.

(ii)   The evolution in a host species of widespread resistance to those pathogenic organisms that are commonly found in that environment. Resistance is determined by genes that enable the host's immune system to make an effective and flexible response to those pathogens.

(iii)   Sexual reproduction may have evolved, at least in part, as an adaptation against pathogens, because it increases genetic diversity among a host's offspring and thus reduces the susceptibility of those offspring to pathogens that infected the parent.

4   Four important factors in destabilising host–pathogen relationships are:

(i)   Mutation, which may give rise to more-virulent or less-virulent varieties of pathogen and to more-resistant or less-resistant hosts.

(ii)   Changes in the proportion of susceptibles and immunes in a host population: new susceptibles are added to the population, by birth and immigration, and susceptibles and immunes are removed through death (from any cause) and emigration. Immunes increase sharply after an epidemic from which most infected people recover and vaccination can dramatically increase the proportion of immunes in a very short time.

(iii)   Pathogens that have been associated with one particular host species may start to infect a new species (zoonotic diseases); typically, the pathogen is much more virulent in the new host species, which has not yet been able to evolve greater resistance.

(iv)   Cultural factors in the history of a host population, which affect its long-term exposure to pathogens, can influence the stability of host–pathogen relationships. For example, the history of exposure to zoonotic diseases derived from domesticated animals was quite different for people in Europe up to the end of the fourteenth century, compared with native Americans.

Chapter 6

1   The evolution of human biology and human culture are continuously interacting. The enormous repertoire of non-self epitopes that the human immune system can recognise has been selected for as a consequence of, and/or has facilitated the evolution of: the longevity of humans and the unusually prolonged juvenile phase before reproduction takes place; the wide range of habitats that humans have colonised; the wide range of foodstuffs that humans can safely eat; the communal living habits of most human populations; and the close proximity of humans with many domesticated species.

2   Each time a person is infected with a particular rhinovirus, a primary *adaptive* immune response results which leaves the person less susceptible to that virus on subsequent encounters. Young children have not developed immunity to any of these viruses from previous encounters, so they are susceptible to all of them and suffer repeated colds, each time with a different

rhinovirus. As time passes, fewer and fewer rhinoviruses remain which have not been encountered before and by old age a person may have developed immunity to all but the rarest rhinoviruses as a result of previous encounters.

3　Three aspects of the biology of HIV contribute to its resistance to destruction by the immune system of the host:

(i)　Like all viruses, it replicates inside the host's own cells, where it derives some protection from the immune system's essential self-tolerance.

(ii)　The genes that code for epitopes on the surface of the virus particle are highly liable to mutate, thereby changing the shape of the epitopes; this 'antigenic drift' prevents an effective *secondary* immune response from developing.

(iii)　Most important of all, the cells that HIV colonises and destroys are the helper T cells, which are essential for the activation and effectiveness of all the other kinds of white cell involved in both innate and adaptive immunity.

HIV infection reveals the extent to which the intact immune system is normally able to protect individuals from 'opportunistic' infections with common pathogens, which cause illness only when the immune system is seriously deficient.

Chapter 7

1　(a)　The stomach muscles contribute to digestion by churning the food, breaking it into fragments and mixing it with acid and a few enzymes secreted by cells in the lining of the stomach. A few molecules (e.g. alcohol) dissolve in the membranes of the cells lining the stomach, but no active absorption takes place there. Sensors in the stomach monitor its contents and thereby regulate the secretion of hormones and neural signals that activate and coordinate the rest of the gut, so it has an indirect role in the digestion and absorption of nutrients into the bloodstream further down the gut.

(b)　The pancreas secretes several different digestive enzymes into the duodenum (first portion of the small intestine). Other cells in this gland are sensitive to the concentration of glucose and other fuels in the blood and synthesise and secrete the hormones insulin and glucagon; these hormones stimulate a variety of metabolic changes in the liver, muscles and adipose tissue, which regulate the concentration of fuels in the blood. The pancreas is not involved in the absorption of nutrients.

(c)　The liver secretes bile into the duodenum, which breaks down fats and oils into small droplets,

exposing a greater surface area to the action of digestive enzymes. The blood supply from the gut passes directly to the liver, which removes from the bloodstream excess nutrients absorbed from the gut (e.g. glucose, amino acids and fats) and stores them until required; it also takes up a variety of non-nutritive molecules such as flavouring substances and toxins, some of which are broken down and made harmless.

(d)　Cells in the lining of the small intestine secrete many different digestive enzymes. The small intestine is the major absorption site in the gut: its lining contains transporters for glucose (and other carbohydrates) and amino acids, and fats pass freely across the lining into the bloodstream and lymphatic system. Muscles in its walls produce peristaltic movements that mix up the food and move it along the intestine.

2　(a)　Muscular movements mix the food and propel it along the gut. Rhythmic movements of the intestine, called peristalsis, are under involuntary control of the nervous and hormonal systems. Swallowing and defaecation are muscular movements which are normally under voluntary control.

(b)　Digestive enzymes attack particular chemical bonds in carbohydrates, fats and proteins, breaking these large molecules into smaller fragments. They are secreted by various kinds of cells lining the gut in the stomach, pancreas and small intestine.

(c)　The principal non-enzymatic secretion is bile, which is mainly emulsifying and neutralising salts. It is secreted by the gall bladder under the control of signals primarily from food sensors in the stomach.

(d)　In humans, symbiotic bacteria are normally present only in and near the large intestine, where they digest many of the materials, particularly carbohydrates, that the human digestive processes did not break down. They also facilitate the uptake of vitamins and may themselves be taken up by endocytosis into cells lining the large intestine, where they are digested.

3　Food selection and appetite are determined by many complex mechanisms including the smell and taste of food and sensations arising from the stomach. Vomiting and diarrhoea prevent the absorption of toxins or parasites by expelling potentially harmful food before digestion is complete, or by accelerating its passage through the small and large intestines. Anorexia (loss of appetite) reduces food intake and so conserves energy normally expended in digestion and absorption of nutrients from the gut, and conserves the large quantities of protein, salts and water in digestive secretions. The body switches from using nutrients absorbed from the gut to using reserves of fuel and protein.

4   (a) Blood glucose is increased by eating a meal rich in glucose or digestible carbohydrate, or by a rise in the level of the hormone glucagon in the bloodstream together with a fall in the level of insulin, which together cause stored fuels (principally glycogen) to be converted into glucose and released into the bloodstream.

(b) Blood glucose falls following strenuous exercise (which breaks down glucose at a high rate to yield energy), and in starvation, or if there is a rise in insulin levels, which promotes its uptake by muscles and the liver for conversion into stored fuels.

5   (a) All suckling mammals can digest lactose, the major carbohydrate of milk, but most human populations and all other mammals lose this ability after weaning, when fresh milk disappears from or becomes a minor component of the diet. Retention after weaning of the capacity to secrete lactase, the enzyme that digests lactose, evolved among humans for whom milk obtained from domesticated animals was (and still is) a major food. Dairy farmers among whom the ability to absorb lactose was rare or absent usually convert milk into cheese or yoghurt, which renders it digestible.

(b) Skin depigmentation probably evolved in people who migrated to cooler, cloudier regions where protection from strong sunlight was less necessary than for ancestor populations living closer to the Equator. Essential precursors of vitamin D are synthesised in the skin during exposure to UV(B) radiation. Less pigment in the skin reduces the shading of the molecules involved in this mechanism, making it more efficient at producing vitamin D at low intensities of UV(B) radiation. Wearing clothes would further promote natural selection favouring individuals who could maintain efficient synthesis of vitamin D in areas of skin that remain exposed.

Chapter 8

1   This argument is not based on the theory of natural selection, which can only operate on individuals. It assumes (incorrectly) that since prevention of overcrowding will benefit the *species*, this will be favoured by natural selection. However, there is no advantage to the individual in ageing and dying, so natural selection cannot favour this process. (You may be interested to know that data for organisms in natural communities suggest that mortality, through predation and disease, is typically so high that overcrowding is a problem only for a few species at certain times, and so cannot provide a general explanation for ageing.)

2   Joints become stiffer and movement more restricted, the lens of the eye becomes less flexible and focusing is more difficult, skin becomes wrinkled (which may be depressing in a youth-oriented culture), and arteries can become hardened, which leads to a rise in blood pressure and an increased risk of stroke or coronary heart disease. All these changes are due in part to the loss of elasticity in collagen as the cells that produce it age.

3   The rate of breakdown of 'old' rigid collagen and the synthesis of new flexible collagen slows with age. The decline in the rates of protein synthesis and turnover may be brought about by a number of factors, including the accumulation of lipofuscin in ageing cells, a somatic mutation in the gene that codes for collagen, the damaging activity of free radicals on that gene or on the collagen itself, or by a combination of these and as yet unknown other factors.

Chapter 9

1   (a) All research on fetal tissue could be claimed to 'increase knowledge of human development' or have the potential to 'improve the human condition', so nothing is ruled out as unethical by this framework. Neither does it suggest how the unique nature of fetal tissue would be 'acknowledged'. However, the 'review panels' mentioned are intended to assess the potential value and ethical implications of research using fetal tissue and bring consistency to decisions about what is sanctioned and what is banned.

(b) The major attraction of fetal implants from the biological viewpoint is that relatively few fetal cells can multiply in the implant recipient to replace a missing cell population, without being attacked by the recipient's immune system.

2   The man's disease is probably due to a new mutation, since neither of his parents were affected. However, he is mistaken about not passing the Huntington's gene to his children; there is a one in two risk of passing on the new mutation to his children.

3   The following important factors should be considered:

(i) Is the disease treatable? If so, population screening of newborn babies could be undertaken, as in the case of PKU. If not, pre-natal diagnosis combined with selective abortion might be considered, but this has ethical implications (see point (v) below).

(ii) Could the at-risk communities be educated effectively about the risks of carrying the gene and the benefits of screening? Are the communities in favour of a programme of population screening, or are there religious, cultural or other objections?

(iii)   How reliable is the screening test? What would be the frequency of false negatives, i.e. individuals who were incorrectly reassured that they or their unborn child did not carry the gene? (False positives are not generated by screening tests that directly detect the presence of a faulty allele in the DNA.)

(iv)   Would genetic counselling be available, so that an individual or couple could learn about and discuss the options available in a supportive and impartial situation?

(v)   What are the ethical consequences of such a screening test being available? For example, would screening be optional or enforced? If pre-natal screening detected an affected fetus, would the parents be pressured to accept an abortion? Would the results of the test be kept confidential, and would employers, insurers or other family members try to obtain the information?

4   The central aim of somatic gene therapy is to insert normal alleles of the affected gene into the appropriate tissues of an individual with a genetic disease and thus permanently correct the disorder. A consequence of the technique is that the frequencies of defective alleles may increase in the population because the normal gene inserted by gene therapy does not enter the germline and the treated person lives to reproduce and pass the defective allele on to succeeding generations.

Chapter 10

1   Many of the gases liberated by industrial processes are known to damage the ozone layer in the upper atmosphere, causing it to become thinner and allow more UV radiaton from the Sun to pass through and reach the Earth (Leaf, 1989). UV radiation can cause mutations (changes in the sequence of nucleotides in DNA) and disrupt proteins; these in turn can lead to skin cancers, cataracts, and depression of the immune system with consequent lowered resistance to infection (Leaf, 1989, and Chapters 8 and 10). These direct adverse effects on human health might, to a small extent, be offset by a small increase in UV levels at higher latitudes (that is further away from the Equator), which enabled more vitamin D to be converted to the active form in exposed skin; this might improve bone density in populations that cannot extract calcium readily from milk, because vitamin D acts as a calcium transporter (Chapter 7). However, UV damage to

phytoplankton in the oceans could cause major disruption of the global food chain which, combined with global warming, could lead to widespread famine in human populations (Leaf, 1989).

2   Cell division always involves the risk of mutations caused by errors in assembling new strands of DNA alongside the template of the original strands (Chapter 4). Although most such mutations are detected and repaired by special enzymes, some persist and may damage either the cell or, indirectly, the whole organism; for example, a mutation may activate oncogenes and lead to the normal cell transforming into a cancerous one (Chapters 8 and 10).

3   The mechanisms involved in an acute inflammatory response to a respiratory-tract infection and an acute hypersensitivity reaction to an inhaled allergen such as pollen are exactly the same: antibodies produced in response to the infection or the allergen bind to mast cells in the mucus membranes of the respiratory tract and trigger the release of iriritant chemicals, including histamine. The difference is that the inflammatory response is an appropriate, short-term defensive reaction against a pathogen, whereas the hypersensitivity reaction is an inappropriate, prolonged and damaging response to harmless material such as pollen.

4   (a)   The drug thalidomide was not toxic to the pregnant women who were prescribed it to relieve morning sickness, but it was highly *teratogenic* to the fetuses, particularly in the first few months of pregnancy. In this example, the young fetuses are a *sensitive group*.

(b)   The exposure and the fetal malformation occurred quite close together in time (although not close enough to be considered an example of acute toxicity; the malformation was usually only discovered several months after the drug had been taken). Limb malformations of the type seen in the babies of women who had taken thalidomide are extremely rare in the absence of exposure to the drug, and (you may recall from news reports at the time) a very high proportion of exposures resulted in malformations. Note that teratogenicity is a special case of chronic toxicity, because the toxic agent has its effect only during a short sensitive period during fetal development.

(c)   The risk to the fetuses of experimental animals may have been much less than it was to human fetuses for two reasons:

(i)   Humans and other mammals may differ in their ability to resist or repair damage from certain chemicals because their different evolutionary history has resulted in adaptation to chemicals to which they have been persistently exposed in their natural environment; for example, the drug did not affect rats, so perhaps they have already adapted to a chemical that resembles thalidomide, whereas humans have no prior exposure to it.

(ii) The experimental animals may have been affected if they had been given a different dose of the drug, or were given it at a different stage of pregnancy, or via another route. (You may be interested to know that the reasons why different species differ in their response to thalidomide during fetal development is still an active area of research; for example, they could differ in whether or to what extent the drug crosses the placenta from the mother to the baby, whether it is broken down in the liver, the speed at which it is excreted, and its effects on cell metabolism.)

Chapter 11

1   (a)   A high degree of genetic diversity in a species should, in theory, enable it to adapt more rapidly and more effectively to sudden environmental change. If the future food supply of human populations becomes unpredictable, and periods of plenty are interspersed with scarcity, then the 'thrifty' genotype will again become advantageous. Individuals with that genotype are likely to leave more offspring than those without it. The Nauruan example illustrates that the same genotype can be expressed in either an adaptive (fat-storing) or deleterious (obese diabetic) phenotype, depending on environmental conditions.

(b)   In times of persistent plenty, the thrifty genotype results in diabetes, which is damaging to the individual and to their reproductive success. It cannot be preserved in the population by natural selection, because characteristics are only favoured (selected for) if they give the individual or their closest kin (who have some of the same genes) a reproductive advantage. Natural selection cannot favour a characteristic that damages the individual, even if it would be 'in the interests of mankind' as a whole. Neither is natural selection capable of 'foresight'; a characteristic cannot be selected for in the expectation that it will become advantageous in the future (e.g. the thrifty genotype cannot be preserved by natural selection 'foreseeing' that food supplies might suddenly change). The only way to preserve it is by medical treatment and dietary counselling of the diabetic Nauruans, so that they have as many children as non-diabetic Nauruans.

Acknowledgements

Grateful acknowledgement is made to the following sources for permission to reproduce material in this book:

Figures

Figure 1.1 (part) courtesy of Dr Caroline Pond; *Figure 1.1 (part)* courtesy of Dr Marion Hall; *Figures 1.1 (part), 4.1* Mike Levers/Open University; *Figures 2.1, 2.2, 4.20* adapted from Jones, S., Martin, R., Pilbeam, D. and Bunney, S. (eds), 1992, *The Cambridge Encyclopedia of Human Evolution*, Cambridge University Press, Cambridge; *Figures 3.4b, 3.5* courtesy of Heather Davies; *Figure 3.9b* Perry, M. M. and Gilbert, A. B., 1979, *Journal of Cell Science*, **39**, p. 266, The Company of Biologists Ltd; *Figure 3.9d* Herzog, V., Sies, H. and Miller, F., 1976, *Journal of Cell Biology*, **70**, p. 698, by copyright permission of the Rockefeller University; *Figures 3.12, 4.2* Science Photo Library; *Figure 3.17a* courtesy of Dr John Williams, London School of Hygiene and Tropical Medicine; *Figure 3.17b* courtesy of Dr J. P. Ackers, London School of Hygiene and Tropical Medicine; *Figure 3.17c* courtesy of Emeritus Professor W. Peters, International Institute of Parasitology; *Figure 4.3* Department of Cancer Studies, The Medical School, University of Birmingham; *Figures 4.4, 4.5* Courtesy of Professor M. A. Ferguson-Smith, Department of Medical Genetics, Royal Hospital for Sick Children, Glasgow; *Figure 4.21* MENCAP National Centre; *Figure 4.22* Strickberger, M. W., 1990, *Evolution*, Jones and Bartlett; *Figure 5.5* adapted from Bradley, D. J., 1977, in *Origins of Pest, Parasite, Disease and Weed Problems*, ed. Cherrett, J. M. and Sagar, G. P., Blackwell Scientific Publications, Oxford; *Figure 5.9* adapted from Yorke, J. A. and London, W. P., 1973, Recurrent outbreaks of measles, chickenpox and mumps, II systematic differences in contact rates and stochastic effects, *American Journal of Epidemiology*, **98**, pp. 469–82; *Figure 6.2* courtesy of Dr S. Gordon and G. G. McPherson, Sir William Dunn School of Pathology, University of Oxford; *Figures 7.4, 7.5* adapted from Durham, W. H., 1991, *Coevolution, Genes, Culture and Human Diversity*, Stanford University Press; *Figure 8.2* reprinted from Shock, N. W. *et al.*, 1957, *Geriatrics*, **12**(40). Copyright 1957 by Advanstar Communications. Printed in U.S.A.; *Figure 8.5a* courtesy of Hemel Hempstead General Hospital, Radiography Dept; *Figure 8.5b* courtesy of Milton Keynes General Hospital, Radiography Dept; *Figure 9.5* Modell, B., Kuliev, A. M. and Wagner, M., 1992, *Community Genetics Services In Europe*, World Health Organization.

Tables

Table 4.1 From *Principles of Human Genetics* by C. Stern. Copyright © 1973, by W. H. Freeman and Company, San Francisco. Reprinted with permission; *Table 5.2* Jones, S., Martin, R., Pilbeam, D. and Bunney, S. (eds), 1992, *The Cambridge Encyclopedia of Human Evolution*, Cambridge University Press, Cambridge; *Table 7.1* adapted from Johnson *et al.*, 1977, Lactose malabsorption in the Pima Indians of Arizona, *Gastroenterology*, Elsevier Science Publishers, Barking, Essex, **73**, p. 1303; *Table 7.2* adapted from Durham, W. H., 1991, *Coevolution, Genes, Culture and Human Diversity*, Stanford University Press.

Un-numbered photographs/illustrations

pp. 9, 23, 170 courtesy of Dr Caroline Pond; *p. 10, 11, 25, 107, 143, 162, 178, 198* Mike Levers/Open University; *p. 22* Wellcome Medical Foundation; *p. 24* Aerofilms; *p. 27* Panos Pictures/Jeremy Hartley; *p. 28* Hulton–Deutsch Collection; *p. 47* A. Barrington-Brown; *p. 91* MENCAP National Centre; *pp. 109, 147* courtesy of Heather Davies; *p. 110* courtesy of Dr Roger Trout; *p. 116* *American Indian Holocaust and Survival: A Population History since 1492*, by Russell Thornton. Copyright © 1987 by the University of Oklahoma Press, Norman, Oklahoma and London; *p. 151* courtesy of Dr H. M. Gilmour, Dept of Pathology, University of Edinburgh Medical School; *p. 154* courtesy of Teaching Aids at Low Cost (TALC), P. O. Box 49, St Albans. Details of TALC materials sent free on request; *p. 160* courtesy of Dr M. J. Cullen, Muscular Dystrophy Group Research Laboratories, Newcastle General Hospital, Newcastle Upon Tyne; *p. 167* courtesy of Professor G. C. Arneil; *p. 169* courtesy of P. W. Keer-Keer; *p. 176* Photographic Unit, Department of Histopathology, John Radcliffe Hospital, Oxford; *p. 186* courtesy of the Salvation Army; *p. 190* Camera Press; *p. 195* courtesy of Milton Keynes General Hospital; *p. 212* Greenpeace; *p. 216a* courtesy of Dr R. E. Church; *p. 216b* courtesy of Dr D. J. Gawkrodger, Royal Hallamshire Hospital, Sheffield; *p. 216c* Royal Infirmary, Sheffield; *p. 217 (top)* AP-Wirephoto; *p. 217 (bottom)* US Army Military History Institute; *p. 218* Hoffman/Greenpeace; *p. 229* Werner Bischof/Magnum; *p. 231* Sebastiao Salgado/Magnum.

Index

Entries and page numbers in **bold type** refer to key words which are printed in **bold** in the text. Indexed information on pages indicated by *italics* is carried mainly or wholly in a figure or table.

ABO blood groups, 79–80
abortion, 195–6, 201–2, 226
absorption of nutrients, **146**, 150–2
Achillea (yarrow), variation, *76*
achondroplasia, 84, 96
Ackers, J. P., *56*
active site, 43
active transport, **40**–1, 151
acute toxicity, **217**–18, 221
adaptations, **63**, 65
    genetic and cultural, 226
    life histories as, 106
    to a novel diet, 161–6
    of parasites, 109, 110
adaptive immunity, **132**–40
ADD *see* adenosine deaminase deficiency
adenine, 48
adenosine deaminase deficiency (ADD), 207
adenosine triphosphate *see* ATP
adipose tissue, 18, 158, *159*, 160
adolescence, 15–16
adolescent growth spurt, **15**
adrenal hormones, 142
age
    and food preferences, 158
    and mutation, 89
    vulnerability to infection, 105, 108, 142
age-1 gene, 184
ageing, 17, 173, **174**, 228
    bodily signs, 177–83
    of cells, 175–7, 183–4
    core mechanism, 184
    and death, 184–7
    evolution, 174–5
    mechanisms, 173, 183–4
Agent Orange, 217, 221
agriculture, **21**–3, 230
    costs and benefits, 23–4
    monoculture, 230
AIDS, 29, 124, 138
    see also HIV (human immunodeficiency virus)
ALARA principle, 222
albino people, 214
alcohol, 149, 155, 183, 213
    effects on fetus, 74
allele frequencies in human populations, 91–2
alleles, **77**–80, 193–4, 196–200, 202, 205, 206, 208–9, 226
allergen, 131, 214
allergies, 131, 152, 214
Alzheimer's disease, 206
American Indians (Amerindians), 24, 116–17
Ames, Bruce, 222–3

amino acids, 33–34, 52–4, 149
    effects of excess, 161
Amish people, 93
amniocentesis, 194, 195
amoebae, movement, 55, *56*
amoebiasis (amoebic dysentery), *101*
ancylostomiasis (hookworm) *101*
Anderson, H. R., *215*
animal cells, **35**, *36*
animal models, 9, 127, 142, 208
    toxicity testing, 220–1, 222
Anopheles spp. (mosquitoes), 26
anorexia, 157
anthrax, 104, 111
antibiotics, 115, 230
antibodies, 43, 130, 131, **136**
    in babies, 142
    and hypersensitivity reactions, 214
    use in cancer treatment, 144
antigen presentation, 140
antigenic drift, 140
antigens, **133**
anti-oncogenes, 185, 186, 209
antisomes, 130
α_1-antitrypsin, commercial production, 205–6
α_1-antitrypsin deficiency, 201, 202, 203
    and sensitivity to environmental factors, 214
    treatment, 204
anus, *148*, 152
apes, 10–11
    fertility of females, 16
    skeleton, *13*
apoptosis, 177n.
appendix, *148*, 152
arthritis, 144, 178
arthropods, 103
ascariasis (roundworm), *101*
Ascaris lumbricoides (roundworm), 140
asexual reproduction, 118
Association of British Insurers, 202
asthma, 214–15
atoms, **6**, 32
ATP (adenosine triphosphate), 44
Australopithecus, 17–18
autoimmune diseases, 135

B cells (B lymphocytes), **137**, 140, 144
babies
    antibodies, 142
    calcium absorption, 171
    food preferences, 158
    gut, 151
    screening for PKU, 197
    sensitivity to environmental factors, 214
bacteria, **35**, 40, *103*, *109*, 120
    and antibiotics, 115, 153, 230
    cyst formation, 150
    DNA, *46*

endotoxins, 141
in large intestine, 153
and lysozyme, 125–6
multi-drug resistant strains, 115, 230
reproduction, 57, 108, 119
toxins, 44, 133
bacteriophages, 102
Barinaga, M., 186
Barnard, Christiaan, 189, *190*
base-pairing rule, **48**
bases (in DNA), 47–8, 53–4
BATNEEC principle, 222
beetroot, 156
Begon, M., *105*, *112*, *115*
Beral, V., 216
Bianchi, D. W., 210
bile, 149, 150
bile duct, *148*
bile salts, 156
bilharzia *see* schistosomiasis
binding site, 43
bioaccumulation, **219**
biodiversity, **120**–2, 132, 230
biological half-life, **219**
biomass, **121**
pyramids, 121–2
bipedality, 11, **12**–14, 63
birth weight, factors affecting, 75
'Black Death' *see* plague
blackflies, 25
blood, 150
control of glucose levels, 158–61
blood groups, 79–80
blood system *see* cardiovascular system
blood transfusions, 189
blood–brain barrier, 214
bloodstream, 61
body height, variation, 80–1, 82
body louse, 21, *102*
body temperature, regulation, 62–3
Bogin, Barry, 16
bone marrow, 139
transplants, 191, 204, 207
see also stem cells
bones
age-related impairment, 178, 181
healing, 213
osteoporosis, 181
Brade, H., 141
brain, 17–18, 62
age-related change, 184
evolution, 17–18, 63
fetal cell implants, 191
interactions with gut, 156–8
bran in diet, 154
Branwell-Booth sisters, *186*
breast milk, 23, 142, 147
breast cancer, 206
breasts, 120
bronchitis, 213
Brown, Michael, 83–4
brucellosis, 110
Brundtland, G. H., 82

calcium, absorption, 151, 171, 181–2
Campbell, N. A., 31
cancer, 64, **185**
development of, 219–20
disease of ageing, 89, 185–6
environmental factors, 186, 222–3
familial types, 206
gene therapy, 206, 209
and immune response, 144
lung, 29
skin, *169*, 214
see also carcinogenic substances
carbohydrates
digestion, 146, 149
in membranes, 39
carbon dioxide accumulation *see* global warming
carcinogenic substances, 186, 219–20, 222–3
cardiovascular system, **60**, 150
human, *61*
Caren, L. D., 142
Carey, J. R., 186
Carney, John M., 184
carriers, **85**
allele frequency in population, 92
genetic disorders, 85–6, 92, 200
infectious diseases, 112
cartilage, age-related impairment, 180
cascade reactions, **130**–1, 141
Caskey, C. T., 207
cataract, 182
cell cycle, **57**–8, *59*
cell membranes, *35*, 37, 38–44, 219
cell metabolism, 44–5, 176
cell wall (bacteria), 35, 36
cells, **35**–45
ageing, 175–7, 183–4
evolution, 34, 55
membranes *see* cell membranes
organelles, 36
protein/lipid turnover, 176–7, 183–4, 213
specialisation, 60
see also cell metabolism
cellulose, 154
Cervus elephas (red deer), reproduction, 108
chance or random processes in genetic inheritance, 93
CHD *see* coronary heart disease
cheesemaking, 163, 166, 169
chemical elements, **6**, 32
chemical industrial environment, effects of, 211–12
childbirth, 12
childhood mortality, 174
chimpanzee, 10, 11, 12
chromosome number, 46
growth, 15
chloracne, 217, 218
chloride absorption, 151, 152
choking, 148
cholera, 110
evolutionary change, 111
toxin, 44
see also Vibrio cholerae
cholesterol, 39, 83–4
see also familial hypercholesterolaemia
chorionic villi sampling (chorion biopsy), 194, 195

chromosomal mutation, **90**, 92
chromosomes, **46**, 68–74
    crossing over, 73, *74*
    homologous pairs, 69–71, 78
    in meiosis, 71–3, *74*, 77–8
    in mitosis, 58, *59*
    sex, 70, 71, 72–3
chronic toxicity, **218**, 221–2
cirrhosis of liver, 213
clonal selection, **135**, *136*
clothing, 19, 20–1, 168, 170
club-foot, 96–7
codominance, **80**
coevolution, **109**–11
    host and pathogen, 114–15, 117, 119, 132, 140, 230
Cohen, S., 142
Coleman, M., 216
collagen, 180–1, 187, 213
colon, 152, 153
colour-blindness (red), 79
commensalism, 100, 111
common cold, 28
competition
    between individuals, 51, 63–4
    between species, 63–4, 100
complement, 130–1
concentration gradient, 40, 129
congenital malformations, 83
consumers (in food web), 120–1
contact dermatitis, 215, *216*
continuous variation, 80–2
cooking, 20, 22–3, 155–6
corneal grafts, 190
coronary heart disease (CHD), 83, 193, 201
Corynebacterium diphtheriae, 27
costal cartilage, 180
Council for International Organisation of Medical Sciences, 208
Cournoyer, D., 207
cousin marriages, 86
Coutelle, C., 208
cretinism, 21
Crick, Francis, 46, *47*, 48
critical group (environmental exposure), **213**, 214n., 224
Crombleholme, T. M., 191
cross-infections (interspecific), **24**, 101
crossing over (chromosomes), 73, *74*
crystallins (lens proteins), 182, 184
Cuatrecasas, P., 162
Cullen, M. J., *160*
cultural adaptation, 226
cultural evolution, 18–24, **225**–26
    and human immune system, 126–7
    impact on resistance to infection, 116–17
culture
    impact on human genetic evolution, 226–8
    impact on human health, 228–31
cysts, 150
cystic fibrosis, 83, 84–5, 97
    family history, *193*, 194
    gene therapy, 207–8
    incidence in populations, 95–6
    location of gene, 196, 206
    screening for, 197–8, 202
    transport protein deficiency, 151

cytoplasm, *35*, **36**
cytosine, 48
cytotoxic cells, **128**–9, 131
cytotoxic T cells, 138, 215

dairying, 23, 165–6
    see also milk
Darwin, Charles, 34, 51
Davies, C. T. M., *179*
Davies, K. J. A., 184
Davies, Laura, 190–1
Dawkins, Richard, 55
death, 174
    ageing and, 184–7
    of cells, 177
    evolution, 106
    timing, 106
defaecation, 153–4, 156
defence mechanisms of body, 212–13
    see also immune system
defoliant (Agent Orange), 217, 221
dental caries, 22, 161
deoxyribonucleic acid *see* DNA
dermatitis, contact, 215, *216*
dermis, 213
detoxification (by liver), 155, 156, 161, 213
diabetes (*diabetes mellitus*), 74, 83, 135, **161**, 204
    genetic involvement, 206
    Nauru epidemic, 227
diagnosis
    pre-natal, 194–6
    pre-symptomatic, 193
Diamond, Jared, 227
diarrhoea, 108, 153–4, 163
diet, 20, 21–3, 156
    and diabetes, 161
    changing, 20, 161–2
    effect of reduced-calorie, 183–4
dietary fibre, 154
diffusion *see* passive diffusion
digestion, **146**–7, 149, 155–6
    defects in, 151–2
    lactose *see* lactose malabsorption and intolerance
digestive enzymes, 147, 148, 149, 152, 156
    inactivation, 155
digestive system, 147–50
    see also gut
dioxin, 215–22
diphtheria, 27
direct genetic screening tests, 197–8
diseases, human, 82, 226
    age-related, 178, 185
    see also genetic diseases; infectious diseases
disposable soma theory, **175**
distal cause, 184n.
DNA (deoxyribonucleic acid), 6, **45**–47, 64
    analysis, and pre-natal diagnosis, 196–7
    bases, 47–8, 53–4
    effect of free radicals, 184
    errors, 186
    and genetic code, 48–50, 52–4
    germline and somatic, 55
    interspecific similarities, 128
    mutation and variation, 50–1
    nucleotides, 47–50

and natural selection, 51–2
repair, 213
structure, 47–8
see also chromosomes
DNA fingerprinting, 64
DNA replication, **48**, *49*, 58
Doll, Sir Richard, 185–6, 222
domesticated species, 21, 117
dominant characteristics, **78**
dominant disorders, **78**, 83–4, 92, 193
dose–response relationship, **221**
Down's syndrome, 89–90, *91*, 92, 195
Dowse, Gary, 227
Dracunculus medinensis (guinea worm), 25, *101*
drug resistance (pathogens), 115, 230
Duchenne muscular dystrophy, 206
duodenum, 149, 150
Durham, W. H., *164*, 165, 166–71
dysentery, 110

East African peoples, 170, 171
ectoparasites, **101**
see also fleas; lice
egg cell, 55
electromagnetic radiation, effects of exposure, 216
elephantiasis, 25, *101*
Ellis–van Creveld disorder, 93
emphysema, and α_1-antitrypsin deficiency, 214
endemic human diseases, **24**
endocytosis, 40, **41**–2
by intestinal cells, 150
by phagocytes, 128, *129*
endoparasites, **101**, 149–50
endoplasmic reticulum, 36, *38*, *54*
endotoxins (bacterial), 141
energy
required by cells, 44
sources in living organisms, 158
Entamoeba histolytica, *56*, *102*
environment, **74**
biological, 229–30
changing, 64–5
chemical industrial, health effects, 211–12
intra-uterine, 74
physico–chemical, 228–9
psycho–social, 230–1
environmental exposure, **211**, 213
environmental factors in disease, 201, 209, 211–23
see also under cancer
Environmental Protection Act 1991, 222
enzymes, 34, 42–3, **44**–5, 146–7
epidermis, 213
epitopes, **133**–6, 138, 140, 144
antigenic drift, 140–1
concealed from immune system, 140
escape mechanisms (pathogens), 140–1
Escherichia coli, 108, *109*
generation time, 108, *109*
virulence, 111
Eskimos, 20, 22, 24, 170–1
ethical issues in medical intervention, 6, 188–9, 190, 192
gene transfer therapy, 208–9
pre-natal diagnosis and genetic screening, 201–4
transplants, 189–92

eukaryotes, 36n.
evolution, 5, **31**, 63, 64–5
of ageing and death, 106, 174–5
of bipedality, 14
of host–pathogen relationships, 108–14, 117, *118*
of immunity, 127–8
of lactose absorption, 165–6, 168–71
of menopause, 178–9
of pathogen virulence, 111
role of mutation, 51
of sex, 63, 118–20
of skin colour, 168–70
of soft tissues, 17–18
time-scale, 31–2, 65n.
see also cultural evolution; genetic evolution; human evolution
Ewald, P. W., 111
exercise
and free radical generation, 184
and immune system, 142–3
exocytosis, 40, **42**–3
exploitation (of another species) *see* interactions *under* species
export of wastes, 223
extinctions, 117
eye
age-related changes, 182, 184
corneal grafts, 190

Factor VIII, 204
faeces, 152, 153–4
false negatives, 198, 221
false positives, 197, 221
familial conditions, 75–6, 193–4
familial hypercholesterolaemia, 83–4, 193
gene located, 206
treatment, 204
family history, 77, 83, 193, 195
see also pedigree charts
fats, digestion, 146, 149, 156
fatty acids, 149
absorption, 150
effects of excess, 161
fatty tissue *see* adipose tissue
fecundity, **23**, 106
fertilisation, 71–2, 77–8
fetal cell implants, 189, **191**–2, 210
fetoscopy, 194–5
fetus, environment, 74
fever, 141
fibre, in diet, 154
Fiennes, Richard, 24
Filaria, *103*
filarial worms, *102*
fire, 19–20
fitness, **51**, 105–6
flatworms, 25
fleas, 20–1, 28, 103, *104*
adaptations, 109
fluid mosaic model (membranes), 39
flukes, 25, 102, 103, *104*, 114, 140
Følling, A., 86
food, 146
see also digestion

'food allergies', 152
food chains, 120, 219
food webs, 120–1
free radical theory, 184
Friedman, D. B., 184
Fries, James, 186

Gage, F. H., 191
gait, effects of ageing, 180
galactose, 147, 149, 158n., 162, 163
gall bladder, *148*, 149
Gallo, M. A., 221
gametes, **55**, 68, 77–8, 88
    formation, 71–3
Gardner, M. J., 216
gene cloning, **205**
gene mutations *see* mutations
gene pool, **92**, 106
gene product, **52**, 86
gene therapy, 189, **206**–8, 209, 226
gene vector, **206**
generation time, **108**–109, 127
genes, **50**, 52, 64, 68
    arrangement on chromosomes, 70–1
    and cellular ageing, 183–4
    cloning, 205
    coding for proteins, 52–4
    interspecific similarity of sequences, 128
    'shuffling', 134, *135*
    see also alleles; anti-oncogenes; oncogenes
genetic adaptation, 226
genetic bottleneck, 117
genetic code, 45, 48, 50, 52–4
genetic counselling, 193, **194**
genetic diseases, **82**–8, 151, 227–8
    family decisions, 193–7
    incidence, 92
        effect of screening, 199–201
    treatment, 204–8
genetic engineering, 144, 189, **204**–6
genetic evolution, **225**
    impact of culture on human, 226–8
genetic isolation, 93
genetic screening
    direct and indirect tests, 197–8
    ethical issues, 201–4
    false negatives and positives, 197–8, 221
    insurance industry, 202–3
    population screening, 197–9
    pre-natal diagnosis, 193–6, 199–200
genetic variation/variability, 64, 72, 73, 91–2, 225
genotype, **52**, 64, 68, 75–6, 78
    mapping of human see Human Genome Project
    modification, 206
    thrifty (hypothesis), 227
gerbils, 28, 184
German measles (rubella), 74
germline cells, **55**, 64, 192
    see also gametes
germline DNA, **55**, 192
germline gene therapy, **206**, 209
giardiasis, *101*
glands, **147**
global warming, 211–12, 229

glucagon, *159*, 160
glucose, 147, 149
    absorption, 151, 163
    regulation of blood levels, 41, 44, 158–61
glycogen, 158, 159, 160
goitre, 21, *22*
Goldstein, Joseph, 83–4
Golgi body, 147, 156
gonorrhoea, 108
gorilla (*Gorilla gorilla*), skull, *17*
graft rejection, **129**, 133, 189–90
graft-versus-host disease, 191
'greenhouse effect' *see* global warming
growth, human, 14–15, 82
guanine, 48
guinea worm, 25, *101*
gut, 147–54
    interactions with brain, 156–8
    see also large intestine; small intestine
gut cells, *35*, 175, 181

haemoglobin, 44, **80**
    sickle-cell, 93–5
    variants, 80
haemophilia, 97, 204
hair, human, 18
Hamilton, W. D., 119
Harper, P. S., 203
Harris, R., 194
hay fever, 214
head louse, 21, *102*, *104*, 112
health
    defined by the World Health Organisation, 226
    in chemical industrial environment, 211–12
    impact of culture on, 226, 228–31
hearing, age-related loss, 182
heart transplants, 189, *190*
Hebb, D. O., 75
helper T cells, 138, 139, 140
herbivore, 99
Herzog, V., *42*
heterozygotes, **78**
heterozygous alleles, 78
HFEA *see* Human Fertilisation and Embryology Authority
hip joint, 12, *180*
histamine, 131, 214
HIV (human immunodeficiency virus), 96, *103*, 111, 112–13, 116, 125, 127, 145
    dormancy, 111
    hypothetical resistance to HIV, 96
    mutations, 119, 125
    test for, 136, 203
    and tuberculosis incidence, 115
    variant strains, 140
    virulence, 110
homeostasis, **57**, 60, 62, 158–61
    age-related impairment, 178
hominids, **11**, 18
    brain, 12, 18
    feet, 12
    growth and longevity, 16–17
    pelvis, 12
Homo erectus, 17–18
    skull, *17*

Homo habilis, 19
Homo sapiens see human evolution
homologous pairs (chromosomes), **70**–1, 78
    crossing over between, 73, *74*
homozygotes, **78**
homozygous alleles, **78**
hookworm, *101, 102*
hormonal system, **62**
hormone replacement therapy, 182
hormones, 42, 43, **62**
    action on gut, 156–7
    adrenal, 142
    see also glucagon; insulin
host (to a parasite), **9**
host density, 114
host–pathogen relationships, 98
    evolution, 108–14, 117, *118*
    human intereference with, 230
    instability, 29, 99, 110, 114–17
    see also coevolution
host-versus-graft response, 191
human conflict, 230
human evolution, **5**–6, 8–30, 11–14, 16–17, 29, 30
    evidence for, 9
    expected slowing, 228
    impact of culture on genetic, 226–8
    see also cultural evolution
Human Fertilisation and Embryology Authority (HFEA), 192
Human Genome Project, 189, **203**
hunter-gatherer societies, 22, 23, 24
    contact with pathogens, 26, 117
    lactose absorption, 165
    present-day, 24
Huntington's disease, 84, 202, 206, 210
hydrochloric acid, 148, 152
hypersensitivity, **214**, *216*
        see also allergies, contact dermatitis

identical twins, 64, 75, 81, 133
ileum, 149, 150, 152
immune response
    medical manipulation, 137, 141, 143–4, 115
immune system, 42, 63, 108, **124**, 126–8
    age-related impairment, 108, 178
    effects of UV radiation, 212
    suppression, 144, 189, 190, 212
immunes (in a population), 112, 113, 114
immunisation, 27n., 113–14, 137
immunity, **108**, 114, 115, **124**
    adaptive, 132–40
    evolution, 127–8
    innate, 128–32
immunology, **124**
immunotoxic substances, 220
indirect genetic screening tests, 197
industrialisation, 228–9
infectious diseases, 124–145
    childhood, 108
    cyclic outbreaks, 115–16
    defences, 125–6
    dynamic properties of, 112–14
    impact on human survival, 105
    mortality and morbidity, 124
    origins, 24–9

physical and chemical barriers, 125–6
    see also resistance to infection
infectious period, 114
infertility treatment, 189, 192
inflammatory response, inflammation, 128, 131, 141, 144, 214
influenza, 117
influenza virus, *37*
    antigenic drift, 140
    variant strains, 140–1
inheritance, 45, 67–74
    multifactorial, 80–2
    single-gene, 77–80
        multiple-allele, 79–80
        sex-linked, 79
innate immunity, **128**–32
insects, parasites, 101–2
insulin, 62, **158**–61, 204, 205
insurance industry and genetic screening, 202–3
interferon, 131
intracellular pathogens, 126
Inuit people *see* Eskimos
invertebrates, 102
iodine, dietary, 21
iron, absorption, 151, 152
isolated populations (and chance mutations), 93

jejunum, 149, 150
Jenner, Edward, 137
Johnson, T. E., 184
joints, age-related impairment, 178, 180–1
Jones, Steve, 51, 204, 208–9, 227–8

kala azar, *101*
karyotypes, **69**, 70, *90, 195, 196*
kidney
    grafts, 190
    reduced function with age, 177, 182
kin selection, 179
Kirkwood, Thomas, 174, 177
knee joint, *180*
Komrower, G. M., 198
Kuliev, A. M., *199*, 200

lactase, 44, 147, 162–4
lactation, 23
lactose, 44
lactose malabsorption and intolerance, **162**–6, 168–72
Lancet, 202
large intestine, *148*, 152–4
latent period, 114
latents (in a population), 112–13
Leaf, Alexander, 211, 229
leeches, 101, *104*
legionnaires' disease, 124
leishmaniasis (kala azar), *101*
leprosy, 143
Lerner, I. M., 92
leucocytes *see* white cells
leukaemia, 191
Libby, W. J., 92
lice, 21, 28–9, 100, *102*, 103
    adaptations, 109
life on Earth, origins, 31, 32–5

life history, 106–8
    human, 14–17
life-history theory, 106, 175
lifespan
    effect of lifestyle, 183
    human, 16–17, 22, 174, 186
ligaments, 12n.
Lilienfeld, D. E., 221
Lindgren, C., 82
lipofuscin, 176–7, 182, 183
lipophilic substances, 219
liver, *148*, 149, 150
    age-related volume loss, 182, 183
    alcohol-related damage, 183, 213
    and blood glucose regulation, 158, *159*, 161
    detoxifying role, 155, 213
liver fluke, *102, 104*
lock-and-key interactions, 43
    antibody–epitope, 131, 132, 138
    of enzymes, 147
    of hormones, 62
    in immune system, 127
    in membranes, 43–4, 127
Loudon, Irvine, 152
Luckinbill, L. S., 183
lung disease, 201
    α_1-antitrypsin deficiency, 201, 202, 203, 214
    bronchitis, 213
    cancer, 29
    emphysema, 214
lymph nodes, 139–40
lymphatic filariasis (elephantiasis), *101*
lymphatic system, 139–40, 150
lymphocytes, 134–9
    see also B cells; T cells
lysosomes, 37, *38*, 128, 177
lysozyme, 125–6, 130

McGue, M., 186
McKeown, Thomas, 27n.
macroparasites, 102–3, *104*, 109, 114, 147
macrophages, 128
Maiden Castle, *24*
malaria, 26, 100, 105, 109, 127
    resistance
        and sickle-cell anaemia, 94–5
        and thalassaemia, 200
    Plasmodium, 26, 94, 101, *102, 103,* 115
    vaccine, 143
males
    sexual characteristics, 119
    value, 119
Mallon, Mary, 112
Martin, G. M., 184
Martin, R. D., *13*
Masoro, E. J., 183
mast cells, 131, 214
May, Robert M., 99
MDR *see* multi-drug resistant strains of bacteria
measles, 26, 98, 108, 114, 115–16, 117
meiosis, 63, 71–4, 77–8, 90, 118–19
Mellanby, Sir Edward, 167
Meltzer, D. J., 116, 117
membranes, *35*, 36, **38**–44, 62, 219

memory, age-related impairment, 178
memory cells, *136*, 137
meningitis, 124
Mennie, M. E., 198
menopause, 16
    as evolutionary adaptation, 178–9
mental retardation
    due to maternal alcohol consumption, 74
    due to PKU, 86–7, 197
    see also Down's syndrome
messenger RNA (mRNA), 53–4
metabolism, 16, 146
    see also cell metabolism
mice (*Mus* spp.), 22, 28
    growth in, *15*
micro-organisms, 9, 26–9
    in food, 147, 148
    in large intestine, 153
microparasites, 104–5
microvilli, 150
'military metaphors', 98–9
milk, 27–8, 147
    antibodies in, 142
    digestion and absorption, 162–6
    see also lactose
minerals, absorption, 146, 152
mitochondria, 36, *38*, *160*, 184
mitosis, 58, *59*, 68, 72
Modell, Bernadette, 199, 200
molecules, 6, 32
    organic, 32
Moltz, H., 141
monoculture, 230
morphology, 67
mosquitoes, 100, *104*, 109
    disease vectors, 26, 95, 101
motor neurons, 179
mouth, digestion in, 148
movement (of protistans), 55, *56*
mRNA *see* messenger RNA
mucus, 148–9, 150, 151, 212
Müller-Hill, Benno, 203
multicellular organisms, 60–3
multicellular parasites, 9, 25–6
multi-drug resistant (MDR) strains of bacteria, 115
multifactorial characteristics, 80, **81**–2, 84
multifactorial diseases, 206, 209
multiple alleles, 79–**80**
multiple lipoma, 77–8
multiple sclerosis, 206
multiple-organ transplants, 190–1
multipotent stem cells, 134, *135*, 191, 207
Mus spp. *see* mice
muscle fibre cells, *35*, 160
muscles, age-related impairment, 178, 179–81
mutagenic substances, 50, **219**–20
mutation rate, 88, **92**, 127
    predicted reduction, 227–8
mutations, 50–1, 80, 88–90, 109, 110, 114–15
    and ageing, 63, 184
    and cancer, 219
    detection, 196
    and genetic diseases, 227–8
    source of variation, 80

mutualism, 99, 100
Mycobacterium tuberculosis, 27–8, 98, *103*, 115
myelin, 87
Myxoma virus, 110–11
myxomatosis, 110–11, 114

natural killer (NK) cells, 129, 144
natural selection, **51**–2, 109, 225
    death as consequence, 106
    DNA variants, 51
    effect of cultural factors, 96
    in humans, relaxation, 226
    of receptors that bind pathogens, 132
    and resistance to infection, 114
    RNA variants, 34
    role of competition, 51, 63
    in shifting environment, 64–5
nature–nurture debate, **75**–6
Nauru diabetes epidemic, 227
nausea, 157
Neanderthal people
    lifespan, 17
    tools, *19*
Neel's thrifty genotype hypothesis, 227
negative feedback, **57**, 160
nematodes, 25, 103, 114, 150
    destroyed by cooking, 20
nephrons, loss with age, 177
nerve cells, *35*, 62
nervous system, **62**
    and digestive system, 156
    repair mechanism, 213
Nessell, C. S., 221
neural-tube defects, 195
neurofibromatosis, 97
neurons *see* nerve cells
neurotransmitters, 42, 43
neutralism, *100*
'non-self' material, 127, 133
normal distribution curve, **80**
nucleotides, **33**, **47**–50, 88–9
nucleus (cell), *35*, 36, *38*
    see also chromosomes
Nuffield Council on Bioethics, 199, 201, 202

obesity, 158
oesophagus, 148
oestrogen, 62
oestrogen replacement therapy, 182
Onchocerca volvulus, 114
onchocerciasis (river blindness), *101*
oncogenes, 185–6, 209
opportunistic infections, 138
organ transplantation, **189**–91
    multiple, 190–1
    for treatment of genetic diseases, 204
    see also graft rejection
organelles, **36**
organic molecules, **32**
organisms, **31**
osteoporosis, 181
ovum, sizes of species compared, *37*
oxidation, 158, 184
ozone

ground-level, 215
in outer atmosphere ('ozone layer'), 50, 211–12

pancreas, *148*, 149, 158, *159*
parasites, **8**–9, **100**–5
    destroyed by cooking, 20
    multicellular, 9, 25–6
parasitism, **100**
Parkinson's disease, 191
passive diffusion, **40**, 60, 150
Passmore, R., *177*
pastoralism, **21**–3
    costs and benefits, 23–4
pathogens, **9**, 98, 100–5, 126
    barriers, 125–6
    body's defence and repair mechanisms, 125–6, 212–13
    drug resistance, 115, 230
    escape mechanisms, 140–1
    non-specific recognition, 131–2
    specific recognition, 133–4
    see also host–pathogen relationships
PCBs (polychlorinated biphenyls), effects of exposure, 216, 218, 220, 222
Pediculus humanus capitis (head louse), 21, 112
Pediculus humanus humanus (body louse), 21
pedigree charts, **84**, 85, *86*, 193
pelvis, in humans and apes, 12, *13*
Penrose, L. S., *90*
peptic ulcers, 149
peristalsis, 149, 153–4, 156
pernicious anaemia, 152
Perry, M. M., *41*
Peters, W., *56*
Peto, Richard, 185–6, 222
pets, 25–6
phagocytes, 128, *129*, 130, 131, 139–40
phagocytosis, **128**, *129*
pharynx, 148
phenotype, **64**, 75–6, 77, 78, 164
    lactose absorption and malabsorption, 164–5
    modification, 204–8
phenylalanine, 53–4, 86–8, 197
phenylketonuria *see* PKU
phospholipids, 38–9, *41*
photochemical smog, 215
phytoplankton, 121, 212
pigment cells, *35*
PKU (phenylketonuria), 83, 85, 86–8, 92, 175
    gene therapy, 207
    screening, 197
    treatment, 87, 204
placenta, 195, *196*
plague, 22, 28, 110, 117
Plasmodium spp., 26, 94, 101, *102*, *103*, 115, 143
platelets, 134
pollution
    effects, 212
    see also industrialisation
polychlorinated biphenyls *see* PCBs
population, **91**
    age structure, 105
    characteristics, 91–2
    human, 24
    mixing, 95–6

population genetic screening, 189, **197**–204
  economic analysis, 198–9
  effect on disease incidence, 199–200
  ethical considerations, 202–4
population genetics, **91**–5
porphyria, 97
posture, erect, 11–14
potassium absorption, 152
predation, 100
pre-natal diagnosis (of genetic disease), **194**–6
  and DNA analysis, 196–7
  ethical considerations, 201–2
pre-symptomatic diagnosis, 193
primary immune response, *136*, **137**, 140
primary producers (in food web), 120–1
primates, **9**–11, 22, 30, 179
'primeval soup', 32, 50, 108
privacy, right to, 203
producers (in food web), 120–1
progeria, 184
prokaryotes, 36n.
prolactin, 62
proteases, 147, 148
protein synthesis, **52**–4
  age-related decline, 183
proteins, **33**, 43, 45
  digestion, 146, 149
  in immune system, 130
  in membranes, 39, 40–1, 44, 151
  replacement, 204
  synthesis, 33–4, 52–4
  turnover in cells, 176–7, 183, 213
  see also enzymes
protistans, 9, **35**–6, 40, 55
  movement, 55, *56*
  parasitic, 100–3, 104–5
  reproduction, 57
proximal cause, 184
psittacosis, 29
puberty, variation in age of, 82
Pulex irritans (human flea), 20
pyloric valve, 149
pyramid of biomass, 121–2
pyramid of numbers, 121

rabbit *see* myxomatosis
rabies, 26, 110
'races', 91–2
radiation effects, 216
  in eyes, 182
  mutagenic, 50
  on mutation rate, 219, 227
  on skin, 168–70, 214
  and vitamin D synthesis, 168–71
Raff, M. C., 177n.
random assortment of chromosomes, 73
random processes
  in genetic inheritance, 93
  in natural selection, 93
rats, 22, 28
  effect of reduced-calorie diet, 183
receptor molecules, **43**, 132–3, 134–5
  in gut lining, 151
recessive characteristics, **78**

recessive disorders, 83, **84**–6, 92, 93, 95–6
  see also cystic fibrosis; PKU (phenylketonuria)
reciprocal benefit, 99
rectum, *148*, 152
red blood cells, 134, 176
red deer, reproduction, 108
Red Queen's hypothesis, 65
reduction division *see* meiosis
regulation of glucose concentration in blood, 41, 44, **158**–61
repair mechanisms of body, 213
reproduction, 31
  cells, 34–5
  multicellular organisms, 63
  sexual, evolution, 63, 118–20
  single-celled organisms, 57
reproductive anomalies, 220
reproductive effort, 107, 175
reproductive 'schedule', 106
reproductive success, affected by parasites, 105
reserve capacity, loss with age, **177**
resistance to antibiotics, 230
resistance to infection, **114**–15
  impact of cultural evolution, 116–17
  see also under malaria
response mechanisms, 57
retinal atrophy, 97
rheumatoid arthritis, 134, 135, 206
rhinoviruses, 28, 111, 145
ribonucleic acid *see* RNA
ribosomes, 36, *38*, 53, 54
rickets, 167
rickettsia, 28–9
Rietschel, E. T., 141
risk assessment, **223**
risk factors associated with CHD, 83
risk management, **223**
risk prioritisation, 222–3
river blindness, 25, *101*, 114
RNA (ribonucleic acid), **33**–4, 45, 46
  messenger (mRNA), 53–4
  variants, 33–4, 46
RNA replication, **33**
Rosenberg, L. E., 207
rotaviruses, *37*
roundworms, *101*, *104*, 149
  age-1 gene, 184
  life cycle, 25
  protective coating, 140
  see also nematodes
Royal College of Physicians, 198, 199
rubella virus, 74
ruff lemur, *9*
Rusting, R. L., 184

Saudi Arabian people, 170, 171
scabies, *102*
scar tissue, 213
Schistosoma, 25, *103*, *104*, 140
schistosomiasis, 25, *101*, 105
screening *see* genetic screening
scurvy, 20
secondary immune response, *136*, 137, 140
secondary sexual characteristics, **15**–16, 119–20
secretion, 42–3, 147, 150

self-maintenance, 31, 57
self-tolerance, 127, 135
senses, age-related impairment, 178, 182–3
sensitive group (environmental exposure), **214**, 221, 224
sensors, 57, 157
Seveso accident, 217, 221, 222
sex chromosomes, 70, 71, 72–3
sex-linked characteristics, **79**
sexual reproduction, evolution, 63, 118–20
sexual selection, 18, **119**–20
sexually transmitted diseases *see* STDs
Sharpe, R. M., 216
shelters, 20–1
shivering, 63, 160
sickle-cell disease, 82, 93–5, 96
    identification of carriers, 200
    location of gene, 196, 206
sickle-cell trait, 94
signalling molecules, 43
Simoons, F. J., 163–4
Simulium spp. (blackflies), 25
single-celled oranisms, 55
single-gene inheritance, 77–80, 84
Skakkebaek, N. E., 216
skeleton, 12–14
skin
    cancer, *169*, 214
    cells, *35*
    colour, 168–70
    healing, 213
skull, *17*, 18
sleeping sickness, 26, 100, *101*
small intestine, *148*, 149–52
smallpox, 26–7, *103*, 117
    eradication, 114, 143
    origin, 27, 117
    vaccination, 137, 143
smog, 215
smoking, 186, 201, 214
sodium absorption, 152
somatic cells, 55, 63–4, 192
s**omatic DNA, 55**
somatic effort, 107, 175
somatic gene therapy, 206–8, 209
somatic mutation theory, 184
Spears, N., 192
specialisation of cells, 60
s**pecies, 8**–9, 99
    interactions, 99–100
    turnover, 65
sperm cell, *35*, 55
spina bifida, 83, 195
spinal column in humans and apes, 12, *13*
spleen, 139
sponges, rejection reaction, 129
Staphylococcus aureus, 140
Stárzl, Thomas, 191
STDs (sexually transmitted diseases), 108, 113, 114
stem cells, 134, *135*, 191, 207
Stern, C., *81*
stomach, 148–9
    in pernicious anaemia patients, 152
stone tools, 18–19, *23*
Strassburg, Marc, 27n., 143

Strehler, B. L., *177*
stress, 142–3, 157
Strickberger, M. W., *94*
strongyloidiasis (threadworm), *101*
'struggle for existence', 51
sunbathing, *169*, 170
sunlight and vitamin D synthesis, 168–71
suppressor T cells, 138, 144
survival curves, 105
susceptibles (in a population), 112–13, 114, 116
swallowing, 148
sweating, 18, 63
symbiosis, 99–100
symbiotic bacteria in large intestine, 153
symptomatic infected (in a population), 112–13
synovial fluid, 180
syphilis (disease), 108
Syphilis (organism), *103*

T cells (T lymphocytes), 136, **138**–9, 214
    cytotoxic, 138, 215
    helper, 138, 139, 140
    suppressor, 138, 144
Taenia (tapeworm), 20, 25, *103*, *104*, 150
Tanner, J. M., *15*, 82
tapeworms, 100, *102*, 103, 104, 114, 149
    destroyed by cooking, 20
    life cycle, 25, 104
    see also Taenia
Tay–Sachs disease, 82, 199, 200
    location of gene, 196
TB *see* tuberculosis
teeth
    evolution, 18, 161
    see also dental caries
temperature and mutation rate, 88
temperature regulation, 62–3
tendons, 12n., 180
teratogenic substances, **220**, 222
testosterone, 62
tetanus, 104
thalassaemia, 97
    bone marrow transplants, 204
    gene identified, 206
    gene therapy, 207
    screening for, 199–200
thalidomide, 74, 220, 224
Thornton, R., *116*
threadworm, *101*
threshold effects (toxicity), **222**
thymine, 48
thymus, 139
ticks, 100, *102*, 103, *104*
tissue culture, 176
tissue typing, 189–90
tools, 18–19, *22*
toxicity testing, 220–1, 222
    see also acute toxicity; chronic toxicity
toxins, 155
    accumulation in cells, 183
    bacterial, 44, 133, 141
    biological half-life, 219
Toxocara, 25, 101, *102*, 150
trachea, 148

Tracy, 205
transplanted tissue, 129, 133
    see also organ transplants
transport proteins, 40–1, 44, 151
Trichinella spiralis, 20, 25
trichinosis, 20
trichlorophenol (TCP), 217
Trichomonas vaginalis, 56
trichuriasis (whipworm), 101
trophic levels, 120
Trypanosoma spp. (trypanosomes), 26, 56, 102, 103
trypanosomiasis see sleeping sickness
tsetse flies, disease vectors, 26
tuberculosis (TB), 27–8, 98, 115
tumour suppressor genes see anti-oncogenes
twins, 97, 107
    identical, 64, 75, 81, 133
    and lifespan, 186
    non-identical, 81
'Typhoid Mary', 112
typhus fever, 28–9, 105
tyrosine, 53–4, 86–8

ultrasonography, 194, 195
ultraviolet radiation
    effects on phytoplankton, 212
    immunosuppressive effects, 212
    mutagenic effects, 50, 88
    and vitamin D synthesis, 167–9, 171
UV(B) radiation, 167–9

vaccination, 27, 143–4
vaccine, influenza, 140
Varecia variegata (ruff lemur), 9
variation, 51
    continuous, 80–2
    environmental factors in, 74, 81–2, 87
    genetic, 64, 72, 73, 91–2, 225
    human, 4, 68
    in immune responsiveness, 141–3
    see also lactose malabsorption and intolerance
Vaupel, James, 186
vectors (of infectious disease), 26, 101, 105, 109, 111
    see also gene vectors
vesicles, 36, 38, 41–2
viability, 64
Vibrio cholerae, 150, 153, 154
    cyst formation, 150
    evolutionary change, 111
villi, 150
virulence, 110–11, 114–15
viruses, 9, 36, 37, 103, 131
    gene vectors, 206, 207

reproduction, 119
resistant envelope, 126
vitamins, 146
    absorption, 150, 152
    A, 150
    B, 153
    C, 20
    D, 150, 167–71, 181–2
    E, 150
    K, 150, 153
vitamin D deficiency, 167
vomiting, 157

Wagner, M., 199, 200
walking see bipedality
warfare, 230, 231
Warner, H. J., 183
Washkansky, Lewis, 189
wastes, export of, 223
water, secretion and reabsorption, 152
Watson, James, 46, 47, 48
weaning, 23, 163
whipworm, 101
white cells, 128–9
    see also lymphocytes
whooping cough, 108
Williams, John, 56
Williamson, G. M., 142
Williamson, R., 197, 198, 201
women
    in agricultural societies, 24
    breasts, 120
    post-menopausal, 106, 179, 182
    secondary sexual characteristics, 15–16
World Health Organisation, 101, 208, 223, 226
worms, parasitic, 100, 103
    see also roundworms; tapeworms

X chromosome, 70
X-linked inheritance see sex-linked characteristics
X-rays, mutagenic effects, 50, 88
xeroderma pigmentosa, 97, 214

Y chromosome, 70
yarrow, variation, 76
yellow fever, 26, 110
yoghurt, 163, 166, 169
Young, S., 184

Zimmet, Paul, 227
zoonoses, 24, 26–9, 110, 116
Zuk, Marlene, 119

DATE DUE

APR 2 4 2004			
APR 2 9 2005			
GAYLORD			PRINTED IN U.S.A.